Special Recreation:
Opportunities for Persons with Disabilities

Dan W. Kennedy, Ph.D.
Pennsylvania State University

David R. Austin, Ph.D.
Indiana University

Ralph W. Smith, Ph.D.
University of Maryland

wcb
Wm. C. Brown Publishers
Dubuque, Iowa

Printed in the United States of America by Wm. C. Brown Publishers
2460 Kerper Boulevard, Dubuque, IA 52001

10 9 8 7 6 5 4 3

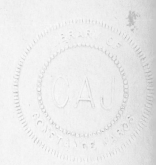

This book is dedicated
to the ones we love.

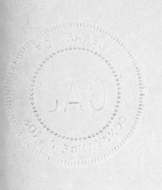

Foreword

All experience is an arch, to build upon.

This statement of Henry Brooks Adams' in *The Education of Henry Adams* reflects on the foundations of knowledge. In *Special Recreation: Opportunities for Persons with Disabilities*, the authors have carefully provided the groundwork that assists the reader in conceptualizing and developing both the special recreation framework and edifice necessary for sound program development.

The authors, Dan Kennedy, David Austin, and Ralph Smith have integrated the prevalent thinking of therapeutic recreation, special recreation, leisure education, and related professions into a pragmatic and realistic compendium. They have reflected the evolution and development of recreation services for the disabled over the past 100 years and have provided a rich source for both the student and practitioner in their quest to work hand-in-hand with individuals with disabilities.

Drs. Kennedy, Austin, and Smith individually have made numerous contributions to special recreation in the past two decades. Their work in curriculum development, mainstreaming, attitudinal assessment, playground development, accessible environments, therapeutic recreation education, and sports for those with disabilities provides the structure necessary for the formulation of this book. The backgrounds and experiences of the authors have enabled them to incorporate prior and existing recreation practices and provoke thoughts and concerns regarding the future direction of special recreation services.

The authors have provided an exciting dimension to the arena of recreation and leisure for individuals with disabling conditions. Their coverage of historical and conceptual approaches, program planning, special program areas, resources, and trends represents the essentials of this thrust. They have built on the cornerstone of special recreation a book for all seasons.

HELEN JO HILLMAN, C.T.R.S.
Program Manager
Therapeutic Recreation Services
D.C. Department of Recreation

Preface

During the past 20 years there have been many dynamic developments in the field of recreation. One of the most exciting is the movement of persons with disabilities out of institutions into the mainstream of recreational involvement. Existing community programs and services have expanded and new opportunities developed to meet the leisure needs of these individuals. From all indications, this growth will continue as the recreation field moves into the 1990s. Thus, we feel there is an acute need for a textbook that, rather than emphasizing disabilities, focuses upon the many facets of Special Recreation programming.

The term "Special Recreation" was selected for use in this textbook in order to distinguish freely chosen recreation participation from Therapeutic Recreation. As described in Chapter 1, we feel that a polarity exists between Therapeutic Recreation and Special Recreation. This textbook, therefore, concentrates upon nonclinical approaches and emphasizes the delivery and value of Special Recreation opportunities for people with disabilities.

It is important to note that this textbook was written primarily for undergraduate students, especially those within their first two years of study. As such, it is appropriate for use in community (or junior) college courses, as well as within four-year baccalaureate programs. Throughout the preparation of this textbook, we have tried to keep the needs, interests, and learning styles of undergraduate students foremost in our minds. Whenever possible, we have included concrete examples to illustrate important points, and we have provided useful references and learning activities at the end of each chapter. We have also attempted to write in a style that is appealing to undergraduate students.

This textbook is organized into four distinct parts, and each part is preceded by an introductory statement highlighting its contents. Part I provides an introduction and overview to Special Recreation. The emphasis of this section is upon the scope of Special Recreation services, including important concepts and terminology. Part I also provides useful facts and techniques related to selected disabling conditions. Part II focuses upon actual program planning and implementation, and includes detailed descriptions of exemplary Special Recreation programs. Part III offers some examples of program areas (or activities) that have proven effective in meeting the recreational needs of people with disabilities. The final section, Part IV, provides valuable information on community resources and legislation that relate to Special Recreation services. This section also outlines current trends in Special Recreation. At the conclusion of this textbook, we have inserted several Appendixes containing materials and resources that should prove useful to Special Recreation students and educators, as well as to practitioners.

Completion of this textbook combined the efforts of three authors with vastly different backgrounds and areas of expertise. As a result, each of us assumed primary responsibility for selected chapters based upon our knowledge of and interest in the topic. Dr. Kennedy had primary responsibility for Chapters 6, 7, 11, and 12; Dr. Austin for Chapters 1, 2, 5, and 13; and Dr. Smith for Chapters 3, 4, 8, 9, and 10. It should be stressed that every chapter was reviewed by each author and the final product is very much a collaborative effort. Nevertheless, readers wishing more detailed information on a given chapter are encouraged to contact the primary author of that chapter.

We would like to express our sincere gratitude to the many people who have assisted in the preparation of this textbook. The reactions, insights, suggestions, and efforts of the following people were instrumental in the completion of this book: Barbara (Sam) Browne, Cincinnati Recreation Commission; Tammy Buckley, formerly of Manor Care Nursing Home, Largo, Maryland; Mary Cece, Lois Gill, and Fred Humphrey, University of Maryland; Peg Connolly, formerly of Florida State University; Cliff Crase, Paralyzed Veterans of America; Michael Crawford, University of Missouri; Mary Crooks and Dorothy Lougee, Parks and Recreation Department, Lincoln, Nebraska; Jeanne (Hap) Feeley, Pennsylvania Easter Seal Society; Catherine Fowler, mother of Claudia Fowler; Gene Hayes, University of Tennessee at Knoxville; Doug Herbert, National Committee, Very Special Arts; Helen Jo Hillman, District of Columbia Department of Recreation; Jerry Kelley, President's Committee on Employment of the Handicapped; Terry Kinney, Temple University; C. Wayne Korinek, Parks, Recreation and Library Department, Phoenix; Stan Labanowich, University of Kentucky; Michal Ann Lord, Austin Parks and Recreation Department; Steven Mason, District of Columbia Special Olympics; John McGovern, West Suburban Special Recreation Association, Elmwood Park, Illinois; Lee Meyer, University of North Carolina; Anna Miller and Glori Steifler, formerly of the League for the Handicapped, Baltimore; Bob Myers, Montgomery County Health Department, Silver Spring, Maryland; Lynn Parfitt, Maine-Niles Association of Special Recreation, Illinois; David Park, National Park Service; Janet Pomeroy, Recreation Center for the Handicapped, San Francisco; Lou Powell, University of New Hampshire; Lawrence Reiner, Northeast DuPage Special Recreation Association, Elmhurst, Illinois; Gary Robb, Bradford Woods, Indiana; Lynn Rourke, Courage Center, Golden Valley, Minnesota; Kevin Smith, Department of Leisure Services, City of Miami; Byron Welker, Central State Hospital, Indianapolis; and many students from Indiana University, The Pennsylvania State University, and the University of Maryland.

Finally, we would like to thank our wives and children for their understanding and support throughout the preparation of this textbook. We sincerely hope that the finished product is worthy of the many sacrifices that were made by our families.

Dan W. Kennedy
David R. Austin
Ralph W. Smith

Contents Overview

Contents

III. SPECIAL RECREATION PROGRAM AREAS

8. Special Camping and Wilderness Experiences   185

9. The Arts—For Everyone   209

10. Competitive Sports for Individuals with Disabilities   241

Contents

xix

1

INTRODUCTION AND OVERVIEW

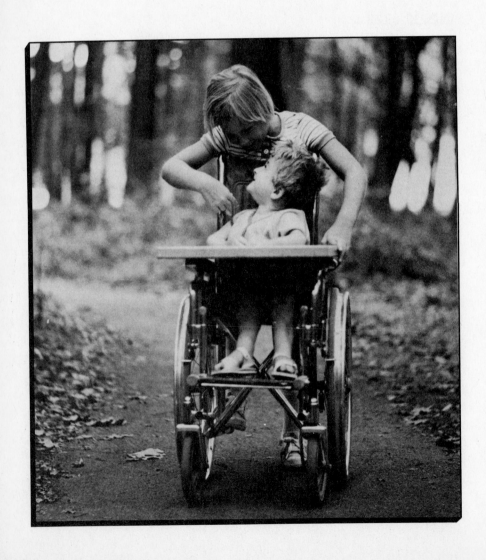

The public parks and recreation profession has long prided itself on its ability to contribute to the well-being and quality of life of the citizenry. Yet, as problems of persons with disabilities have become increasingly more visible in society, it has become apparent that this profession has had only a tenuous grasp on the nature of the problems that citizens with disabilities must face during their leisure and their need for the provision of special recreation programs. Fortunately, today there is an emerging movement among those in the parks and recreation profession to establish services that meet the recreational needs of persons who are disabled.

Although special recreation is a comparatively new area of interest for public parks and recreation, one can see origins of concern with recreation for members of special populations dating back to the beginnings of organized recreation in America. Chapter 1, *Introduction to Special Recreation Services,* reviews both historical and philosophical bases for special recreation services. Views of authorities such as Carter, Kelley, Meyer, Robb, Pomeroy, and Stein and Sessoms are presented and conclusions are drawn that suggest that a harmonious arrangement for cooperation of general park and recreation professionals and specialists in therapeutic recreation can become a reality.

Chapter 2, *Concepts and Attitudes Underlying Special Recreation Services,* presents concepts and attitudes basic to understanding the delivery of special recreation services. Concepts surrounding the terms *disability, handicap, special populations, mainstreaming, normalization,* and *advocacy* are discussed. Chapter 2 concludes with an in-depth approach to attitudes as they relate to serving persons who have disabilities. A major segment of the section on attitudes is devoted to alternatives proposed by the Easter Seal Society to avoid stigmatized language when referring to individuals with disabilities.

Although it is critical that we avoid the trap of labeling those with disabilities, we may find information concerning various disabling conditions to be useful. Chapter 3, *Disabling Conditions,* begins with a discussion of the potential pitfalls and hazards involved in labeling people who have disabilities. This is followed by helpful facts, tips, and techniques associated with specific types of disabilities.

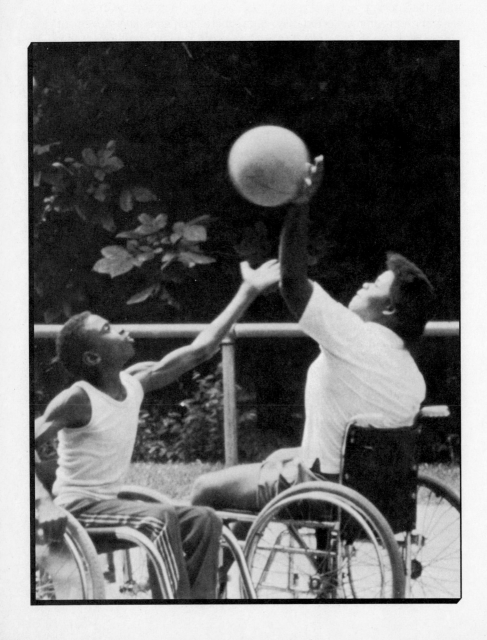

1

Introduction to Special Recreation Services

Organized recreation in the United States grew out of social concern for persons attempting to cope with a rapidly changing world created by the Industrial Revolution. Most authorities cite the establishment of a sand play-area for disadvantaged children in Boston in 1885 as the beginning of the recreation movement in America. This play area became known as the Boston Sand Gardens. The provision of wholesome recreation was also a central part of the settlement-house movement established to ease the transition to urban living for thousands of persons immigrating to the cities of America during the Industrial Revolution. Settlement houses, such as Jane Addam's Hull House in Chicago, provided playgrounds for children and recreational opportunities for adults to help them adapt to an urban life characterized by overcrowding and poor living conditions.

The beginnings of organized recreation in our nation thus evolved from a humanistic concern for the welfare of those whose found themselves with few resources in inhospitable circumstances. Wholesome recreation was viewed as necessary for those disadvantaged individuals who were, indeed, members of special populations with special needs.[1]

---

[1]The term *special populations* broadly describes those who have special needs because of some social, physical, mental, or psychological difficulty. In contemporary usage it has come primarily to describe persons with physical and mental disabilities and those who are elderly.

Murphy (1975) has written the following account of the growth of the recreation movement:

> The initial impetus of the Recreation Movement came from social and civic workers who provided funds for the establishment of the first playgrounds and began building up public opinion favorable to governmental support and direction for public recreation facilities. At the time the Playground Association of America was started in 1906, there were some 41 cities that were maintaining municipally supported and operated playground programs. By 1915, 83 communities reported public recreation departments, and the number had increased to 465 by 1920. (p. 43)

However, as community recreation grew, it began to lose its focus on meeting the special needs of those who were disadvantaged. The more affluent sections of cities demanded and received recreation services as well. Community recreation took on the cause of "recreation for all." Recreation was perceived not as a social instrument but as an end in itself, an experience all should enjoy.

Gray (1969), in a widely cited article titled "The Case for Compensatory Recreation," has written:

> The recreation movement was born with a social conscience. It grew up with the settlement house movement, the kindergarten movement and the youth movement that fostered the great youth agencies of the nation. Its earliest practitioners had a human welfare motivation in which the social ends of human development, curbing juvenile deliquency, informal education, cultural enrichment, health improvement and other objectives were central. Gradually the social welfare mission weakened and a philosophy which sees recreation as an end in itself was adopted; this is the common view in public recreation agencies throughout the country. (p. 23)

In a similar vein Sessoms and Stevenson (1981) have written:

> Adult education, recreation, and social group work all have a common heritage. Each is a product of the social welfare reforms that occurred in our cities and industries at the turn of the nineteenth century. Their founders shared a similar belief—they were concerned with the quality of life and believed that through the "proper" use of leisure, it could be achieved. (p. 2)

Like Gray, Sessoms and Stevenson observed that the organized parks and recreation movement has deviated from its original mission. They have written:

> With both adult education and social work establishing their turf, recreation services did the same. Although some recreation specialists

were concerned with the therapeutic or socially rehabilitative activities or with teaching and developing leisure skills and attitudes, the recreation profession set as its primary concerns the management of recreational environments and the offering of free-time activities. Outdoor recreation and sports programs became its program focus. (pp. 2, 3)

Although having its roots in socially purposeful programs for special populations, the recreation profession appears to have moved away from its initial focus. As community recreation has grown, it has broadened its scope to "recreation for all." However, as Carter and Kelley (1981) have suggested, the idea of recreation for all may have in reality become "recreation for the norm." As community park and recreation departments have attempted to spread their resources to meet everyone's recreational needs, concern for special populations has been lost as a central feature of public parks and recreation.

WHY THE LACK OF LEISURE SERVICES FOR SPECIAL POPULATIONS?

As might be anticipated, there have been pleas for a return to an extensive concern for leisure services to members of special populations. These have come during the 1970s and 1980s from a number of individuals and groups. For example, early in the 1970s, Kraus (1971) wrote of the need for recreation and park administrators to take leadership for socially purposeful programs, including those to serve the elderly and persons with physical and mental disabilities. From another perspective, in 1980 the International City Management Association in its publication, *Managing Municipal Leisure Service* (Lutzin, 1980), called for the development of leisure services for special populations. In a chapter devoted to services for persons who are disabled or elderly it was stated, "A goal of the municipal leisure service agency is to serve the leisure needs of all in the community, including special populations, on an equal basis" (p. 152).

Yet today we find that persons with physical or mental disabilities, individuals who are old, and other members of special population groups are still largely underserved by community public recreation and parks departments. Why is this? Why have so many departments, which owe their very existence to the social welfare motive, failed to respond to the needs of special populations?

Perhaps the lack of services for special populations has simply reflected the history of neglect of society in general for those who have not fit society's norms. During the first half of the twentieth century we systematically excluded indigent people and persons with physical or mental disabilities from community participation. Indigent old people were sent to "old folks farms" or "county poor homes." Mentally retarded individuals were placed in large institutions located in rural areas. Likewise, individuals with serious problems in mental health were taken away to "insane asylums." In short, those who deviated from society's norms were effectively removed from the mainstream of society. In light of this, it is not surprising that as the recreation and parks movement expanded across the United States and Canada, it lost its dedication to individuals from underserved groups.

In recent years, however, we have become more enlightened as a society to the needs of special populations. Through social institutions such as schools we have made a concerted effort to bring members of special population groups into the mainstream of society. Why have public park and recreation departments been slow to return to their heritage of concern for special populations?

Pragmatic Reasons for Lack of Service

Surveys of public park and recreation departments have revealed a number of reasons for the absence of services for special populations. Reasons include insufficient budgets, inadequate facilities, lack of skills and knowledge necessary to establish a program, the feeling that other community agencies already provide programs, and an unawareness of the need for programs for special populations. Assistance, these agencies felt, would be helpful to them in establishing programs by providing financial aid, additional staff, specially trained staff, additional accessible facilities, in-service training, consultation, and transportation (Austin, et al., 1978; Edginton, et al., 1975).

Vaughan and Winslow (1979) identified for community park and recreation departments five major problem areas in the provision of recreation programs for special populations. These included: (1) transportation (listed by 78.9% of the agencies), (2) budget allocations (50.4%), (3) the identification of members of special population groups (45.2%), (4) insufficient numbers of program personnel (40.7%), and (5) architectural barriers (32%).

In general, the reasons identified as blocks to programming for special populations are practical considerations. These include appropriating adequate budgets, training staff and volunteers, readying facilities, identifying participants, and organizing transportation. While these problems are formidable, Vaughan and Winslow (1979) have presented a number of specific solutions for dealing with each of them. Given the motivation, these problems can be overcome. Of greater apparent significance are the reported lack of awareness of the need for these programs and the feeling that other agencies already provide such programs. These cognitions on the part of administrators of park and recreation systems allow them to remove themselves entirely from the responsibility of providing recreation for special populations. Perhaps the broadening of the concept of *therapeutic recreation*, discussed in the next section, has prompted administrators to feel less responsible for the provision of recreation for special populations.

A Broadening Concept of Therapeutic Recreation

In the United States during the 1940s and 1950s there developed recreation services within hospitals and institutions serving persons with various physical and mental disabilities. In some instances those who provided these services were known as "hospital recreation workers." They identified themselves primarily with the Hospital Recreation Section of the American Recreation Society. Their approach was that of "recreation for the sake of recreation." They believed that recreation existed within their hospitals to promote the general well-being of the patients. Another segment employed in hospitals and institutions identified themselves as "recreation therapists." They formed the National Association of Recreation Therapists. To them recreation was more than a wholesome activity—it was a tool to treatment and rehabilitation.

These two contrasting groups formed together in the 1960s under the banner of a then relatively new term, *therapeutic recreation*. Therapeutic recreation was used as an umbrella term to generally encompass the perspectives of both the American Recreation Society and the National Association of Recreation Therapists. Ultimately, therapeutic recreation came to be broadly interpreted as including any recreational service to individuals with mental or physical disabilities, either in the hospital or community, whether for the purpose of providing treatment or a recreative experience.

Carter and Kelley (1981) have made a persuasive case that the broadening of the concept of therapeutic recreation has led to difficulty in establishing community-based park and recreation services for persons with disabilities. They have written:

> This expanded concept of therapeutic recreation that included
> community services has had two major consequences for disabled
> adults and children, consequences that are not necessarily regarded as
> positive. First, because most disabled and impaired individuals are now
> living in a noninstitutional setting or are in the process of being

mainstreamed back into community life, they do not need, nor do they have any desire to have, "therapy." Furthermore, they have no wish to carry the stigma of being recipients of "therapeutic" recreation services. Therefore, the broadened service delivery perspective that has maintained a "treatment" image runs counter to the desires of many disabled adults and young people to seek a "normal" range of experiences like their nondisabled peers.

Secondly, the therapeutic recreation field claims to be the primary professional group delegated the exclusive responsibility to serve disabled populations. The longer this image is promoted, the more difficult it becomes to convince the community recreation specialist that he must assume responsibility to provide recreation to *all* persons in his community regardless of the extent of their disabilities. (pp. 64, 65)

Carter and Kelley's points seem to be well founded. Most persons with disabilities who live in the community do not require the therapy normally associated with therapeutic recreation, nor do they wish to be stigmatized as being recipients of therapeutic recreation services. Like other citizens, the vast majority of members of special population groups and their families simply desire to have the opportunity to take part in recreation experiences.

The twin concepts of mainstreaming and normalization call for helping disabled populations to take part in the mainstream of society within the most normative and least restrictive environment possible. Most persons in our society are not served by therapeutic recreation

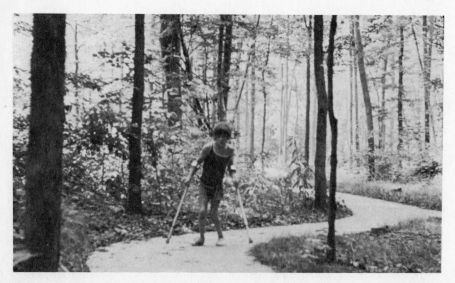

Figure 1–1. To enjoy nature: A recreative experience to be enjoyed by all children.

specialists but by community recreation personnel. It is then the responsibility of community recreation professionals to provide recreation services for those who are disabled. Carter and Kelley feel that only when the therapeutic recreation profession steps aside and acknowledges that community recreation for persons with disabilities is the domain of public parks and recreation will the full responsibility be born by those who have the obligation to meet the recreational needs of our citizens. It seems quite possible that by claiming to be primarily responsible for the entire spectrum of recreation for special populations, therapeutic recreation specialists may be allowing community recreation systems to relinquish their rightful duty to serve persons with disabilities.

At the least, Carter and Kelley (1981) have brought out the fact that unless there is a clear determination of the domain of therapeutic recreation, confusion will reign regarding who should be ultimately responsible to provide community programs for persons from special population groups. There is a natural tendency to associate therapeutic recreation services with health and social welfare agencies and, therefore, to assume that these agencies should be the major providers of recreation for individuals with special needs.

It is necessary to briefly examine the field of therapeutic recreation in order to understand the controversies surrounding special recreation services. In doing so it may be possible to better grasp the difficulties raised by Carter and Kelley.

WHAT IS THERAPEUTIC RECREATION'S RELATIONSHIP TO RECREATION FOR SPECIAL POPULATIONS?

The Purpose

The purpose of therapeutic recreation has been long debated. In order to clarify the situation, early in the 1980s the National Therapeutic Recreation Society (NTRS), a branch of the National Recreation and Park Association (NRPA), developed a philosophical position in which it was stated that, "The purpose of therapeutic recreation is to facilitate the development, maintenance, and expression of an appropriate leisure lifestyle for individuals with physical, mental, emotional, and social limitations" (Philosophical Position Statement of the National Therapeutic Recreation Society, 1982).

This purpose is based upon the assumption that:

> Leisure, including recreation and play, are [sic] inherent aspects of the human experience. The importance of appropriate leisure

involvement has been documented throughout history. More recently, research has addressed the value of leisure involvement in human development, in social and family relationships, and, in general, as an important aspect of the quality of life. Some human beings have disabilities, illnesses, or social conditions which limit their full participation in the normative social structure of society. These individuals with limitations have the same human rights to, and needs for, leisure involvement. (Philosophical Position Statement of the National Therapeutic Recreation Society, 1982)

The NTRS position is strikingly similar to that taken originally by the Hospital Recreation Section of the American Recreation Society (ARS). In the 1950s, ARS had championed the cause of recreation as a need and right of all individuals, including persons with illnesses and disabilities. You may recall that those affiliated with ARS viewed therapeutic recreation as the provision of wholesome recreation experiences for ill and disabled persons. In contrast, the National Association of Recreation Therapists (NART) viewed therapeutic recreation as the provision of recreation as a means to treatment. Those taking the ARS position were very much tied to the recreation movement that stood for "recreation for all." Those affiliating with NART had little association with organized recreation but were more closely aligned with the health and rehabilitation community. Their cause was not recreation; it was health restoration and promotion.

Although the National Recreation and Park Association has since replaced the American Recreation Society, similar arguments can be heard. Those supporting the NTRS/NRPA position still champion the "recreation for all" philosophy of the ARS. Other therapeutic recreation specialists argue just as strongly that the purpose of therapeutic recreation is to use recreation as a purposeful intervention to help clients relieve or prevent problems and to assist them in personal growth in an effort to allow achievement of as high a level of health as possible. Although they realize the tremendous benefits to be achieved in recreation, the therapeutic recreation specialists see recreation as a means to an end, not an end in itself.

The forming of the American Therapeutic Recreation Association (ATRA), in 1984, may be perceived as an attempt by clinically orientated therapeutic recreation specialists to break away from NTRS/NRPA to form a professional association that would foster the delivery of treatment services. In many respects, ATRA seems to have picked up where the National Association of Recreation Therapists left off. The expressed concern of ATRA is with the application of intervention strategies using recreation to promote independent functioning and to enhance the optimal health and well-being of clients (*American Therapeutic Recreation Association Newsletter*, 1984).

A Model for Therapeutic Recreation

The NTRS philosophical statement is fashioned after a model originally proposed by Gunn and Peterson (1977, 1978) and which later appeared in Peterson and Gunn (1984). These authors believe the purpose of facilitating leisure experiences for persons with limitations should be carried out through a continuum of services. They divide the continuum into three components: therapy, leisure education, and recreation participation. Therapy is directed toward improvement of functional behavior that may impede leisure involvement. Leisure education teaches new recreational and social skills, and allows for the pursuit of various issues in leisure counseling. The last component, recreation participation, concerns the provision of self-directed leisure participation for members of special population groups. Thus the continuum ranges from client dependence during therapy that will remove barriers to leisure behavior, at one end, to independent leisure functioning at the other.

When examined closely it becomes apparent that the therapy and leisure education components merge together. Both deal with facilitating change. Thus, as Meyer (1981) has proposed, the model is essentially made up of two components—treatment and recreation. Meyer has identified five resulting implications of the model: (1) Two different types of practitioners (therapists and adaptive or special recreators) are represented; (2) The adaptive recreators operate within the jurisdiction of community recreation; (3) Therapeutic recreation is a title that describes a service continuum; (4) Therapeutic recreation is not an occupation in itself but a field that represents at least two occupational specialities; and (5) The uniqueness of therapeutic recreation is related primarily to whom it serves (i.e., people with limitations), rather than what is provided or how it is provided.

Meyer (1981) goes on to elaborate on these points. He has written:

> The dual representation of therapists and special recreators by NTRS seems to present some ideological as well as practical difficulties. Ideologically, this position suggests that therapeutic recreation is not an occupation per se, which seems to imply that therapeutic recreation is a "field." This same position also seems to suggest that the uniqueness of therapeutic recreation is not so much in what it provides or how it is provided, but rather to whom it is provided. This is less an issue in the treatment component of therapeutic recreation. But, in the special

recreation component it approaches a categorical orientation: adapted recreational opportunities for a mentally retarded child, eight years old, is therapeutic recreation . . . while recreation opportunities for a pre-school child, four years old, is considered to be "community or general" recreation. . . . Both children require some type of adaptations to facilitate recreation participation. What makes one set of adaptations TR (special recreation) and another set of adaptations general recreation? The purpose of service is the same in both cases. (pp. 13, 14)

Elsewhere, Meyer (1980) has concluded:

Some might argue there are not two cadres of practitioners, only one—therapeutic recreators. To reason in this fashion is to ignore the obvious differences between these two subspecializations in regard to purpose, work setting, accountability structure, etc. Therapists and special recreators function in different worlds. Given such significant differences it is only a matter of time (if it is not already here) when one or the other of these specializations seeks independence from the other. (p. 37)

Others have also taken issue with the concept that therapeutic recreation should be all encompassing, including both the use of recreation as a purposeful intervention and the provision of opportunities for recreation participation. It is their position that any philosophical approach must establish clear boundaries for the field. Carter and Kelley (1981), for example, draw a distinction between recreation and therapeutic recreation. They have written:

The primary purpose of recreation is to provide programs and services to make possible individualized recreation experiences. . . . The primary purpose of therapeutic recreation is to assist the individual in achieving optimal healthy functioning and independence through interventions designed to bring about a desired change in behavior. To the community recreation specialist, the recreation experience can be viewed as an "end unto itself," requiring no other justification. To the recreation therapist the recreation activity is a means by which remediation, restoration, or rehabilitation objectives can be achieved. (p. 65)

Austin (1982), like Meyer (1980) and Carter and Kelley (1981), has also questioned the inclusion of the special recreation component under the domain of therapeutic recreation. He has written:

I object to the suggestion that a *primary* role of the therapeutic recreation specialist is that of "a recreator for special populations" [Gunn & Peterson, 1978, p. 23]. If the major function of special recreation is the provision of opportunities for self-directed leisure, then those charged with the responsibility for the delivery of leisure service—

community recreation personnel—should operate recreation programs for special populations. (p. 59)

Austin concludes by stating that therapeutic recreation specialists are not "recreators for special populations," but rather helping professionals who intervene in their clients' lives through purposeful intervention directed through the application of the *therapeutic recreation process*, involving: (1) individual client assessment, (2) individual program planning, (3) implementation of the program, and (4) evaluation of the effect of the program.

A parallel point of view has been taken by Carter, Van Andel, and Robb (1985). In their introductory textbook, they have written that therapeutic recreation:

> ... refers to the specialized application of recreation for the specific purpose of intervening in and changing some physical, emotional, or social behavior to promote the growth and development of the individual. Therapeutic recreation may be viewed as a process or systematic use of recreation activities and experiences to achieve specific objectives. This process is not limited to certain categories (of individuals) or a particular setting. (pp. 15, 16)

Robb (1980) has expressed a similar view. He has stated:

> The position (defining therapeutic recreation as the application of the therapeutic recreation process) seems to be the best approach ... to enhance organizational understanding, eliminate encroachment, and spell out jurisdictional boundaries. In my discussion with leaders of the park and recreation field, I believe many would welcome this delimitation. Acceptance of this position would eliminate conflicts within the TR field. Persons currently working with special populations in a service capacity through recreation experiences ... could identify with the general recreation field. Perhaps this identification would provide the impetus and leadership needed for the broader field to accept the responsibility of serving all people. (p. 46)

Thus, Robb believes therapeutic recreation should maintain a singularity of purpose by employing the therapeutic recreation process as a means to helping clients. By so restricting therapeutic recreation, he expects the general field of parks and recreation would react by assuming its rightful responsibility for the provision of recreation for special populations.

Summary and Conclusion

Two philosophical points of view have emerged within the field of therapeutic recreation. One defines therapeutic recreation primarily as

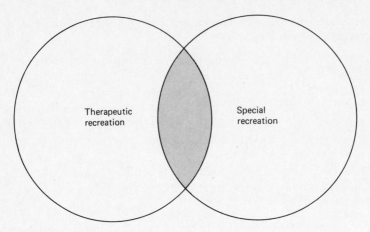

Figure 1–2. Therapeutic recreation and special recreation as two separate entities that sometimes overlap.

the provision of leisure services for those people who have some type of limitation. This position has been adopted by the National Therapeutic Recreation Society, a branch of the National Recreation and Park Association. The other view holds that therapeutic recreation should restrict itself to the application of purposeful interventions employing the therapeutic recreation process, and should, therefore, relinquish the provision of community recreation for special populations to community recreation personnel.

At this point, we, the authors of this book, take the position that a polarity does exist. We believe therapeutic recreation and special recreation (or recreation for persons with disabilities) stand as two separate entities that occasionally overlap. Overlap occurs when a therapeutic recreation program (directed primarily toward a specific therapeutic outcome through a planned intervention) offers the client an accompanying benefit of a recreative experience, or when a special recreation program (aimed primarily toward the provision of a recreative experience) serves as an intervention, bringing about a desired therapeutic benefit.

This book examines special recreation services, *not* therapeutic recreation. Its focus is in line with actual special recreation program developments and services being delivered in many of our communities today. That is, like contemporary special recreation programs, it deals principally with recreation for persons who have disabilities. It covers programs that allow participation in certain kinds of recreation activities by persons who have the type and magnitude of impairments that necessitate accommodations above and beyond those generally provided by public park and recreation systems.

It is our intent, as authors, to bring about an appreciation of the importance of recreation services for persons with disabilities, as well as a knowledge of how to develop and deliver special recreation services. When clinically oriented examples are used, they should be viewed as part of a transition to special recreation participation. In addition, the reader should be warned that some of the references cited in relation to recreation services for persons with disabilities offer comments on therapeutic recreation service (which may reflect the current state of the literature). However, we, the authors, have made a concerted effort to provide a nonclinical textbook that deals with the provision of special recreation services to persons with disabilities.

LEADERSHIP WITH SPECIAL POPULATIONS

Stein and Sessoms' (1977) *Recreation and Special Populations* has been an important book in the movement to bring recreation services to special populations, including persons with disabilities. In the view of Stein and Sessoms, professionals from the general recreation and parks field should provide community-based recreation services for members of special populations. They have written:

> . . . if such concern (for special populations) is to be converted into new and expanded community service, it must be accompanied by a growing cadre of professional recreation leaders and volunteers who have gained some awareness and understanding of the leisure problems of these disadvantaged people and who are oriented to the possibilities of providing leisure opportunities aimed at resolving their needs. Here, it is important to understand, our focus is on present and future recreators who are trained for general community service rather than on those leaders who might be considered specialists in working with a specific population. (pp. 15, 16)

Stein and Sessoms go on to state:

> Experience has demonstrated that a professional recreator who is effective in working with people in general can be equally effective in working with people from a special population. The only provisions beyond his professional skills and understanding are 1) that he be properly oriented to any unique psychological, social, or physical difficulties and possible limitations that may sometimes be faced by persons within a given population; and 2) that he be endowed with the attitudinal capacity to work with such people. Remember, we are discussing the ability to work with *people*—nothing more! Therefore,

we should recognize that such orientation and attitudinal capacity are essential in working with *any* segment of a general population, whether considered special or not. (p. 16)

Janet Pomeroy is well known as the Founder and Director of the Recreation Center for the Handicapped in San Francisco, California. Since its inception in 1952, the Center has served thousands of children and adults with all types of disabilities. Most of those who have participated in the Center's program could be classified as having severe disabilities.

Pomeroy, like Stein and Sessoms, has expressed the view that general community recreators should provide the leadership in special recreation programs. Pomeroy (1974) has stated:

We've found that general community recreation leaders have the essential skills needed, and that the best leaders are those who have leadership skills that they use successfully with non-handicapped. In addition to the essential skills and professional qualifications required of all recreation personnel, we feel that they should also have a number of special qualities, desirable attitudes and attributes. Some of these have been emphasized by the Center staff, and are listed here in line of importance:

■ Stamina and physical energy.
■ Enthusiasm and a sense of humor.
■ Ingenuity, resourcefulness, creativity and innovativeness.
■ Exceptional patience, understanding and tact.
■ A capacity for accepting limited and slower progress, and the ways in which affection and hostility may be expressed.
■ A strong commitment to health, physical education and recreation as integral parts of the total educative process.
■ A willingness to experiment or pioneer with new activities, attitudes and approaches.
■ A willingness to do custodial tasks, such as feeding and lifting, toileting and handling of wheelchairs, beds and cots. (pp. 9, 10)

Vaughan and Winslow (1979), in their *Guidelines for Community Based Programs for Special Populations*, have suggested the establishment of an in-service training of general community recreators as a means to provide staffing for recreation and park departments wishing to serve special populations.

Such a program [of in-service training] would train regular recreation program personnel to work effectively with the handicapped program participants and would also help them to work with any handicapped participants that they might have in their regular recreation programs. The comprehensiveness of the in-service training program should be dependent upon the extent to which the personnel will be involved in the special populations program and upon the functional level of the handicapped persons with whom they will be working. (p. 10)

Finally, Bullock, et al. (1982), have similarly suggested that existing general recreation staff can be given training to enable them to work with participants who have disabilities. Specific areas of training prescribed by Bullock and his colleagues include:

1. Characteristics of various disabilities, noting possible limitations and special considerations (emergency and health care procedures should also be outlined here).
2. General activity and equipment modification techniques.
3. Overview of the least-restrictive-environment concept and how it is being implemented in the department.
4. Assessment of existing attitudes of recreation professionals toward individuals with handicapping conditions.
5. Creation of peer acceptance.
6. Use of instructional aides and volunteers.
7. Location of additional resource information for a specific disability. (pp. 106, 107)

Thus, several authors have proposed that general community recreation professionals can and should assume responsibility for special recreation opportunities. Pomeroy (1974) and Bullock and his colleagues (1982), respectively, have submitted characteristics and broad training areas for community recreators serving special populations. But what specific skills and knowledges are needed to work in community recreation for special populations? Perhaps a study covered in the next section will help to answer this question.

COMPETENCIES NEEDED TO SERVE SPECIAL POPULATIONS

Austin and Powell (1980) conducted an investigation to determine what competencies entry-level general community recreation professionals should possess in order to enable them to serve participants from special populations. They first detected 142 colleges and universities in the United States and Canada that offered a course on recreation for special populations for general recreation and park students. Instructors of the special populations course at 62 of the institutions of higher education, along with 27 administrators of community-based recreation programs for special populations, participated in a competency identification

Table 1–1
Areas of Competency

Cluster	Mean Score
Attitudes	4.26
Facility Design and Accessibility	4.17
Orientation to Recreation for Special Populations	4.15
Leadership and Supervision	4.09
Mainstreaming	3.94
Program Design	3.92
Aids, Appliances, Safety Procedures	3.89
Trends and Issues	3.84
Leisure Education	3.80
Professionalism	3.79
Resources and Services	3.75
Advocacy and Legislation	3.75
Training	3.73
Equipment and Supplies	3.69
Characteristics of Special Populations	3.50
Funding Sources	3.26

Source: Austin, D. R., and Powell, L. G. Competencies needed by community recreators to serve special populations. In Austin, D. R., ed., *Directions in Health, Physical Education, and Recreation; Therapeutic Recreation Curriculum: Philosophy, Strategy, and Concerns* (Bloomington: Indiana University School of Health, Physical Education and Recreation, 1980), p. 34.

study. These instructors and administrators identified 86 competencies they felt were necessary for entry-level recreation personnel to serve special populations.

The 86 competencies identified by Austin and Powell were organized according to clusters of similar competencies. The highest-ranked cluster dealt with competencies related to attitudes (rated 4.26 on a 5-point scale). Other high-ranking areas of competence were facility design and accessibility (4.17), orientation to recreation for special populations (4.15), leadership and supervision (4.09), mainstreaming (3.94), and program design (3.92). The rankings for all 16 clusters of competencies are shown in Table 1–1.

In order to present the nature of specific competencies, a representative sample has been listed under each of the highest ranked clusters. First, under the *attitudes cluster* are competencies such as:

- Understands how positive attitudes toward the handicapped may be developed within recreational programs.
- Demonstrates awareness of personal attitudes toward ill, handicapped, and disabled individuals.

■ Understands various societal attitudes toward special
  populations.

Under the cluster on *facility design and accessibility* are competencies such as:

■ Understands the frustrations experienced in an inaccessible
  environment.
■ Describes physical barriers to accessibility and how they can
  be eliminated.
■ Identifies resources available on the design of barrier-free
  recreational environments.

Representative of the cluster on *orientation to recreation to special populations* are competencies dealing with philosophical understandings, including:

■ Develops a personal/professional philosophy of recreation for
  special populations in community settings.
■ States a rationale for the provision of community recreation
  for special populations.
■ Knows role of recreation services for special populations in
  the community recreation department.

The *leadership and supervision cluster* contains competencies such as:

■ Recognizes the importance of considering individual needs
  and interests during program leadership.
■ Knows principles of instruction useful for executing recreation
  activities for special populations.
■ Knows how to facilitate integrated recreational groups (create
  an atmosphere conducive to mainstreaming).

The *mainstreaming cluster* contains the following competencies, among others:

■ Understands concepts of mainstreaming.
■ Understands concepts of normalization.
■ Describes approaches to mainstreaming special populations in
  community recreation.

Austin and Powell also analyzed their data to determine which specific competencies were seen to be the most critical by both the college instructors and the community recreation administrators. The results of this analysis formed the basis for the article, "What You Need to

Know to Serve Special Populations," which appeared in *Parks and Recreation* (Austin and Powell, 1981).

The analysis by Austin and Powell indicates a high level of congruence between educators and administrators on what these two groups of experts judge to be the most important competencies. Examination of the data reveals 16 competencies that both the educators and administrators deem "highly desirable" (i.e., rated 4.20 or above on a 5-point scale). These critical competencies follow with the average rating for each listed after the competency statement.

1. *Knows first aid and safety procedures and practices as these relate to special populations.* (4.67)
   It is essential that community recreation professionals acquire a basic knowledge of first aid and safety. Applying proper lifting techniques when helping transfer persons with physical disabilities, reacting appropriately to epileptic seizures, and responding to diabetic reactions are examples of necessary abilities.
2. *Understands how positive attitudes toward special populations may be developed within recreation programs.* (4.66)
   Society's attitudes and expectations toward special populations are likely to be of critical importance in mainstreaming efforts. Many opportunities can be designed within recreation programs to induce attitude change if recreators know how to attempt to produce positive attitude change.
3. *Recognizes the importance of considering individual needs and interests during program leadership.* (4.63)
   Individuals make up special population groups. Each of these individuals has his or her own personal needs and interests. Leaders must consciously work on the development of an approach that considers each participant to be unique. Professionals need to be particularly aware of the dangers of stereotyping.
4. *Understands the concept of mainstreaming.* (4.56)
   More and more, individuals from special populations are moving out of institutions and into the community. They do not, however, necessarily enter into the mainstream of society. By understanding the concept of mainstreaming, the community recreator can begin to develop ways to enhance the opportunity and the ability of special population members to increasingly become a part of the mainstream of society.
5. *Knows the role of recreation services for special populations in the community recreation department.* (4.48)

Recreation services for special populations cannot simply be relegated to health and social agencies but must be seen as a community responsibility. Special populations have the same right as others to receive recreation and leisure services. Community recreation professionals should assume their role of providers of services for all populations within the community.

6. *Demonstrates awareness of personal attitudes toward special populations.* (4.46)

Effective professionals must become aware of the personal attitudes they hold toward members of special populations. All possible means should be used to become conscious of these attitudes. Those who become aware of their attitudes have moved toward overcoming any negative feelings regarding members of special population groups.

7. *Understands the impact the leader can have on a handicapped individual.* (4.38)

Community recreators need to develop an understanding of the personal influence they can have on clients from special population groups, especially with regard to self-worth and feelings of acceptance.

8. *Understands the concept of normalization.* (4.37)

It is necessary to understand the concept of normalization in order to remove barriers to normal living for special populations.

9. *Understands the frustrations experienced in an inaccessible environment.* (4.37)

Community recreators should be knowledgeable of design features for parks and recreation facilities that permit accessibility. They should also develop sensitivity for the frustrations persons with disabilities encounter in dealing with inaccessible facilities.

10. *Describes approaches to mainstreaming special populations in community recreation.* (4.31)

Many levels of mainstreaming exist in community recreation programs, and diverse techniques are employed to facilitate mainstreaming. Knowledge of practical approaches to mainstreaming can allow recreation professionals to select the best approaches for their community situations.

11. *Knows principles of instruction useful for executing recreation activities for special populations.* (4.31)

It is critical that recreators become aware not only of what they are instructing but also of whom they are instructing, and the most successful methods of dealing with various types of participants.

12. *Understands various societal attitudes toward special populations.* (4.31)

Recreators need to understand society's attitudes as they attempt to serve special populations in the community. Understanding societal attitudes is a first step toward dealing with them.

13. *Knows potential community resources (human and physical) that may be utilized for recreation for special populations.* (4.30)

Professionals' conceptions of the community guide their selection of actions in regard to serving the recreational needs of special populations that reside there. In order to guide practice decisions, professionals need to be able to complete community analyses, including relevant subsystems.

14. *States general objectives for recreation programs for special populations.* (4.23)

Defining the objectives for recreation programs for special populations allows community recreators to interpret their program to others and to evaluate the program to see if the objectives are being reached.

15. *Understands how the handicapped individuals' attitudes about themselves influence recreational behavior.* (4.23)

Self-attitudes in regard to our abilities and self-esteem can directly affect our behavior. While disabilities are usually thought to bring about negative self-attitudes leading to behaviors such as withdrawal, this does not have to occur. Recreators need to understand the influences of self-attitudes on behaviors in order to help facilitate healthy adjustments on the part of participants.

16. *Identifies activities that are appropriate to age and functioning level of the handicapped person.* (4.22)

It is necessary to match participants with appropriate activities so that they are not frustrated by their pursuits but, rather, are challenged by reasonable activity demands.

Austin and Powell (1981) had the following comment on the 16 aforementioned competencies:

> It is interesting to note that four of the competencies deal with attitudes. Three others concern normalization and mainstreaming, indicating agreement among experts that those entering the field of community recreation should have training in: attitudes as they relate to

special populations and the twin concepts of normalization and mainstreaming.

It also seems that community recreators will be asked to give increased attention to humanistic concerns in their service to special populations. Concepts such as the individuality of the participant, the impact of the leader upon self-worth and acceptance, and human interaction in instruction merit special consideration in this regard.

Several areas are conspicuous by their absence from the list of highly desirable competencies. Nowhere was the community recreator called upon to become expert on the characteristics of particular special populations, nor was the knowledge of special equipment or supplies demanded. Also absent was any reference to the history of community therapeutic recreation services. Perhaps these areas are less important than some might have us believe. (p. 42)

The competencies identified by Austin and Powell's (1981) experts constitute a listing of basic skills and knowledges necessary for entry-level professionals assuming positions in recreation and park departments. (The entire list of 86 competencies is found in Appendix B.) This information, coupled with that provided by others such as Pomeroy (1974) and Bullock (1982), could serve as a basic foundation for pre-service and in-service training of community recreation professionals.

COMMENT ON LEADERSHIP RESPONSIBILITY IN COMMUNITY RECREATION FOR SPECIAL POPULATIONS

It appears to us that public park and recreation agencies must return to their professional heritage of concern with recreation for special populations. As the suppliers of public park and recreation services, it seems clear that they have the responsibility to offer recreation services for persons with disabilities since it is their duty to serve the recreational needs of their jurisdictions at large. But it is particularly important, in our view, that public park and recreation agencies reach out to underserved segments of the population, including persons with physical or mental disabilities and aging persons. Therefore, we urge students preparing for careers in parks and recreation to ready themselves for the important task of providing special recreation services.

Further, we agree with Pomeroy (1974), Stein and Sessoms (1977), and other experts that special recreation programs should be largely organized and led by general recreation professionals. If such programs are to be an integral part of the agency offerings, they should be provided by the regular professional staff. The exception to this would be in programs with therapeutic intent. These are programs directed toward facilitating change through meeting specific objectives. Utilization of the therapeutic recreation process to effect specific outcomes calls for the knowledge and skills possessed by a professional prepared as a therapeutic recreation specialist. Therefore, we envision therapeutic recreation specialists working in park and recreation agencies in programs that are aimed at therapeutic objectives, with general recreation professionals delivering opportunities for leisure experiences. There appears to be no reason why general recreation professionals and therapeutic recreation specialists should not function together in the cause of providing necessary services for special populations.

———————————— SUMMARY ————————————

The organized recreation movement grew out of a social welfare concern reflected by the establishment of the Boston Sand Garden and recreation programs in settlement houses. Eventually, however, public recreation lost its focus on individuals with special needs as a new philosophy developed that viewed recreation as an end in itself, rather than a means to reach social ends.

It has been suggested that a broadened concept of therapeutic recreation, which viewed TR as encompassing all recreation for persons with disabilities, has further contributed to a perception that public parks and recreation does not have a responsibility for special recreation since this service is provided by those identified as therapeutic recreation specialists. This broad view of therapeutic recreation has been challenged by a number of authors who have taken the position that special recreation services rightfully fall within the domain of public parks and recreation. The final segment of the chapter discussed in-service training needs and necessary competencies for recreation professionals to offer leisure opportunities for those persons who have disabilities.

Suggested Learning Activities

1. Prepare a two- to four-page paper in which you provide support for the idea that organized recreation evolved out of humanistic concerns.

2. Within a discussion group, list reasons why communities fail to offer leisure services to special populations. Which reason(s) does the majority of the group consider most prominent?

3. Interview a park and recreation administrator in your home town on the subject of community recreation for special populations. Ask why the community offers (or fails to offer) leisure services for special populations. Prepare a two- to three-page report on your interview.

4. Prepare a two- to three-page paper on the relationship between therapeutic recreation and special recreation services. Arrive at your own personal position regarding the relationship.

5. Prepare a two-page paper in which you agree or disagree with the statement that "existing general recreation staff can be given training to enable them to work with participants with disabilities."

6. Examine the sixteen critical competencies listed in the chapter. Then do a three- to five-page self-assessment paper based on the critical competencies.

7. In class, discuss how you feel general recreation professionals and therapeutic recreation specialists can function together in the provision of community recreation for special populations.

References

American Therapeutic Recreation Association Newsletter 1(1): 2, 1984.

Austin, D. R. *Therapeutic Recreation Processes and Techniques.* New York: John Wiley & Sons, Inc., 1982.

Austin, D. R., J. A. Peterson, and L. M. Peccarelli. The status of services for special populations in park and recreation departments in the state of Indiana. *Therapeutic Recreation Journal* 12(1): 50–56, 1978.

Austin, D. R., and L. G. Powell. Competencies needed by community recreators to serve special populations. In Austin, D. R., ed. *Directions in Health, Physical Education, and Recreation, Therapeutic Recreation Curriculum: Philosophy, Strategy, and Concepts.* Bloomington, IN: Indiana University School of Health, Physical Education, and Recreation, 1980, pp. 33, 34.

Austin, D. R., and L. G. Powell. What you need to know to serve special populations. *Parks and Recreation* 16(7): 40–42, 1981.

Bullock, C. C., R. E. Wohl, T. E. Webreck, and A. M. Crawford, eds. *Leisure is For Everyone Resource and Training Manual.* Chapel Hill: University of North Carolina Curriculum on Recreation Administration, 1982.

Carter, M. J., and J. D. Kelley. Recreation programming for visually impaired children. In Kelley, J. D., ed. *Recreation Programming for Visually Impaired Children and Youth.* New York: American Foundation for the Blind, 1981, pp. 63–79.

Carter, M. J., G. E. Van Andel, and G. M. Robb. *Therapeutic Recreation: A Practical Approach*. St. Louis: Times Mirror/Mosby College Publishing, 1985.

Edginton, C. R., D. M. Compton, A. J. Ritchie, and R. K. Vederman. The status of services for special populations in park and recreation departments in the state of Iowa. *Therapeutic Recreation Journal* 9(3): 109–116, 1975.

Gray, D. E. The case of compensatory recreation. *Parks and Recreation* 4(4): 23, 24ff, 1969.

Gunn, S. L., and C. A. Peterson. *Therapeutic Recreation Program Design: Principles and Procedures*. Englewood Cliffs, NJ: Prentice-Hall, Inc., 1978.

Gunn, S. L., and C. A. Peterson. Therapy and leisure education. *Parks and Recreation* 12(11): 22ff, 1977.

Kraus, R. *Recreation and Leisure in Modern Society*. New York: Appleton-Century-Crofts, 1971.

Lutzin, P. B. Serving the handicapped and elderly. In Lutzin, S. G., ed. *Managing Municipal Leisure Services*. Washington, DC: International City Management Association, 1980, p. 152.

Meyer, L. E. Three philosophical positions of therapeutic recreation and their implications for professionalization and NTRS. In *Proceedings of the First Annual Post-Doctorate Institute*. Bloomington: Indiana University Department of Recreation and Park Administration, 1980, pp. 28–42.

Meyer, L. E. Three philosophical positions of therapeutic recreation and their implication for professionalism and NTRS/NRPA. *Therapeutic Recreation Journal* 15(2): 7–16, 1981.

Murphy, J. F. *Recreation and Leisure Service*. Dubuque, IA: Wm. C. Brown Company Publishers, 1975.

National Therapeutic Recreation Society. Philosophical position statement of the National Therapeutic Recreation Society, 1982.

Peterson, C. A., and S. L. Gunn. *Therapeutic Recreation Program Design: Principles and Procedures* (2nd ed). Englewood Cliffs, NJ: Prentice-Hall, Inc., 1984.

Pomeroy, J. One community's effort. Paper presented at the Institute on Community Recreation for Special Populations sponsored by North Texas State University and the Texas Recreation and Park Society, Arlington, TX, July 19, 1974.

Robb, G. M. A practitioner's reaction to three philosophical positions of therapeutic recreation and their implications for professionalization and NTRS. In *Proceedings of the First Annual Post-Doctorate Institute*. Bloomington: Indiana University Department of Recreation and Park Administration, 1980, pp. 43–52.

Sessoms, H. G. and J. L. Stevenson. *Leadership & Group Dynamics in Recreation Services*. Boston: Allyn and Bacon, Inc., 1981.

Stein, T. A., and H. D. Sessoms. *Recreation and Special Populations* (2nd ed). Boston: Holbrook Press, Inc., 1977.

Vaughan, J. L., and R. Winslow, eds. *Guidelines for Community Based Recreation Programs for Special Populations*. Arlington, VA: National Therapeutic Recreation Society, 1979.

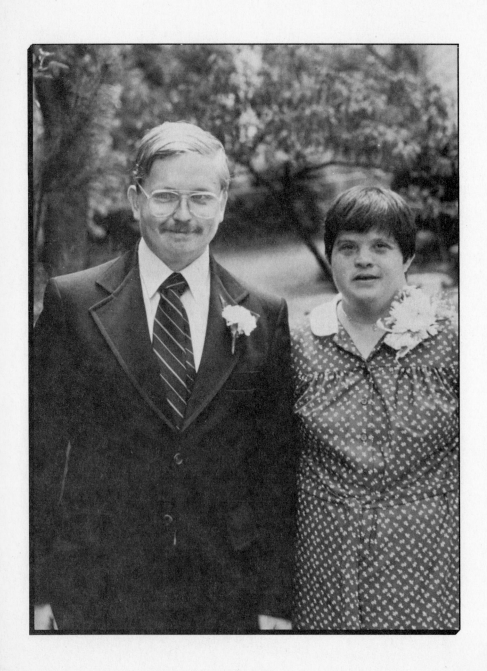

2

Concepts and Attitudes Underlying Special Recreation Services

This chapter deals with concepts and attitudes basic to understanding the delivery of special recreation services. The chapter begins with a review of terminology related to special recreation services. Reviewed are terms often used without precise definition in the parks and recreation literature. This discussion is offered with the hope that it will make clear the terms that appear not only in this textbook but throughout literature dealing with special recreation services.

Also contained in this chapter is a discussion of attitudes toward the provision of recreation programs and services for individuals with disabilities. Attitudes are important to our understandings since our attitudes influence our behavior toward providing programs and services for members of special population groups.

TERMS

It is not surprising that students are often confused by the terms "disabled" and "handicapped." These terms are regularly used without definition in the parks and recreation literature. Many authors use the terms interchangeably; others distinguish between them.

Disability/Handicap. A useful distinction between the terms *disability* and *handicap* is that the word disability refers to a specific impairment or disorder, whereas a handicap results from actions of the person with the disability or by society. That is, persons with a specific disability can handicap themselves by believing that they cannot do something when, in fact, they could function given the right conditions. Or, society can handicap persons with disabilities by refusing them opportunities.

The distinction between the terms disabled and handicapped is reflected in the following quote from *The Source Book for the Disabled*, edited by Hale (1979).

> Then there are the words "disabled" and "handicapped" themselves, which are used interchangeably, as if they meant the same thing and, by usage, have come to mean the same thing. But a physical disability, no matter how or by what it was caused, is a medically determined fact that can be defined and described explicitly. The word "handicap," originally used to denote a disadvantage in sports, is in effect a concept that's open to change as well as to interpretation.
>
> Sometimes a handicap can be minimized or even completely eliminated. A man whose legs are paralyzed and depends totally on a wheelchair, is very handicapped if he lives and works in inaccessible buildings and cannot use public transportation. If, however, he moves to a ranch style house, gets a job in a building which has an elevator and buys a car with hand controls, he is no longer handicapped. . . . There are, too, disabilities which will seriously handicap a person in one situation and not in others. A concert pianist who loses two fingers is severely handicapped as far as her career is concerned, although she may not be particularly handicapped in most of the other areas of her life. (pp. 2–3)

Society can cause persons to be handicapped, as indicated by Lord (1981). He has stated:

> Being handicapped is a social phenomenon. Our society handicaps many people. Examples include individuals with physical disabilities because of lack of accessibility to community facilities; persons with mental retardation or learning disabilities because of poor teaching or low expectations; single parents because of limited child support and narrow definitions of what constitutes a family; older adults because of stereotyped and inappropriate programming; and all of the above because of negative attitudes, economic deprivation, segregation, and denial of human rights. (p. 4)

Thus, the terms disabled and handicapped have singular meanings. At the same time, however, the reader must remain aware that in popular usage the terms are often employed to mean the same thing.

Special Populations. A related term, that may be familiar to students in parks and recreation, is *special populations*. Austin and Powell (1980) define members of special populations as: "Individuals who are not typically included in the mainstream of society. . . . " The International City Management Association's publication, *Managing Municipal Leisure Services* (Lutzin, 1980) states, "The term 'special populations' often is used to encompass both the handicapped and elderly—and sometimes other groups as well" (p. 140).

The term special populations has been used consistently in the literature to cover a broad range of persons, including those with disabilities. In general, we can say the term describes those who have special needs because of some social, physical, mental, or psychological difficulty. Because of its encompassing nature, it is popularly used to describe those who have not been served traditionally by leisure service delivery systems, including public park and recreation departments and voluntary and youth serving agencies. Within this textbook, we have purposefully reserved the use of the term *special populations* for instances when a broad, encompassing term seemed to be necessary.

Special Recreation. The term *special recreation* has recently emerged to describe recreation and leisure provisions that accommodate recreation participation by members of special population groups, and particularly by persons with disabilities. The term may have originated in the special recreation associations formed in Illinois during the 1970s. Special recreation services allow participation by individuals who have disabilities that necessitate special accommodations (modifications of activities, altered environments, personal assistance, etc.) above and beyond the kinds of accommodations generally provided. *Special recreation* deemphasizes categorizing people by placing the emphasis on the special nature of the accommodations required (Meyer, 1984).

Advocacy. During the 1970s a movement developed that emphasized the rights of persons with disabilities. This movement to some degree resembled the civil rights movement of the 1960s. However, its concern was with the rights of disabled persons, rather than the rights of black Americans. It was during the period of the 1970s that the term *advocacy* came into the vocabulary of many concerned helping professionals and parents of children with disabilities. Hillman (1972) has defined *advocacy* and has called on therapeutic recreation specialists to assume the role of advocates for disabled persons. Hillman has written:

> Advocacy is defined two ways in the dictionary. "One that pleads the cause of another" is the meaning given to the legal advocate, the lawyer. Another definition is "one who argues for, defends, maintains, or recommends a cause or a proposal." The latter definition should be of interest to the therapeutic recreation profession because of its generic

quality. As the TR specialist becomes more involved in community affairs with a social group, he will increasingly be thrust into an advocate role. (p. 50)

During the 1970s advocacy did become a role not only of therapeutic recreation (TR) specialists but also of many professionals from health and human service organizations, the federal government, and even some public park and recreation agencies, who argued for the causes of persons with disabilities. As the movement grew, professionals were joined by persons who were themselves disabled. Those advocating for their own rights were said to engage in *self-advocacy*. Today the role of disabled people has grown to the point that they themselves assume much of the advocacy leadership.

SELF-ADVOCACY STATEMENT BY KATE HOFFMAN:

"I" became a "We." I experienced others' pain in being different. We realized that collectively we could bring about changes in our own lives and for others. To me, the disability movement means the right to have and express a positive identity. Each of us must choose that identity. (Roth, 1981, p. 34)

Mainstreaming. Along with the terms disabled, handicapped, special populations, special recreation, and advocacy, *mainstreaming* and *normalization* are words that should become part of the vocabulary of park and recreation personnel. The term *mainstreaming* has been defined by Project Head Start (Kieran, et al., 1978) as follows:

"Mainstreaming" means helping people with handicaps live, learn, and work in typical settings where they will have the greatest opportunity to become as independent as possible. (p. 4)

Another definition of mainstreaming has been offered by Stein (1985):

Mainstreaming refers to providing individuals with handicapping conditions opportunities for appropriate education, physical education, recreation, and sport services and activities in settings as near to traditional practice as possible. (p. 3)

Mainstreaming then concerns the provision of opportunities for persons with disabilities to join in the mainstream of society. All of society's services, including parks and recreation, are a part of the mainstream that should be accessible to every citizen.

It has been said that mainstreaming is both a goal and a process (Austin & Powell, 1980). As a goal, mainstreaming involves integrating people with special needs into the mainstream of society. It is based on the concept that all persons deserve to participate in the *least restrictive environment* possible so that they can function at their optimal level of independence.

The term *mainstreaming* is also used to indicate the process by which alternatives are created so that persons with special needs can experience the least restrictive environment possible. It is the process by which individuals move from a segregated program toward an integrated one. This process is not the wholesale moving of persons with disabilities from segregated settings to regular programs but allowing individuals to progressively move toward their optimal level of functioning. For example, an individual might begin participation in a certain activity, say bowling, while institutionalized in a facility for persons with developmental disabilities. After gaining basic skills, the person may take part in a league for staff and residents of the institution. Later, he or she may take part in a special bowling league for persons with mental retardation run by the local park and recreation department. Finally, the bowler may be able to move into a league sponsored by his or her church, place of work, or other community organization. This process of progressive movement toward independent community participation may properly be referred to as mainstreaming. Of course, some individuals will be able to progress farther and faster than others since potential for independent functioning is individual.

It is important that a *continuum of services* be provided that offers opportunity for progressive skill development. Such a continuum gives participants a chance to move from being dependent on others toward being independent, as they develop their recreational and social skills. Thus, services along the continuum range from those requiring a great deal of staff assistance to those in which the participants take charge.

Several continua of services are detailed in Chapter 13, where the provision of various levels of programming is discussed as a trend. Typical of these is a continuum by Beck-Ford and Brown (1984), which has five phases: (1) *remedial programs* to improve physical and social skills needed in leisure pursuits; (2) *interest development and skill acquisition*

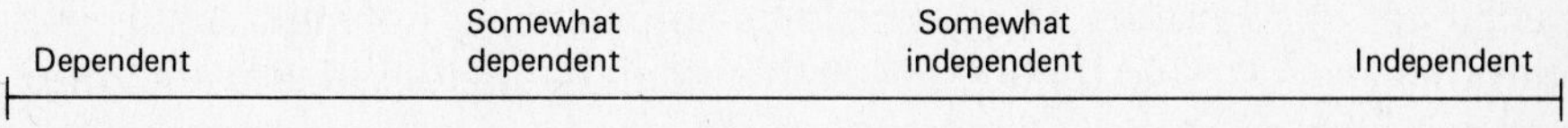

Dependent	Somewhat dependent	Somewhat independent	Independent

Figure 2–1. Continuum of services. Participants move toward becoming independent.

to expose participants to a number of leisure pursuits and to develop skills in specific activities; (3) *special programs* to develop the social and interpersonal skills needed for community participation; (4) *transition to community recreation programs* to develop knowledge of community resources and to obtain leisure counseling in preparation for community participation; and (5) *independent leisure management* to provide a minimal level of guidance sought at the initiative of the participant who functions relatively independently.

Park (1979) has summed up the concept of mainstreaming very well in the following statement. Park writes:

> Mainstreaming, in its fullest sense means, first of all, assuring that handicapped individuals who are ready and able to participate in mainstreamed settings are not denied that opportunity, and secondly, that individuals who are not ready and able are provided services which do prepare them for integrated participation. (p. 4)

Normalization. Another important term is *normalization*. This term refers to the provision of relatively normal experiences so that individuals with disabilities can maintain or develop traits and behaviors that are as culturally normative as is possible (Wolfensberger, 1972). In Wolfensberger's words, normalization is:

> . . . the utilization of means which are as culturally normative as possible, in order to establish and/or maintain personal behaviours and characteristics which are as culturally normative as possible. (p. 28)

The term *normalization* does not imply that *all* members of special population groups should be participating in regular community recreation programs. Following the concept of normalization does not preclude the provision of special, segregated programs. Normalization does, however, imply that special recreation programs be as normal as possible and that relatively normal behaviors be expected from participants, to the greatest possible degree.

For example, segregated athletic participation should be as close as possible to the way the sport is normally played. Modifications need to be minimal so that as normal an athletic experience as possible may be gained by the participants. Another example involves planning activities to fit the age range of participants. Activities should be age appropriate. Adults who are mentally retarded should not be expected to take part in childish games. They should be able to enjoy normal adult activities that are suited to their skills, rather than being forced into activities designed for children.

As a general rule, the least possible modification of activities is best. Ideally, activities should not be modified at all, or should be changed as

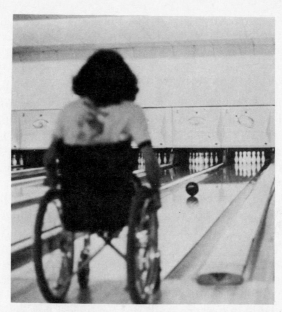

Figure 2–2. Bowling is an activity that may require no adaptations. Wheelchair users only need to gain access to the approach.

little as possible. At the same time, appropriate behavior should be expected from participants, to the greatest extent possible. In so doing they will be able to develop skills that allow them to fit into regular recreation activities in the community. The expectation of socially normative behavior allows participants to adjust to normal community programs.

We would hope that ultimately there would be a diminished need for special recreation programs as persons with special needs are able to take part in regular community programs. In regard to this point Spinak (1975) has written:

> The long term objective for recreation programming for the disabled would hopefully be a gradual phasing-out process of "special" programs—but not to the point of termination. As disabled citizens begin to get a better grip on independence and integration, their need for special group programs should diminish. This idea is based on the belief that many handicapped individuals will be able to accept the normalizing process. Undoubtedly, there will be those who are incapable of taking on full or even semi-independence for any one of many reasons. For these individuals, special recreation programs will

have to be retained. Many of those who become self-sufficient will still maintain a need for generically-focused social and recreation activities. For them as well, special recreation programs should be kept available. These are reasons why community sponsored recreation activities for the disabled will probably never disappear altogether.

Integration. The ultimate goal of special recreation would be the total *integration* of persons with disabilities into regular, ongoing programs. Even though this is the ideal, as Spinak has suggested, it is a goal that will likely never be reached. Instead, by offering various types of special recreation programs for members of special population groups, the community-based agency can allow mainstreaming to occur in the most normal and least restrictive environment appropriate for each participant. *Segregated programs* can offer opportunities for participants to develop skills that may be useful in moving into transitional programs. *Transitional programs* may help participants move into traditional, ongoing programs, should this be something that they desire and that is appropriate for them. Still other special recreation programs provide opportunities for individuals to take part in activities not traditionally available to persons with unique needs. For example, wheelchair sports may provide recreational outlets for individuals who have lower extremity disabilities.

ATTITUDES AND SPECIAL RECREATION SERVICES

What Are Attitudes?

Attitude theorists almost inevitably include an affective component in defining the term *attitude*. That is, they see attitudes as reflecting the degree of favorableness, or unfavorableness, an individual feels toward an attitude object. Said another way, our attitudes are a gauge of our liking for someone or something (Ajzen & Fishbein, 1980).

Attitudes are generally thought to be based on beliefs, thoughts, or ideas held toward attitude objects, whether the objects are persons, groups, places, or things. Although attitude theorists once included a behavioral component in their definitions, Fishbein and Ajzen (1975) have recently presented persuasive evidence that leads to the conclusion that attitudes are a separate entity from behavior. Individuals' attitudes are not necessarily displayed in their behavior. While attitudes may certainly influence behavior, they deal exclusively with how individuals *feel* toward an object, not with how they act.

Thus, in summary, we may say that attitudes rest on learned beliefs and reflect an individual's degree of liking for the attitude object, whether the object is a person, group, place, or thing. While attitudes may have a strong effect on behavior, there does not appear to be a one-to-one correspondence between attitudes and behaviors. Attitudes deal with the degree of liking for an object. Behaviors deal with our actions.

Language and Attitudes toward Persons with Disabilities

The words we use in our everyday language tend to reflect our attitudes. The use of the terms "the disabled" or "the handicapped" are offensive to many persons because their use implies that those individuals placed in these categories are not unique human beings but are all the same as others so categorized. It is just as misleading to categorize people with disabilities as "the disabled" as it would be to categorize those enrolled in elementary schools, high schools, vocational schools, and colleges as "the students." Of course, all are students but there the similarity ends. Their only similarity is that they are studying in educational institutions. Yet once labeled one of "the students," a young adult may be perceived differently when encountered by university personnel or the local police, or when attempting to cash a check at a place of business or obtaining housing in the community.

Likewise, the only similarity among those with disabilities is that they differ from others in having a disability. Even in regard to their disabilities there is a tremendous degree of variability among those who are disabled. Certainly orthopedic disabilities are very different from learning disabilities or mental impairments. Hearing impairments differ greatly from emotional disturbances, and so on. However, once we label a person "handicapped," there is a tendency not to think of him or her as an individual with unique potentials. Instead we restrict our thinking about the individual to the labeled condition. Our stereotyped thinking minimizes our perceptions of the person's uniqueness as a human being. We focus our perceptions on categorical differences, rather than on the individual.

Because labeling a person does tend to restrict everyone's thinking, within this book we have attempted to avoid using the terms "the handicapped" or "the disabled." Instead, we have used phrases such as "persons with disabilities," "persons with special needs," and "members of special population groups." In so doing we hope to remind ourselves and the reader of the fact that those who have a disability are first, and foremost, individual human beings much more similar to us than different.

Further guidelines for portraying persons with disabilities have been provided by the National Easter Seal Society (1981). The Easter Seal guidelines are:

1. Out of respect for the uniqueness and worth of the whole individual and because a disabling condition may or may not be handicapping, use the word disability rather than the word handicap, but give reference to the person first.

Following this guideline, phrases such as "person with a disability" or "individual who has a disability" are appropriate since these place the person or individual first. It would be inappropriate to refer to persons with disabilities as "the disabled" since this places the emphasis on the noun "disabled" and implies the person's total identity is tied to his or her disability. Also, this guideline suggests avoiding the use of the term "disabled" as an adjective, such as in "disabled persons." Within this book the expression "disabled persons" is used. Its use is hopefully restricted to occasions when it would be awkward to employ a phrase referring to the person first.

2. Because the person is not the condition, reference to the person in terms of the condition he or she has is inaccurate as well as demeaning.

We should never refer to someone as an "epileptic" or a "C.P." Instead, we should state "a person who has epilepsy" or "a person who has cerebral palsy." The individual is, of course, much more than a person who happens to have epilepsy or cerebral palsy or any other disorder.

3. Some categorical terms are used correctly only when communicating technical information—for example, hard of hearing, deaf, partially sighted, and blind.

Rather than using expressions such as "partially sighted," or "deaf," it is more appropriate to use the expressions "persons who have partial vision" or "individuals who have a partial hearing loss." Such expressions not only place the emphasis on the person but more accurately reflect the disabilities.

4. Avoid all terms carrying negative or judgemental connotations and replace them with objective descriptors.

Terms such as "afflicted with," "crippled," "invalid," "lame," "wheelchair-bound," and "victim" should be avoided. Instead of saying "afflicted with," say the individual "has." Instead of using "crippled," use an expression such as "the person with a disability," and so on.

5. Be careful with certain words that, if used incorrectly, can reinforce negative misconceptions of persons who have disabilities.

Words such as "defect" or "defective," for instance, certainly can reinforce negative ideas concerning persons with disabilities. As the

Easter Seal Society guidelines stipulate, it is permissable for us to use the terms "defect" or "defective" in describing an object—but not in describing human beings. Instead of "birth defect," we can say "disability present at birth" or "born with ( )." Rather than describing persons as "normal," use "persons without disabilities" to avoid language demeaning to individuals who have disabilities. Other terms that may cause difficulty if used incorrectly are *diagnose*, *disease*, and *patient*.

Means to Attitude Change

Attitude change is generally perceived to be brought about through two means. One is through the use of *persuasive communication*. The second is *exposure*.

Persuasive Communication

Authorities generally agree that attitude persuasion is equal to the communication, plus the communicator's characteristics, and the audience's identity and reaction (Eagly & Himmelfarb, 1978; Worchel & Cooper, 1979). The *communication* needs to transmit information that can be integrated into the judgments of those receiving the message. To be persuasive, the communication needs to be understandable to those who hear it. Otherwise, it may not be integrated into their thinking. If the message is associated with a positive emotion, it will be more likely to be persuasive. Secondly, the *communicator* needs to be credible and to present a positive image (Eagly & Himmelfarb, 1978). In addition, the communicator who is characteristically similar to the audience is more likely to alter attitudes that are value-oriented. Experts, on the other hand, are more successful in altering beliefs about facts (Worchel & Cooper, 1979). Finally, the communication should be directed toward already existing attitudes of the *audience*. If the thoughts expressed are vastly discrepant from those held by the audience, there is a greater possibility of rejection of the communication, unless the presenter is seen as highly credible (Worchel & Cooper, 1979).

Therefore, to alter attitudes toward serving persons with disabilities, certain principles should be followed. The message regarding serving individuals with disabilities should be clearly presented and, if possible, linked with something that is related to a positive emotion. The presenter should be chosen carefully since the attributes of the communicator may have a significant effect. Knowledge of already existing beliefs about serving persons with disabilities can aid in knowing what should be stated in the message. The message should not be too discrepant from the beliefs of the audience or it may be dismissed as too extreme. A knowledge of prior-held beliefs also provides direction in order to add or delete beliefs. In short, if we know the beliefs our audience holds toward serving those with disabilities, we can direct our communication in ways to positively influence their attitudes.

A related strategy is to ask audience members to *role play*. If persons are asked to play the role of someone who holds a position differing from theirs, they often will alter their beliefs to correspond with the role taken. Some research has found that role-playing produces greater attitude changes than receiving a presentation (Worchel & Cooper, 1979). Although there is a lack of empirical evidence in the literature indicating the use of role-playing in changing attitudes toward serving members of special population groups, it would appear to be an effective method.

Altering Attitudes toward Persons with Disabilities. Both role-playing and presentations have been successfully employed to alter general attitudes toward individuals with disabilities. Researchers at the University of Illinois (Clore & Jeffery, 1972) found that role-playing a wheelchair user by traveling on the campus for an hour brought about more positive attitudes toward disabled persons. Such realistic experiences should not be confused, however, with simulations where nondisabled individuals take part in recreational activities while simulating disabilities. Donaldson (1980), after reviewing the research, has stated, " . . . the present fad of game-type disability simulations may have little effect in helping participants see handicapped persons in less stereotypic ways."

Presentations have sometimes been effective in changing global attitudes toward disabled persons. One study (Austin, Powell, & Martin, 1981) involved the use of a class presentation that positively influenced the attitudes recreation and leisure studies students held toward individuals with disabilities. Results of studies involving such presentations, however, have been equivocal. To date, the exact factors that contribute to positive changes have not been identified. Further research is needed to more precisely determine the factors that facilitate positive changes resulting from presentations directed toward altering attitudes toward persons with disabilities.

Attitudinal Effects of Exposure

Zajonc (1968) conducted the now classical "black bag" social psychology study. Zajonc exposed university students in a speech class to an unknown person covered by a large black bag. The person in the black bag sat quietly on a table in the rear of the classroom during the entire semester. At the beginning, students were hostile toward the black bag but grew to like it by the end of the term. It was reasoned that mere exposure to an object (in this case, the black bag) was sufficient to bring about attitude enhancement. In other words, attitudes are supposedly enhanced by mere exposure to, or contact with, an attitude object.

Exposure as a Means to Altering Attitudes toward Persons with Disabilities. Research has revealed that mere contact with disabled individuals, unlike black bags, does not necessarily produce more positive attitudes toward them. In fact, negative attitudes may result if nondisabled persons experience tension or anxiety or perceive information that reinforces existing stereotypes (Donaldson, 1980). Since uninitiated people may feel uncomfortable with persons who have disabilities, it is of utmost importance to structure the situation so that nondisabled persons experience pleasant feelings during their exposure to persons with disabilities. It is likewise important that old stereotypes are not reinforced but, instead, are changed as a result of the contact. Recreational situations should provide an ideal setting for altering attitudes through exposure to persons with disabilities. A pleasant recreation environment offers an ideal situation in which nondisabled persons can interact with individuals who provide healthy, positive images of disabled persons. An example would be college students working in recreational sports programs with skilled athletes who are disabled.

Austin and Lewko (1979) reported that camp staff working with campers who were disabled became markedly more positive in their attitudes from the beginning to the end of a six-week summer camp. They attributed their results, in part, to the positive environment. They wrote:

> The positive social-recreational climate normally found in the informal camp setting would seem to facilitate the development of positive attitudes toward the handicapped. (p. 5)

In retrospect, while the mere contact hypothesis was perhaps naive, it has led us to future research that has revealed that under certain conditions contact with persons who have disabilities can lead to more positive attitudes. Nevertheless, even though exposure may produce a positive effect on general attitudes toward disabled people, global attitudes have not been found to correlate with specific behaviors, such as providing recreation services for special populations. The following section covers work by Fishbein and Ajzen (1975) that questions our traditional thinking regarding attitudes and behavior.

A Myth?

A number of authors in the field of leisure and recreation (e.g., Kraus, 1978; Lutzin, 1980; O'Morrow, 1980) have proclaimed that negative attitudes toward disabled persons cause barriers to the provision of recreation services for these persons. Fishbein and Ajzen (1975) have argued convincingly, however, that attitudes toward any given object (e.g., persons with disabilities) can predict only a *general pattern* of behavior, and not a *specific* behavior. Thus a general measure of attitude (i.e., a score on a scale measuring attitudes toward disabled persons) would not be useful in predicting a specific behavior, such as providing recreation services for persons with disabilities.

Following the conceptual framework provided by Fishbein and Ajzen (1975), it would be unwise to believe that if we alter attitudes toward disabled persons in a positive way we can expect those holding more favorable attitudes to be more likely to provide services for disabled persons. Fishbein and Ajzen stipulate that to predict a *specific behavior* one needs to know the *specific attitude* related to that behavior. In order to predict whether a community park and recreation professional would provide services designed for persons with disabilities, we would need to know his or her specific attitude towards serving them, not what general attitude he or she holds toward disabled individuals.

There are of course factors other than attitudes that could influence whether persons with disabilities would be served by community park and recreation specialists. Factors such as social norms, influences from other people, consequences of the behaviors, and personality traits have been utilized in predicting behavior (Ajzen & Fishbein, 1980; Eagly & Himmelfarb, 1978; Wicker, 1971). Another factor influencing behavior is the amount of experience a person has had with the attitude object (Regan & Fazio, 1977; Fazio & Zanna, 1978). Findings suggest that behaviors can be predicted from attitudes when the person has had previous experience with the attitude object. For example, an individual who has had experience in the provision of recreation for special populations would be more apt to act in accord with his or her attitudes toward serving persons with disabilities than a person without previous experience.

Thus the traditional model in which it was supposed that improvement in general attitudes toward disabled persons would result in increased provision of recreation services to disabled persons has not found support in modern attitude literature. The level of specificity of the attitude and other factors (e.g., social norms, previous experiences) need to be taken into consideration when attempting to predict any behavior, including the provision of recreation services to persons who have disabilities.

A New Theoretical Model

Fishbein (1967) has developed an attitude model to extend theoretical understandings of the relationship between attitudes and behavior.

Wicker (1969) claims Fishbein's work was the first to combine several factors into a systematic formulation. Fishbein's theory holds that both the *attitude toward the specific behavior* and the *subjective norm* (the influence of significant others and the person's motivation to comply with their desires) combine to bring about a *behavioral intention.* Knowledge of the behavioral intention can then be used to predict *actual behavior.* There is no direct correspondence between the behavioral intention and behavior since other factors may interfere with the intention being carried out.

For example, even though an administrator may intend to initiate a special recreation program, an emergency may occur that could divert resources from being used to begin the program. While the administrator may wish to initiate a plan, outside interferences may prevent that behavior. The behavioral intention may not be carried out.

Nevertheless, without a positive attitude toward establishing the service and social norms that support the action (such as support from the board and staff), there would be no behavioral intention to initiate the service. Thus, the critical nature of developing positive attitudes toward *serving* disabled citizens is apparent. While it may be meritorious to attempt to create more positive general attitudes toward persons with disabilities, there is apparently no reason to believe that this will bring about increased services for these individuals. Therefore, the focus of the discussion will be on the specific attitude of service to persons with disabilities, rather than upon general attitudes toward disabled persons.

Changing Attitudes toward Serving Persons with Disabilities

How then do we bring about changes in attitudes toward serving persons with disabilities? Because our attitudes rest on learned beliefs, our efforts should be aimed toward altering the most prominent, or salient beliefs related directly to the behavior of serving persons with disabilities. There are four means to altering beliefs on which an attitude is based, using the Fishbein model. We can (1) delete old beliefs, (2) add new salient ones, (3) alter their strength (how much we believe them), or (4) change their evaluation (how negative or positive we are) (Austin & Austin, 1982).

To alter beliefs, we must first identify them. Once identified, we may develop strategies to persuade the individuals to alter their belief system. For example, it might be discovered that the person holding a negative attitude toward serving individuals who have disabilities believed that carrying out the service would cause a great deal of inconvenience on his or her part. Information could be provided to show that a minimum amount of inconvenience would be involved for the comparatively large rewards to be received. Hopefully this would help to delete the old belief in regard to inconvenience. Another example would be adding beliefs related to the enjoyment the person might receive in setting up a new service. If it is found the person is not aware of positive benefits, such as getting to travel to other recreation and park departments to meet with colleagues already offering a program, or the good will created in the community as a result of establishing a program, these might be pointed out to him or her (Austin & Austin, 1982).

Subjective Norms. Since subjective norms are similarly based on beliefs, they too are subject to change. Beliefs in regard to perceived social norms can be added, deleted, or changed in strength. Motivation to comply to the norm can also be changed.

For example, beliefs toward serving persons with disabilities might be made more positive if the individual learns that a highly regarded administrator in a neighboring community is initiating a special recreation program. The impact of this knowledge could be multiplied if it were learned that several influential citizens had recently made public statements favoring the establishing of recreation services for special populations and that the mayor, who once opposed any park and recreation program expansion, came out for special recreation programming. The motivation to comply with what significant others desire would likely be increased if the individual saw that his or her compliance might be viewed in a positive way by influential citizens on whom the department relies for support. Thus, by altering beliefs and providing the motivation to comply with significant others, a subsequent increase in the overall subjective norm would be anticipated.

Summary. It has been suggested that any change in attitude toward the behavior, or in subjective norms, can facilitate change in behavioral intentions. In turn, this may bring about changes in behavior. The application of this model in parks and recreation has been discussed in regard to the specific behavior of establishing services for persons with disabilities. Once beliefs toward serving persons with disabilities have been identified, it is possible to design strategies to alter the information base underlying the attitudes and social norms of policy makers.

The popular notion that general attitudes (such as attitudes toward disabled persons) can be used to predict specific behaviors (such as the provision of special recreation services) has been seriously questioned. Research and theory by Fishbein and Ajzen on attitudes has been presented as an alternative to traditional thinking about attitudes. Both attitudes and social norms purportedly influence behavioral intentions.

Further, attitudes and social norms are based on salient beliefs held by the individual. Therefore, attitudes and social norms may be changed by altering beliefs.

SUMMARY

Critical to understanding the provision of services for members of special population groups is a knowledge of concepts and attitudes that underlie special recreation services. Within this chapter, terms were covered that relate to special recreation. To comprehend these terms is to begin to form a foundation for grasping concepts related to special recreation services. Also integral to these understandings is the application of modern attitudes theory to the relationship between attitudes and behavior in serving persons with disabilities. Knowing how attitudes are formed and changed provides park and recreation professionals with means to bring about positive attitudes toward serving individuals who have disabilities.

Suggested Learning Activities

1. Define the following terms in your own words: disabled, handicapped, special populations. Then compare your definitions with those of other students.

2. Within a small group, discuss how you can be an advocate for disabled persons. Do you see any conflict of interest on your part as a recreation professional, as opposed to parents of children who are disabled or those who are themselves disabled?

3. Discuss distinctions between normalization, mainstreaming, and least restrictive environment within a one- or two-page paper.

4. Within a small group, discuss the term *attitudes*. Then discuss what you feel to be the attitudes of recreation students on your campus toward the provision of leisure services for special populations.

5. List practical strategies you might use as a recreation professional to alter attitudes toward serving persons with disabilities. Bring your list to class to compare it with those of other students.

References

Ajzen, I., and M. Fishbein. *Understanding Attitudes and Predicting Social Behavior*. Englewood Cliffs, NJ: Prentice-Hall, Inc., 1980.

Austin, J. K., and D. R. Austin. An attitude theory to enhance understanding of behavior regarding mainstreaming blind and visually impaired persons in recreation activities. Unpublished paper. Bloomington, IN, 1982.

Austin, D. R., and J. Lewko. Modifying attitudes toward handicapped persons in a camping environment. *Therapeutic Recreation Journal* 13(3):3–6, 1979.

Austin, D. R., and L. G. Powell. *Resource Guide: College Instruction in Recreation for Individuals with Handicapping Conditions.* Bloomington: Indiana University, 1980.

Austin, D. R., L. G. Powell, and D. W. Martin. Modifying attitudes toward handicapped individuals in a classroom setting. *The Journal for Special Educators* 17(2):135–41, 1981.

Beck-Ford, V., and R. I. Brown. *Leisure Training and Rehabilitation.* Springfield, IL: Charles C Thomas Publishers, 1984.

Clore, G. L., and K. M. Jeffery. Emotional role playing, attitude change, and attraction toward a disabled person. *Journal of Personality and Social Psychology* 23:105–111, 1972.

Donaldson, J. Changing attitudes toward handicapped persons: A review and analysis of research. *Exceptional Children.* 46:504–14, 1980.

Eagly, A. H., and S. Himmelfarb. Attitudes and opinions. *Annual Review of Psychology* 29:517–54, 1978.

Fazio, R. H., and M. Zanna. Attitude qualities relating to the strength of the attitude-behavior relationship. *Journal of Experimental Social Psychology* 14:398–408, 1978.

Fishbein, M. Attitudes and the prediction of behavior. In Fishbein, M., ed., *Readings in Attitude Theory and Measurement.* New York: John Wiley, 1967, pp. 477–492.

Fishbein, M., and I. Ajzen. *Belief, Attitude, Intention, and Behavior: An Introduction to Theory and Research.* Reading, MA: Addison-Wesley Publishing Company, 1975.

Hale, G., ed. *The Source Book for the Disabled.* New York: Bantam Books, Inc., 1979.

Hillman, W. A. Therapeutic recreation specialist as advocate. *Therapeutic Recreation Journal* 6(2), 50, 1972.

Kieran, S. S., F. P. Conner, C. S. von Hipple, and S. H. Jones. *Mainstreaming Preschoolers: Children with Orthopedic Handicaps: A Guide for Teachers, Parents, and Others Who Work with Orthopedically Handicapped Preschoolers.* Washington, DC: U.S. Department of Health, Education, and Welfare, Head Start Bureau, 1978.

Kraus, R. *Therapeutic Recreation Service: Principles and Practices,* 2nd ed. Philadelphia: W. B. Saunders, 1978.

Lord, J. Opening doors, opening minds! *Recreation Canada,* Special Issue, 1981, pp. 4, 5.

Lutzin, S. G., ed. *Managing Municipal Leisure Services.* Washington, DC: International City Managers Association, 1980.

Meyer, L. E. Personal communication. July, 1984.

National Easter Seal Society. Guidelines. Portraying persons with disabilities in print. *Rehabilitation Literature* 42:284, 285, 1981.

O'Morrow, G. S. *Therapeutic Recreation: A Helping Profession*, 2nd ed. Reston, VA: Reston Publishing Company, Inc., 1980.

Park, D. Mainstreaming—implications for therapeutic recreation. *Therapeutic Recreation Journal* 1979, 13(4), 4.

Regan, D. T., and R. H. Fazio. On the consistency between attitudes and behavior: Look to the method of attitude formation. *Journal of Experimental Social Psychology* 13:28–45, 1977.

Roth, W. *The Handicapped Speak*. Jefferson, NC: McFarland, 1981.

Spinak, J. Normalization and recreation for the disabled. *Leisurability* 2(2):31–35, 1975.

Stein, J. U. Mainstreaming in recreational settings: It can be done. *Leisure Today* (pp. 3, 52). In *Journal of Physical Education, Recreation and Dance*. 56(5), 1985.

Wicker, A. W. Attitudes vs. actions: The relationship of verbal and overt behavioral responses to attitude objects. *Journal of Social Issues* 25:41–78, 1969.

Wicker, A. W. An examination of the "other variables" explanation of attitude-behavior inconsistency. *Journal of Personality and Social Psychology* 1971, 19(1), 18–20.

Wolfensberger, W. *Normalization*. Toronto: National Institute on Mental Retardation, 1972.

Worchel, S., and J. Cooper. *Understanding Social Psychology*, rev. ed. Homewood, IL: The Dorsey Press, 1979.

Zajonc, R. B. Attitudinal effects of mere exposure. *Journal of Personality and Social Psychology* 9(2):1–27, 1968.

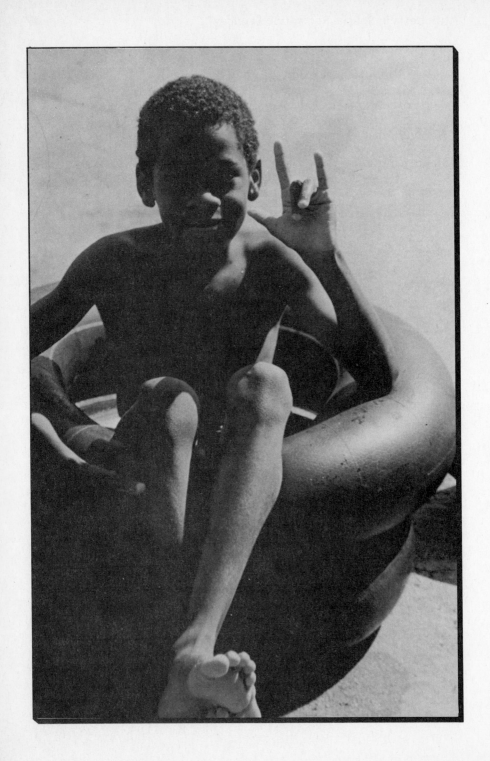

3

Disabling Conditions

Beginning at a very young age, people are capable of observing different objects and recognizing properties that make these objects similar. Tables, for example, are recognized as a large flat surface usually supported by four legs. Doors have handles and open to provide access to the outside or another room. This ability to categorize objects based on common characteristics is essential to human functioning. It not only enables us to recognize things that are essentially the same, but it also allows us to distinguish between items that have different qualities and/or functions. Failing to make such judgments could be catastrophic; i.e., it is essential to recognize that a chair is for sitting and a stove is for cooking, rather than vice versa.

LABELING

Categorizing, therefore, is a useful and necessary process in everyday life. It also presents problems, however. Categorizing can result in overlooking the uniqueness of each item within a category or class of objects. This is particularly troublesome when people, rather than objects, are categorized. Each human being desires to be recognized for his or her own talents and assets. However, placing a categorical label upon people with similar disabilities, a process known as *labeling*, interferes with recognizing the unique qualities of each individual with a disability. Furthermore, stereotypes may be formed, and these generalizations accentuate the differences (real or imagined) from so-called "normals."

Rosenthal and Jacobson (1968) demonstrated that labeling not only creates expectations that a member of a group will behave in a predictable way, but also can result in a "self-fulfilling prophecy." In other words, a person, once labeled, may actually behave in a certain way *solely* because such behavior is expected of him or her. As a consequence of a self-fulfilling prophecy a child labeled mentally retarded may fail to achieve according to his or her cognitive capabilities because others *expect* failure. An adult with a disability may remain physically dependent upon others because he or she *expects* such behavior.

Figure 3–1 summarizes the sequence described above. Placing a categorical *label* on an individual results in formation of a *stereotype*. This stereotype results in *expectations* regarding the individual's behavior. Because of these expectations, the labeled individual actually behaves as predicted. Thus, a *self-fulfilling prophecy* has occurred that appears to confirm the stereotype. It is a vicious cycle that many authorities feel precludes the use of labels for people with disabilities. Hutchison and Lord (1979) noted:

> The problems with a label are: 1) we tend to focus upon the person's disabilities rather than abilities, and 2) we make generalizations about the whole person based upon misconceptions regarding that label; in other words, a disability tends to have a spread effect in the minds of others. For example, a person who is mentally retarded may be considered unfeeling. (p. 18)

Perhaps the self-fulfilling prophecy results because the individual, also, focuses upon the disability and makes generalizations about himself or herself. Consequently, it is sometimes difficult for a person with a disability to develop a positive self-concept. He or she may view himself or herself as different, and somehow less worthwhile, than nondis-

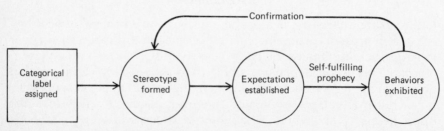

Figure 3–1. Self–fulfilling prophecy.

abled others. His or her concept of "self," and perhaps perceptions of the entire world, is distorted by an overemphasis upon the disabling condition. This overemphasis is exaggerated, if not caused, by the labeling process.

Special Population—A Label

The term *special population* results from categorizing people according to similar physical and/or behavioral characteristics. As such, its use constitutes a label. In addition to the possible consequences previously discussed, labeling someone as a special-population member has conceptual problems. The following questions clarify that identifying special population members is not as easy as one might expect:

1. How severe does a disability or behavioral disorder have to be in order to be classified as belonging to a special population? For example, do people have to be legally blind before they are a special-population member?
2. Is it the degree of disability or the functional limitation that qualifies a person to be a member of a special population? For example, is a person who is categorized "mentally retarded" a special-population member even if he or she functions as well as most nonretarded people?
3. Should the situation or task be taken into account in categorizing a special-population member? For example, is a wheelchair user considered to be a special-population member when playing basketball, but not while eating or playing cards?
4. Does the generic term *special populations* imply that people with different disabilities have common needs and/or problems? Should people with multiple sclerosis (who need cooler water to swim effectively) be classified under the same general term as people with cerebral palsy (who function best in warmer pool temperatures)?

The answers to these questions are by no means clear-cut. Rosenhan (1973) provided evidence that a person may be classified as a special-population member *even if he or she has no disability or functional limitation.* Rosenhan's eight nondisabled subjects admitted themselves to psychiatric hospitals and, once on the wards, behaved normally. Despite exhibiting no signs of psychological disorders, these "pseudopatients" were not detected as imposters by medical personnel. To the staff members of these institutions, Rosenhan's nondisabled subjects were special-population members. Ironically, a few "real" patients were the only ones to recognize that Rosenhan's subjects did not truly belong in a psychiatric facility. It is often said that beauty resides in the eye of the beholder. Whether someone is classified as a special population member may likewise depend upon the beholder.

The Paradox of Labels

The authors of this text recognize the many shortcomings and problems of labeling individuals with disabilities. It seems paradoxical, therefore, that we find it necessary to discuss people in terms of their disabilities. When used in this textbook, terms like *special populations* or *people with disabilities* are *not* meant to imply that all people who have disabilities are alike. On the contrary, the uniqueness of each person, whether disabled or nondisabled, is a concept which recurs throughout this text. For example, people who are classified as deaf (or hearing impaired) have similar, but not identical, limitations which may result in some common problems and/or needs. These same individuals, however, will have widely varied personalities, attitudes, functional behaviors, etc. As with all human beings, people with disabilities are alike in some ways, but in other ways they are quite dissimilar.

If emphasis is placed upon individual differences within categories, many authorities contend that labels may prove useful. Labanowich and Hoessli (1979), for example, have pointed out that categorizing people with similar disabilities may serve as a "starting point for a deeper understanding" by the rest of society. Mandell and Fiscus (1981) gave two additional advantages of labeling according to disability characteristics: (1) professionals can recognize and dispel any negative stereotypes they may have regarding specific disabling conditions, and (2) individuals with special needs can be referred to appropriate alternative services. It seems clear, therefore, that recreators must have some understanding of the nature of disabilities if they are to work effectively with *all* of their constituents. While the authors of this textbook fully recognize the potential problems of labeling, we do believe it is necessary to include selected information on a number of disabling conditions.

CONDITIONS AND CHARACTERISTICS

The remaining portion of this chapter provides selected factual statements about a variety of disabling conditions, including visual impairments, hearing impairments, learning impairments, motor impairments, and psychological and behavioral disorders. Although not a disabling condition, per se, aging has been included in this chapter because of the increasing importance of providing recreational opportunities to older persons.

It must be emphasized that the list in the prior paragraph does not include all possible categories of disability, nor are the factual statements that follow comprehensive in their content. The intent of each set of statements is to provide basic and applied information that may enhance the general understanding of recreators. Medical definitions, as well as etiologies (causes), prognoses (expected outcomes), etc., are *not* provided. The limited scope of this chapter does not allow for such depth; nor do most recreators who work in nonclinical settings require such detailed knowledge. Those desiring more depth on one or more disabling conditions are encouraged to refer to the references cited, or seek assistance from local volunteer health organizations, therapeutic recreation professionals, consumer groups, or information and referral sources.

Visual Impairments

Selected Facts

- Legal blindness is defined as having measured vision of 20/200 or less, in the better eye with corrective lenses. In other words, a legally blind person is able to see at 20 feet or less what a person with average vision can see at 200 feet. A person with a visual field of less than an angle of 20 degrees is also legally blind.
- Most people with visual impairments have some vision. Only about 5 percent of people classified as legally blind have no vision or light perception (total blindness).
- Most visual impairments are present at birth, but people who have adventitious (after birth) visual impairments will generally be able to create mental images of unseen objects based upon prior sight.
- Language, motor, and cognitive skills are not significantly impaired by visual deficits, providing the person's environment has been structured to enhance development of these skills.
- Most people with visual impairments are not able to read Braille; those who do generally read much more slowly than a sighted person. Few Braille readers exceed 150 words per minute.
- Some visually impaired people, particularly children, exhibit mannerisms known as "blindisms." These may be small or

large body movements including head shaking, eye pressing, body rocking, etc.

Tips and Techniques

- Try to involve *all* senses in recreational activities; using sounds, tastes, smells, and textures of materials can be enjoyed by everyone.
- Glare and other lighting conditions may create difficulties for some people with visual impairments. Since optimum conditions for vision will vary from person to person; consult with visually impaired participants to determine the correct type and amount of lighting to provide.
- Placing information on audio tapes is generally preferable to Braille. Some commercial tapes offer "compressed speech," which results from electronically "cropping" speech signals; thus, the speed of a recording is increased without distorting the sound.
- When walking with a visually impaired person who needs assistance, ask how he or she wishes to be guided. One preferred method is for the person with the visual impairment to hold on to your elbow and walk to your side and slightly behind. Verbal cues can help to avoid obstacles.
- Be sure all directions are clear and concise, and demonstrate physical tasks. Allow individuals with visual impairments to be close enough to see or touch demonstrations. Utilize verbal instructions to create mental images for people with adventitious visual impairments.
- Orientation to play and recreational areas is important. Prior to participation, encourage individuals to walk around the area with a guide so they become comfortable with their surroundings. Tactile maps and signs may also allow individuals who are blind to orient themselves to unfamiliar surroundings.

Hearing Impairments

Selected Facts

- Only a small percentage of people with hearing impairments have extreme hearing loss (greater than 90 decibels in the better ear). Those who do, however, are unable to understand amplified speech; they experience sound through vibrations from loud noise.

■ Hearing impairments occurring at birth, or shortly afterward, often result in delayed language development and difficulty with conceptual thinking. This is probably the greatest limitation experienced by people with hearing impairments.

■ Many hearing impaired people communicate by use of sign language and fingerspelling. Not all people with hearing impairments know and understand such communication methods, however, particularly those who developed hearing loss after early childhood.

■ Hearing impaired children often appear to be hyperactive, but their behavior frequently results from difficulty communicating with a "hearing world."

■ Some hearing impaired people have damage to their semicircular canals, which help control balance. Activities requiring balance, therefore, may prove difficult for these individuals.

Tips and Techniques

■ Whenever a deaf individual attends a recreational event, an interpreter should be provided to facilitate communication. Sign language and fingerspelling skills (see Figure 3–2) would

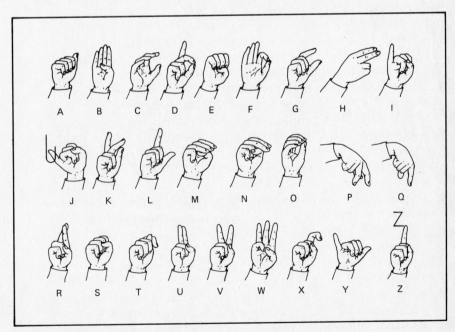

Figure 3–2. Fingerspelling alphabet.

also prove useful for community recreation professionals. As a last resort, write messages on a pad of paper.

- When using sign language or fingerspelling, wear solid, dark-colored clothing to serve as a suitable background. Also, ensure that adequate lighting is provided.
- To gain the attention of a person with a severe hearing impairment, tap the person on the arm or wave your hand (not arm) near his or her visual field.
- When using speech to communicate with a person who has a hearing impairment, always face him or her and do not slow or exaggerate your speech pattern.
- Written instructions should be expressed in short, clear sentences, and difficult vocabulary words should be avoided.
- When working with children who have hearing impairments, have several alternative activities prepared; in order to maintain their interest, it is sometimes necessary to redirect attention to a new activity.

Learning Impairments

Selected Facts

- People with mental retardation have subaverage cognitive functioning, but they *are* able to learn. Their rate of learning is generally slower than that of nondisabled people, however. Deficits in decision making and problem solving may also accompany this delayed learning pattern.
- Mental retardation and other learning impairments encompass a wide range of cognitive and behavioral functioning. Most people with mental retardation are capable of obtaining jobs and functioning independently within the community. The greater the retardation, however, the greater the chance that a person will need some form of assistance with requirements of daily living.
- The majority of people with mental retardation do not differ in physical appearance from their nonretarded peers. In general, the higher the cognitive functioning of a person with a learning impairment, the less likely he or she will have accompanying disabilities, motor deficits, or physical abnormalities.
- Socioeconomic conditions have been found to be associated with some learning impairments; for example, lower socioeconomic environments generally produce higher-than-average percentage of people with mild mental retardation.

- Children with mental retardation and other learning impairments usually experience delays in their physical, cognitive, and social development; they exhibit behavior that is characteristic of children considerably younger in chronological age.
- People with learning disabilities, unlike individuals who have mental retardation, have average-to-above-average intelligence, but do not function up to their cognitive potential.
- The signs of a learning disability vary widely. Problems in following directions, retaining information, performing paper and pencil tasks, and paying attention to *appropriate* cues are a few characteristics that may indicate the presence of a learning disability.

Tips and Techniques

- The wide range of behaviors and functional abilities of people with learning impairments necessitates careful consideration of *each* person's abilities. Assumptions about the individual, based upon a categorical designation, must be avoided.
- Activities should be divided into manageable parts and carefully sequenced to offer a progression of skills. Repetition of important tasks may also facilitate learning. Whenever possible, it is helpful to provide a demonstration so participants with learning impairments can model the desired behavior.
- Assist participants with mental retardation in selecting activities that are age-appropriate and require skills that are useful in community living. Some learning-impaired people have inaccurate perceptions of their own capabilities; try to ensure that the challenges of an activity correspond with the skills of the participants.
- Small group and cooperative activities may facilitate social development for those with deficiencies in adaptive behavior.
- Use verbal instructions that are clear and easily understood. Provide careful supervision of all activities, especially those in which accidents or injuries are possible. Be careful not to overprotect participants, however.
- Start an activity at the participant's current skill level, rather than the lowest possible level.
- With learning disabled individuals it is especially important to reduce extraneous stimuli; the leader should limit the quantity of materials, directions, verbal suggestions, and choices. Care should be taken *not* to limit opportunities for creativity.

- For most children with learning impairments, especially those with learning disabilities, activities should involve as many of the senses as possible. Abstractions are often difficult for such children to grasp, so visible evidence of success, such as certificates of achievement, should be used.

Motor Impairments

Selected Facts

- The diversity of motor impairments makes the use of generalizations exceedingly difficult, if not impossible. Some are easily identified and have reasonably predictable physical effects (e.g., amputations). Others, however, manifest themselves in many ways and result in a wide range of functional limitations (e.g., cerebral palsy).
- Some motor impairments are present at birth (congenital) and others occur after birth (adventitious). Most remain stable or improve, but a few are progressive; as a result, the person's functional abilities may decrease across time (e.g., muscular dystrophy).
- Motor impairments may affect practically the entire body or may impact one specific area, such as the lower extremities. Common terminology for localized paralysis (partial or complete) includes *monoplegia* (one extremity), *hemiplegia* (extremities on one side of the body), *paraplegia* (both lower extremities), and *quadraplegia* (all four extremities, perhaps including head and trunk involvement).
- Some people with motor impairments may have accompanying disabling conditions such as learning impairments, speech difficulties, or seizure disorders. Most people with motor impairments do not have multiple disabilities, however.
- Some children and young adults who have motor impairments experience an overly protective home environment, which places additional limits on their physical and/or social functioning.

Tips and Techniques

- Most people with motor impairments can fully integrate into community recreational activities *if* an accessible environment is provided (see Chapters 4 and 5).
- The wide variety of functional abilities of people with motor impairments dictates careful attention to the needs of

individual participants. Generalized programming tips for people with such diverse abilities are impossible, so seek advice from the participants who have disabilities.

- Ask participants with motor impairments if there are any specific conditions or techniques to avoid during recreational activities. For example, people with spastic cerebral palsy may have an exaggerated jerking response (stretch reflex) to a loud or unexpected noise. It would be unfortunate to have an art project ruined because the instructor was unaware of this reaction.
- Because some people with motor impairments have been overprotected at home, encourage challenging, but safe, activities. During such activities, keep in mind that balance difficulties are common among people with mobility limitations.
- Participation in specific activities and/or exposure to certain weather conditions may be inadvisable for some people with motor impairments. Try to discuss the demands of an activity with participants in advance, and consult a therapeutic recreation specialist (or another knowledgeable professional) if there are any doubts about the advisability of participation.

Aging

Selected Facts

- It is generally accepted that old age begins at 65 years of age, but the physical, cognitive, psychological and social functioning of older people vary considerably. Many people are chronologically old, yet exhibit few signs of advanced age. Conversely, some people display physical attributes associated with advanced age well before their 65th birthday.
- Most older individuals are self-sufficient in all aspects of their lives. Some, however, do experience a "role reversal" situation. This happens when their offspring begin (or attempt) to make important life decisions for the older person. Such situations are extremely frustrating and may lead to feelings of futility and personal ineffectiveness.
- Approximately 95 percent of older people in the United States live and function within the community, rather than in hospitals or nursing homes.
- Advanced age is usually accompanied by decreased visual acuity, some hearing loss (especially higher-pitch sounds), and

decreased motor performances. Generally, however, these declines do not place limits on most activities until a person is well into his or her 70s, or beyond.

- In metropolitan areas, fear of crime and lack of financial resources are two major factors that may limit recreation and leisure participation among elderly individuals. Other factors include health considerations, lack of companionship, and transportation difficulties.

- Contrary to stereotypes held by many, older people *are* interested in sex. They can, and frequently do, engage in satisfying sexual relationships.

Tips and Techniques

- It is essential that older people be given opportunities to maintain personal control over their own life activities. Citizens' councils and other organizations should be used to provide direction for community programs with elderly participants.

- Utilize the skills that older people possess. Provide opportunities for elderly individuals to serve as activity leaders, and try to offer a chance for them to share their life experiences with children, as well as with people of all ages.

- Opportunities to socialize with age cohorts (those in the same stage of life) are important; flexible programs in a relaxed atmosphere should facilitate social interaction. Activities should encourage older participants to proceed at their own pace and desired level of involvement.

- Older people are very capable of learning new information and skills. Many welcome the chance to participate in adult education classes; identify topics, subjects, and skills of interest and provide opportunities for learning.

Psychological and Behavioral Disorders

Selected Facts

- Disruptive or abnormal behavior is manifested in a wide variety of ways and may result from one or more factors. Heredity, learning, physiological malfunctions, and/or environmental (situational) factors are often identified as contributing to problem behavior.

- For an individual to be considered to have a psychological or behavioral disorder, his or her behavior must be viewed in

terms of its degree and/or duration. Extreme outbursts or
withdrawal, or consistently inappropriate behavior over time
may indicate that professional intervention is necessary.
- Some popular and/or prescription drugs may result in
behaviors that appear to be signs of psychological or
behavioral disorders.
- The primary concern of most group leaders is the person
whose actions distract group members or disrupt group
processes. Some behaviors, however, are not disruptive but
may warrant similar attention, including: extreme
withdrawal, excessive shyness, submissiveness, frequent and
prolonged daydreaming, fearfulness, and/or lack of interest in
or response to environmental surroundings.
- The context in which abnormal behavior occurs, as well as
the life situation of the individual must be considered.
Behavioral deviance is based upon culturally defined norms
and values. Much behavior that appears abnormal can be
rationally explained by the heritage or life circumstances of
the individual.

Tips and Techniques

- Group leaders should become familiar with behavior
management techniques, and use them when necessary. Some
specific techniques for dealing with problem behavior in
children are included in Chapter 8.
- No single technique of behavior management has been found
effective with all people. Regardless of the technique used,
consistency and empathy are essential.
- The presence of appropriate behavioral models in a warm
and understanding environment may do a great deal to reduce
or eliminate inappropriate behavior. Patience and acceptance
of individual differences are also important.
- Learn to identify the physiological and psychological effects of
popular drugs.
- If an individual's behavior appears to warrant outside
intervention, seek the assistance of a qualified mental health
professional.

SUMMARY

The traditional approach to special populations is to focus extensively
upon characteristics that distinguish people with special needs from

the general population. Medical terminology, facts and figures, and therapeutic interventions are often stressed. The authors of this textbook, however, feel that this traditional approach often overlooks the uniqueness of each person with a disability. Rather than give detailed characteristics and data for all disabling conditions, we have presented applied information that should be useful to any recreational professional. Readers interested in additional information regarding data, characteristics, and terminology associated with specific disabling conditions are encouraged to consult the following resources:

Adams, R., A. Daniel, and L. Rullman. *Games, Sports and Exercises for the Physically Handicapped.* Philadelphia: Lea and Febiger, 1983.

Atcheley, R. C. *The Social Forces in Later Life.* Belmont, CA: Wadsworth Publishing, 1977.

Basmajian, J. V., ed. *Therapeutic Exercise.* Baltimore: Williams & Wilkins, 1984.

Batshaw, M. L. and Y. M. Perret. *Children with Handicaps: A Medical Primer.* Baltimore: Paul H. Brookes, 1981.

Bernstein, E., ed. *1985 Medical and Health Annual.* Chicago: Encyclopaedia Britannica, 1985.

Bleck, E. E. and D. A. Nagel. *Physically Handicapped Children: A Medical Atlas for Teachers.* Orlando: Grune & Stratton, 1982.

Carmi, A., S. Chigier, and S. Schneider. *Disability.* New York: Springer-Verlag, 1984.

Kelley, J. D., ed. *Recreation Programming for Visually Impaired Children and Youth.* New York: American Foundation for the Blind, 1981.

Mandell, C. J. and E. Fiscus. *Understanding Exceptional People.* St. Paul, MN: West Publishing, 1981.

Peterson, C. A. and P. Connolly. *Characteristics of Special Populations: Implications for Recreation Participation and Planning.* Champaign, IL: Office of Recreation and Park Resources, 1978.

Stein, T. A. and H. D. Sessoms, ed. *Recreation and Special Populations.* Boston: Holbrook Press, 1977.

Stolov, W. and M. Clowers. *Handbook of Severe Disability.* Washington, DC: U.S. Department of Education, Rehabilitation Services Administration, 1981.

Suggested Learning Activities

1. Explain the concept of a "self-fulfilling prophecy." How do you think expectations could cause behavior?

2. Write a two-page paper that gives your personal opinion on the topic "Should Labels Be Used to Identify People with Disabilities?"

3. Learn the fingerspelling alphabet pictured in Figure 3–2. Practice this alphabet by fingerspelling a message to friends (they can use Figure 3–2 to interpret your message).

4. Research one disabling condition and:
   a) add two facts to the *Selected Facts* listed in the chapter.
   b) add two suggestions to the *Tips and Techniques* provided in the chapter.

References

Hutchison, P. and J. Lord. *Recreation Integration*. Ontario, Canada: Leisurability Publications, 1979.

Kelley, J. D., ed. *Recreation Programming for Visually Impaired Children and Youth*. New York: American Foundation for the Blind, 1981.

Labanowich, S. and P. Hoessli. Module 2: Knowing the campers. In Vinton, D. A. and E. M. Farley, eds. *Camp Staff Training Series*. Lexington, KY: University of Kentucky, 1979.

Mandell, C. J. and E. Fiscus. *Understanding Exceptional People*. St. Paul, MN: West Publishing, 1981.

Rosenhan, D. L. On being sane in insane places. *Science, 179*, 250–253, 1973.

Rosenthal, R. and L. Jacobson. *Pygmalion in the Classroom: Teacher Expectations and Pupil's Intellectual Development*. New York: Holt, Rinehart & Winston, 1968.

PROGRAM AND
FACILITY PLANNING

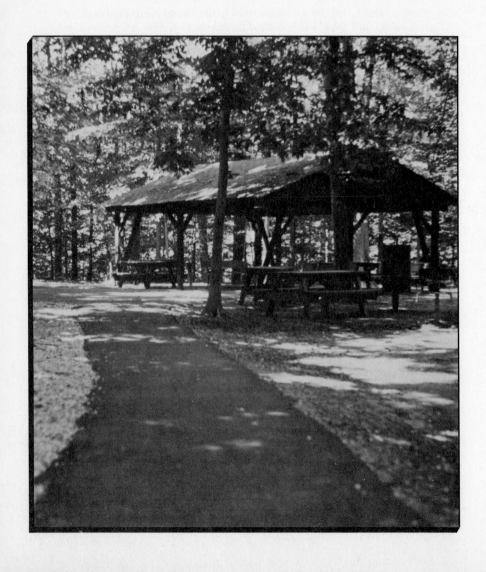

Equal access to recreation programs and facilities is the thrust of Chapter 4, *Barriers to Recreation Participation.* This chapter discusses intrinsic, environmental, and communication barriers that prevent leisure participation by individuals with disabilities, along with means to overcome these barriers.

Chapter 5, *Design of Accessible and Usable Recreation Environments,* concerns designing appropriate recreation environments for all people, including persons with disabilities. A major portion of the chapter is devoted to guidelines and recommendations for creating accessible and usable public park and recreation facilities. A special section on playground design concludes Chapter 5.

Featured in Chapter 6, *Program Planning Processes,* is a discussion of needs assessment and goal formulation. Activity analysis is covered and guidelines are suggested for the selection and modification of activities for persons with disabilities.

The final chapter in this section is Chapter 7, titled *Special Recreation Programs—Exemplaries and Standards.* This chapter begins by presenting information on several outstanding community-based special recreation programs. Each program is highlighted and the philosophy and goals of each are outlined. This unique approach to the study of special recreation offers the reader information never before gathered in one place. The chapter concludes with a discussion of standards for the provision of special recreation services.

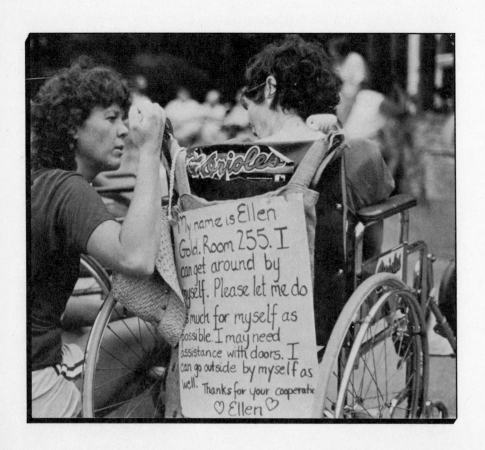

4

Barriers to Recreation Participation

There are many factors that shape an individual's recreation and leisure behavior. People who live in Florida, for example, are much less likely to experience snow skiing than people living in Colorado. Individuals with limited financial resources may find it impossible to afford recreational luxuries such as vacation homes or resort trips. People from specific regions or cultural backgrounds may refuse to participate in activities that others, from different backgrounds, find very acceptable and enjoyable. As with this last example, some of these factors provide a framework for *choice*. The individual freely chooses either to participate or not to participate in an activity that is both available and attainable. Many factors exist, however, that may deny this freedom of choice. In the first two examples above, location and lack of money serve as barriers to participation. Everyone experiences such barriers, but there is no doubt that people with disabilities experience greater and more barriers than nondisabled people. The following expression, based upon a quote from George Orwell's *Animal Farm*, summarizes the situation: "We are all created equal but some of us are more equal than others." When it comes to the opportunity to participate in recreation and leisure activities, people without disabilities are clearly "more equal" than their disabled peers.

James F. Murphy has emphasized the importance of barriers to participation. Describing the delivery of leisure services within a humanistic framework, Murphy (1980) listed two general goals:

1. Making available through an event or series of experiences, opportunities for human expression which enables a person to grow in dignity and self-worth and develop to the fullest of one's capacity.
2. Removal of barriers which impede or prohibit participation because of social, physical, racial or sexist discrimination. (p. 202)

Murphy recognized that merely offering a service program is not enough. It is the obligation of the service provider to ensure that an individual's failure to participate is based, as much as possible, upon personal choice. The decision not to participate should *not* result from barriers that systematically deny participation to specific groups of people.

One single step can deny wheelchair users the right to enter a building independently. The absence of an interpreter may prevent a deaf person from understanding a play. Individuals who have mental retardation may be eliminated from participation in many events unless an effort is made to include tasks appropriate to their cognitive abilities. As noted by Bowe (1978), these and other barriers "impose limitations and exact penalties far greater than do the disabilities themselves" (p. xii). Yet, if recreation professionals are going to assist in the effort to improve lives by removing barriers to recreation and leisure activities, they must be able to recognize more than the obvious barriers previously cited. They must constantly be alert to the *many forms* that barriers take, and attempt to eliminate or minimize the impact these barriers have upon individuals with disabilities.

TYPES OF BARRIERS

The multitude of barriers preventing individuals with disabilities from full leisure participation can be divided into three major categories: (1) *intrinsic* barriers, which result from the individual's own limitations and may be associated with a physical, psychological, or cognitive disability; (2) *environmental* barriers, which are composed of the many external forces that impose limitations upon the individual with a disability; and (3) *communication* barriers, which block interaction between the individual and his or her social environment.

Intrinsic Barriers

Like everyone else, individuals with disabilities face constraints that result from their own physical, emotional, or cognitive limits. These intrinsic barriers may be associated directly with their disabilities, but they also may arise from other factors such as parental overprotection

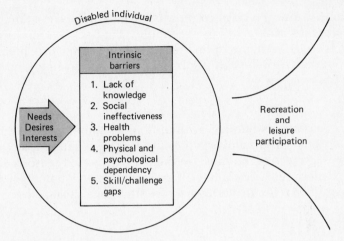

Figure 4–1. Intrinsic barriers.

or inadequate educational opportunities. Regardless of their causes, intrinsic barriers are permanent or temporary limitations that reside within the individual. As illustrated in Figure 4–1, such barriers may block fulfillment of the individual's needs, desires, and interests. The following are intrinsic barriers that may reduce a person's ability to participate in recreation and leisure activities.

Lack of Knowledge.

Many people are not able to realize their maximum leisure functioning because they lack essential information. Knowledge of programs, facilities, and other recreation and leisure resources, for example, is needed in order to make informed choices. Knowledge of support services, such as modes of transportation, also may be necessary in order to participate in a particular recreational activity.

In some cases, people with learning disorders or mental retardation may be incapable of learning about recreational opportunities. Usually, however, knowledge deficits arise from inadequate information or a lack of opportunities to learn about recreation resources. Matthews (1980) found that parents and guardians of mentally retarded individuals "demonstrated a lack of awareness of activities offered in their area; they did not know about particular activities or were ignorant of the fact that their children could participate in recreational activities" (p. 49). Likewise, Hutchison (1980) found that the people in her study with physical disabilities considered lack of information on available services to be an important barrier to recreation participation.

Obviously, an individual cannot participate in a recreational activity if he or she is unaware of its availability. This lack of knowledge can impose a severe restriction upon the recreation behavior of anyone, but especially upon people with disabilities who face so many other barriers to participation.

Social Ineffectiveness.

For many reasons, individuals with disabilities sometimes have ineffective social skills. Parental overprotection and segregation from nondisabled peers are two of the most frequently mentioned reasons. In addition, youngsters with disabilities often receive inadequate feedback on appropriate behavior in various social situations. Regardless of their

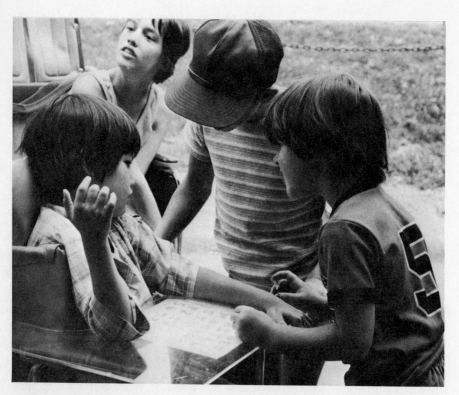

Figure 4–2. Effective communication requires *active* participation by both the sender and receiver of a message. For physically disabled people with speech difficulties, pointing to letters on a "letter board" may facilitate this two–way interaction process. (Courtesy of the League for the Handicapped, Baltimore, MD.)

origin, however, ineffective social skills have a profound effect upon an individual's participation in leisure activities.

People often form their own self-images from their interactions with others. How others react to them provides cues that combine to produce a stable view of their own self-worth. A person who lacks the social skills that are needed to get positive and consistent feedback from others may encounter interference with his or her vital process of self-concept formation. This is especially true if skill deficits in other areas of a person's life limit his or her feelings of personal control and effectiveness. Bowe (1978) noted the impact of poor self-concepts among recently disabled individuals. He wrote that a "vicious cycle" results, in which "damaged self-concepts ... lead to lowered aspirations and increased isolation, further handicapping the disabled individuals" (p. 35).

Health Problems.

Most people with disabilities do not "suffer," but lead relatively pain- and illness-free lives. Still, some types of disabilities do present recurring health problems. Rheumatoid arthritis, for example, is accompanied by frequent and often severe episodes of pain. The pain, plus a limited range of movement within affected joints, may make participation in certain activities impossible. Some types of disabilities also have "contraindications," a term meaning that a particular behavior may result in medical complications or injury. Rough or contact-type activities may be contraindicated for a child with hemophelia, and lengthy exposure to the sun may be contraindicated for people taking certain types of medication.

The following statement by Gunn (1978) emphasizes that health problems in very young children with disabilities may have negative impacts upon their ability to play:

> Physically and mentally handicapped individuals most often have had additional blocks to spontaneous play behavior imposed on them. Some handicapped children suffer much physical pain as infants. Often it is impossible to grant them the comfort for which they cry. Additionally, some are hospitalized and institutionalized, which jeopardizes the healthy symbiotic relationship between infant and mother. (p. 106)

One word of caution should be noted here. Recreators must remain aware that giving *too* much attention to health-related matters may result in overprotection. Care must be given to ensure the *optimum* level of attention to health-related barriers so that maximum participation is encouraged.

Physical and Psychological Dependency.

As any child grows into adulthood, there is a gradual progression toward physical and psychological independence. Total independence from others is neither achievable nor desirable, of course, but most people strive for a level of independence that allows them to feel at least partially in control of their environment. Unfortunately, many people who have disabilities do not achieve their potential for independent functioning. Some are genuinely limited by the effects of their disability, but others "learn" to be dependent in situations they have the capacity to control. From the moment a disability occurs or is discovered, the disabled person may be overprotected and overassisted by others. As time goes on, this situation renders the individual physically and/or psychologically incapable of achieving a desired level of independence.

When a disability makes an individual physically dependent upon others, the limits imposed are obvious. In some cases, an attendant or aide may be necessary. This is reflected in the following statement by Carpenter (1977):

> With the severely handicapped person, such as I, a person is also needed who is able and willing to put on his jacket, help him to the washroom and so on. This required help can prevent many from attending recreation programs. (p. 110)

Psychological dependency is not always as obvious as physical dependency, but it can be even more limiting. Family members, friends, and rehabilitation professionals are all capable of fostering an atmosphere of psychological dependency for people with disabilities. Often this situation is reciprocal, meaning that the person with a disability receives feelings of satisfaction from being protected and patronized, while the nondisabled person enjoys being needed by someone viewed as "less fortunate." Thus, both have their needs met by the other.

When psychological dependency occurs, the disabled person's capacity for personal growth and self-development is severely limited. Many of the barriers that are faced by people with disabilities require personal initiative, creative thought, risk taking, and perseverance in action. These qualities do not develop fully in an atmosphere of psychological dependency. The fact that some rehabilitation professionals encourage their clients to be dependent also compounds this problem. As noted by Illich, et al. (1977), "Life is paralyzed in permanent intensive care" (p. 27).

Skill/Challenge Gap.

Csikszentmihalyi has studied enjoyment of activities for many years. In his book, *Beyond Boredom and Anxiety* (1975), he proposed that enjoyment of an activity is most often possible if the participant perceives that the challenges of an activity are in balance with his or her skills. If the challenges are thought to be too great, worry or anxiety may limit the chance for enjoyment. If the challenge is considered too easily achieved, boredom often results. Many individuals with disabilities do not possess skill levels appropriate for enjoying a number of leisure pursuits. Sometimes the nature of their disabilities limits skill development, but often they do not get the opportunity to develop skills that could enhance participation. As a result, they correctly perceive that many activities are too challenging for their present skills. The result is usually nonparticipation.

This skill/challenge gap barrier has many implications for recreation professionals. Proper progression in teaching specific skills may enable a disabled individual to gain the expertise necessary for participation. Also, an activity may be modified to accomodate the current skills of a participant with a disability (see Chapter 6). It is very important to keep in mind that the participant's *perception* of his or her skill level is a critical factor. Underestimating one's own skill may result in withdrawal from participation, whereas overestimating one's own skill may prove embarrassing or even dangerous. Many overconfident skiers, for example, have ended up in the hospital because they thought they were ready for the advanced slopes. As Bregha (1980) observed, the ability to select appropriate leisure pursuits requires more than knowledge of what is available or permissible. "Something deeper is required: the knowledge of oneself as well as one's milieu. . . ." (p. 31).

Environmental Barriers

No matter how successfully a person with a disability copes with intrinsic barriers to recreation participation, he or she will also be faced with external forces that limit participation. Figure 4–3 illustrates the idea that these external forces, known as environmental barriers, may block the actions that a person takes toward participation in recreation and leisure activities. Unlike intrinsic barriers, environmental barriers are imposed upon the individual by societal and/or ecological conditions. Thus, the person is less likely to feel that he or she can overcome such barriers through individual action. Many intrinsic barriers can be partially or completely overcome through personal efforts, i.e., physical rehabilitation, educational programs, counseling, etc. The solution to environmental barriers is much more complex and, therefore, more frustrating for individuals with disabilities. The following environmental barriers limit recreation and leisure participation for many persons with disabilities.

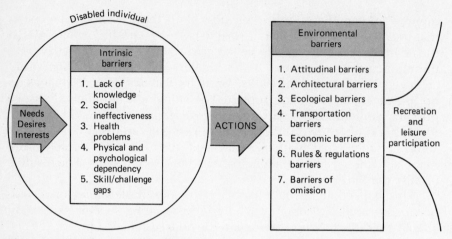

Figure 4–3. Environmental barriers.

Attitudinal Barriers.

Of all the barriers to participation faced by individuals with disabilities, attitudinal barriers are probably the most limiting. They are also the most difficult to overcome. The attitude concept is discussed in depth in Chapter 2, but it is important here to examine the types of behaviors that reflect barrier-producing attitudes. These behaviors, which may be exhibited by family and friends or by strangers, can be divided into three categories: (1) *negative* behaviors; (2) *paternalistic* behaviors; and (3) *apathetic* behaviors. In order to achieve a better understanding of these behaviors, we will examine each type.

(1) Negative Behaviors. From time to time, every person with a disability is subjected to behaviors that arise from negative attitudes toward people who are "different." Some of these behaviors are obvious, but others are subtle. They all, however, clearly inform the individual that he or she has less value than a nondisabled person. One obvious sample of negative behavior is ridiculing or mocking the person with a visible disability. Less obvious, though, is avoidance of people with disabilities. Whether from fear, dislike, or discomfort, many nondisabled people avoid eye contact and maintain exaggerated social distance when in the presence of people with visible disabilities (Langer, et al., 1976). Obsolete and derogatory labels, such as "cripple," "deaf and dumb," and "crazy," are also examples of negative behaviors. Such terms are not only demeaning, but their use encourages others to behave negatively toward people with disabilities.

(2) Paternalistic Behaviors. Many nondisabled people treat adolescents or adults who have disabilities like children. (They often treat children with disabilities like infants!) Unlike negative behaviors, paternalistic actions frequently arise from a desire to show a "favorable" view of disabled people. Unfortunately, the message conveyed by paternalistic behavior is that people with disabilities lack competence, maturity, and the capacity for independence. Head patting, giving undue or excessive praise, and providing help when it is not needed are all examples of paternalistic behavior. The importance of *not* overhelping individuals with disabilities was highlighted by Karol Davenport, a world-class wheelchair athlete from Pennsylvania. Upon returning from her first wheelchair track and field competition, Karol was glowing from her success and the camaraderie she shared with others. Finally, she said, "But you know what I liked best of all? People *didn't* help me when I said I didn't need help!"

(3) Apathetic Behaviors. People who are apathetic toward individuals with disabilities express no feelings of sympathy, understanding, or caring toward people who have disabilities. Rather than being negative or paternalistic, such people totally ignore the needs and concerns of people with disabilities. They behave as if such people did not exist. Doug Wakefield, who is blind, talked about one personal experience with public apathy. Doug and his guide dog were using Washington's Metro (subway) system. They got off of the train at an unfamiliar station, thus Doug did not know the direction of his exit. His guide dog, which is trained to keep him from dangerous situations, preceded Doug as he paced back and forth on the landing trying to determine the appropriate direction. Despite the fact that it was obvious Doug and his dog were pacing aimlessly, none of the passengers and bystanders offered assistance. Some people may have failed to help because of negative feelings, but Doug felt that most were simply apathetic toward his dilemma. Ironically, public apathy prevented him from climbing out of a Washington subway station, but in 1981, Doug Wakefield and 10 other individuals with disabilities scaled Mt. Rainier.

Architectural Barriers.

Manmade structures, such as buildings, walkways, and so on, that are usable by nondisabled people but present obstacles for people with disabilities are known as architectural barriers. These barriers limit mobility and often deprive individuals with disabilities access to worthwhile leisure activities. David Park (1977), the National Park Service's Chief of Special Programs and Populations, noted, "A major reason many handicapped persons do not participate in existing recreation programs is simply that facilities are not physically accessible and barrier-free" (p. 129).

Not all people with disabilities are inconvenienced by architectural barriers, but it is estimated that at least 21 million Americans are affected (Socio–Techological Instrumental Modules Project, 1978). Architectural barriers give an unspoken message to these 21 million people. The message is that society is not concerned with the needs of individuals who have disabilities. In effect, they are second-class citizens. The result is often frustration, anger, and alienation. As one person expressed, "I am not a shut in, I am a shut out" (Bruck, 1978, p. 21).

Despite some progress toward eliminating architectural barriers during the past decade, there is still much to be done. Freedom of mobility and access to programs are rights that should be assured to *every* citizen. (See Chapter 5 for an indepth examination of architectural barriers.)

Ecological Barriers.

Physical obstacles that occur in the natural environment may be termed ecological barriers. Hills, trees, sand, rain, snow, and wind are some examples. The physical impact of such barriers is roughly the same as architectural barriers (discussed above), but there are two important differences. First, ecological barriers are much less frustrating for individuals who have disabilities because they are not man-made. Therefore, they are not reminders of societal insensitivity toward people with disabilities. "I have to accept the fact that I will never backpack unassisted through the wilderness," commented one wheelchair user, "but I deserve the right to go to the store independently!"

The second difference between ecological and architectural barriers is that legislation cannot be used to counteract ecological barriers. Rather than eliminating ecological barriers, the main emphasis must be upon minimizing their impact upon people with disabilities. Careful advance planning may help minimize or avoid ecological barriers. For example, prior to participating in a nature walk, the individual with a disability can ensure that the program leader selects an access route that avoids ecological barriers, such as gullies or large tree roots. Sometimes, however, overcoming rather than avoiding an ecological barrier may offer a greater reward. Satisfaction and pride are feelings that we *all* receive when we face and overcome nature's obstacles.

Transportation Barriers.

The lack of usable and affordable methods of transportation often prevents individuals who have disabilities from benefiting from recreation services. As Labanowich (1979) noted, more and more individuals with disabilities are searching "for a solution to the problem of moving about the neighborhood, city, and between cities conveniently and effectively in pursuit of normal life activities" (p. 3). Automobile or van modifications are expensive, mass transportation is often inaccessible or inconvenient, and specially arranged (dial-a-ride) programs are few and have many restrictions. Some recreational programs do offer transportation services, but these are usually segregated programs that do not meet the needs of all people who have disabilities. Too often, the person with a disability faces the choice of either staying home or imposing upon family and friends by requesting transportation to recreational activities.

The following quote from an American Bar Association (1979) publication highlights the impact transportation barriers have on recreational pursuits:

> It is estimated that with the present transportation system the disabled travel about half as much as the rest of the population, with the largest difference being in social/recreational, work and shopping excursions. If an accessible transportation system were available the number of trips made by disabled persons would increase significantly. (p. 1)

Despite an obvious need, the United States government has no national policy on transportation for disabled individuals. Until such a policy is formulated, and accompanied by a commitment to fund it, many people with disabilities will continue to face difficulties in finding and affording transportation to recreational programs.

Economic Barriers.

Even in times of low unemployment, job opportunities are more limited for people who have disabilities. Furthermore, when they are able to find employment, individuals with disabilities frequently find themselves in low-paying positions with limited opportunity for advancement. These difficulties are compounded by higher-than-average expenses, such as for special transportation arrangements. The end result is less discretionary money to spend on leisure pursuits.

In addition to having less money for leisure than their nondisabled peers, many individuals with disabilities have seen two recent developments further limit their ability to participate in recreational activities. These developments are: (1) increased acceptance of the normalization concept (See Chapter 2, page 34), and (2) the popularity of commercial recreation and fees-for-service public recreation.

Richler (1984) noted that Canadian efforts to institute normalization principles have resulted in economic resources lagging behind the philosophical and legal acceptance of these principles:

> We are currently witnessing ambivalence in Canada between the
> old order and the new. The principle of normalization and its corollary
> of social integration including access to community resources has been
> well thought out and articulated, accepted and has even gained a some-
> what limited legal base. However, resources are still overwhelmingly
> committed to categorical and segregated programs. (p. 9)

Nevertheless, normalization has been a very positive concept for
people who have disabilities. It promotes optimal independent functioning and encourages integration into the mainstream of society. Normalization strives to have individuals with disabilities function by the
same norms as the rest of society. Such individuals, therefore, are
expected to pay for the things that other people have to pay for. The
right to earn money goes hand in hand with the obligation to spend it
wisely. One of the expenses of nondisabled people is recreational activities, so normalization principles justifiably discourage "free" tickets,
and so on, that are often donated out of pity for people with disabilities.
The end result, however, may be less opportunity for leisure participation by individuals who have disabilities.

Just at the time when more people with disabilities are expected to
pay for recreation services, the cost of these services has skyrocketed.
Public recreation programs are increasingly finding it necessary to
charge participants for their services. At the same time, commercial
recreation (i.e., theme parks, vacation resorts, etc.) is becoming more
and more popular, attracting record numbers of participants at inflated
prices. It is also becoming more expensive to enjoy traditional recreation pursuits at home. Cable and pay TV, for example, have increased
the choices, but they have increased the costs of television viewing as
well. More expensive leisure activities, plus the obligation to pay for
most of them, have compounded the economic barriers to participation
faced by many individuals with disabilities.

Rules and Regulations Barriers.

In the early 1970s, a popular song complained about the number of
rules and regulations in our society. The words included, "Signs, signs,
everywhere a sign . . . 'Do this,' 'Don't do that,' everywhere a sign." Historically, people with disabilities have faced many "signs" that limited
their ability to participate in all aspects of our society. Educational
opportunities were systematically denied to people with severe disabilities; literacy tests prevented many capable people with disabilities
from voting; and employers overtly discriminated against people with
disabilities by establishing requirements that were unrelated to job
performance.

Fortunately, legislation has reduced or eliminated many discriminatory policies. Rules and regulations often die hard, however. In 1978, for example, the New York City Marathon Committee turned down the applications of two wheelchair users. The decision was eventually overturned, but not without controversy. Barbara Kevles, who has published many articles on running, supported the original decision. Kelves wrote to the New York Times, "I believe the disabled racers lack the basic qualifications for the sport.... As race director, let [Fred Lebow] exercise his right mandated by the A.A.U. to protect the safety of all participants. Since Lebow wants to bar wheelchair racers from the New York Marathon they should be kept out" (October 7, 1979, Section 5, Page 2).

Rules and regulations are necessary if society is to function effectively. At the same time, they must not be used as an excuse to exclude people with disabilities from participation in leisure activities. In 1979, Tom Turner remained in his wheelchair to watch a Baltimore Orioles baseball game. When he refused to move from the aisle, Turner was arrested and fined $50 as a fire hazard! Such incidents provide evidence that fair rules and regulations, plus sensible envorcement, are needed if individuals with disabilities are to have equal access to recreational activities.

Barriers of Omission.

Most environmental barriers to participation are actions or obstacles that limit people who have disabilities. Sometimes, however, what is *not* done creates barriers as well. The failure of society to provide for the needs of individuals who have disabilities results in barriers of omission. The following are examples of such barriers:

- Lack of appropriate education opportunities, including education for leisure.
- Lack of available recreation services that provide for people who have disabilities. Specifically, individualized services are needed to allow an individual with a disability to function at his or her maximum level.
- Failure to publicize adequately those programs that could offer appropriate services to people who have disabilities.
- Failure to include participants with disabilities in the planning and implementation of leisure services.
- Lack of appropriate technology to maximize the leisure functioning of individuals with disabilities.
- Failure to enforce existing legislation that would reduce other barriers to participation.

■ Lack of adequate leisure role models for youngsters with disabilities and newly disabled adults.

Communication Barriers

The locus of intrinsic barriers is primarily within the individual. Environmental barriers are external forces. Communication barriers, however, cannot be thought of as either primarily intrinsic or extrinsic to the individual with a disability. Communication barriers result from a reciprocal interaction between individuals with disabilities and their social environment. There is an old expression that it "takes two to tango." It also takes two to establish effective communication—a message needs to be sent, but it must be received as well.

If communication is to occur, the sender *and* the receiver must be active participants in the process. This is true whether the message is spoken or written. If the message sender is not able to make the message clear enough to be understood by others, an *expressive* block limits communication. On the other hand, if a clearly expressed message is not received correctly, a *receptive* block interferes with the communication process.

Communication barriers are rarely caused exclusively by expressive blocks or receptive blocks, however. An individual with speech difficulties may find it impossible to pronounce words clearly. This difficulty could be an expressive block to communication. The listener, however, may not concentrate on what is said or take the time to ask for unclear words to be repeated. Thus, the listener could be responsible for a receptive block. Most communication barriers between disabled and nondisabled people result from a combination of expressive blocks and receptive blocks. If effective communication is to occur, *both* individuals with disabilities and society at large must make an effort to overcome expressive and receptive blocks to communication.

People with hearing impairments are probably the most familiar special population affected by communication barriers. To varying degrees, however, most special population members experience communication barriers. Many problem youth feel that their parents don't listen to them. Their parents, in turn, may complain that they don't even speak the same language. Some people with physical disabilities claim that politicians do not listen to their complaints. At the same time, these politicians express frustration because they feel physically disabled activists do not want to discuss the problem of funding social programs.

The importance of communication barriers, such as those just discussed, cannot be overemphasized. Communication links the disabled individual with his or her environment. A two-way dialogue needs to exist between persons with disabilities and the rest of society, including individuals and societal institutions. If blocks are allowed to interfere with this communication, there is little hope of overcoming the many barriers to participation.

OVERCOMING BARRIERS

Barriers to participation prevent many people with disabilities from fully realizing their potential as human beings. Not only do barriers limit recreation participation, but they also impede the personal growth that accompanies recreational activities. As a result, recreation professionals have the *obligation* to work for the reduction or elimination of these barriers. Witt (1977) emphasized this obligation in the following statement:

> The group of individuals who we need to deal with when we consider overcoming attitudinal barriers often also includes 'ourselves' as well, i.e., those of us who feel committed to 'helping' but may place limits on how much help we are willing to give; how far rights really extend; and how much we are prepared to go beyond what is easy and obvious. (p. 17)

Despite this obligation, there are so many barriers to participation that working for their removal may seem like an overwhelming task. Most recreators rightfully feel that their jobs are so time consuming that they have little time for additional efforts. Much of what needs to be done to remove barriers, however, can be accomplished within the scope of a recreator's job. The following concepts may help recreation professionals to provide the proper atmosphere for reducing or eliminating barriers to participation.

Adopt a "Life. Be in It." Philosophy

One way that recreation professionals can help eliminate barriers is by adopting a "Life. Be in it." philosophy. This concept, developed and copyrighted in Australia, has been used extensively by the National Recreation and Park Association. As noted by Miller (1979), "Life. Be in it." incorporates the idea of reducing or eliminating barriers. This includes "providing positive experiences, encouraging choice and alternatives, and advocating modification of activities to suit individual needs" (p. 25). The concept of "Life. Be in it." implies that recreation and leisure are essential aspects of life, and it encourages everyone to participate in activities they enjoy. By adopting a "Life. Be in it." philosophy, recreation professionals can become role models for the rest of society.

Provide Accessible Programs

It is essential that recreation professionals plan and implement programs that are accessible to persons with disabilities. This means more than simply providing ramps into buildings; it involves planning programs that avoid as many barriers to participation as possible. The following suggestions may assist with this process:

- Offer activities that (a) include a range of cognitive and physical skill requirements, (b) allow for proper skill progression, (c) give opportunities for both formal and informal involvement, and (d) encourage cooperative interaction between disabled and nondisabled participants.
- Coordinate activities offered with public transportation schedules, and consider establishing car or van pools to activities.
- Ensure that buildings and facilities, including parking lots, comply with American National Standards Institute (ANSI) specifications for accessibility.
- Develop ways for economically disadvantaged individuals to "pay" for services that require fees; volunteer work could be used, for example.
- Coordinate programs with agencies and organizations that specialize in services to special population members, thus assuring that a continuum of services is available within the community.
- Publicize programs thoroughly and advertise that they are accessible to people with disabilities (including interpreters for participants with hearing impairments.)

Establish Priorities for Action

The traditional approach to overcoming barriers to participation has been for the recreation professional to concentrate on intrinsic barriers. This approach involves using recreation participation to improve the person's social, physical, or cognitive functioning. Emphasis may be on improving a person's disability or "problem," or it may be on strengthening the person's abilities. Regardless, this traditional approach means that the recreation professional focuses upon changing the participant.

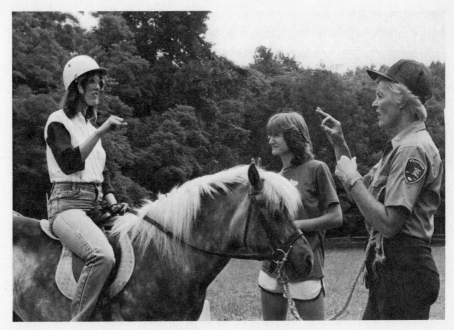

Figure 4–4. Providing accessible programs means more than eliminating architectural barriers. It requires avoiding as many barriers to participation as possible, such as ensuring that interpreters are available for deaf participants. (Courtesy of the League for the Handicapped, Baltimore, MD.)

A number of authorities (Witt, 1977; Bowe, 1978; Wright, 1980) have challenged this traditional approach, however. They contend that professionals should not focus solely upon changing special population members, but should work toward reducing or eliminating environmental barriers. In 1980, Hutchison developed and used a Barriers to Community Involvement scale to determine the impact of 13 intrinsic and environmental barriers. Her results "suggest that disabled persons largely see barriers to community involvement as lying beyond themselves" (p. 10). She stated that this was a "noteworthy finding and should be analyzed further, since much of the focus in rehabilitation, education, and vocational services is upon changing disabled persons rather than the community" (pp. 10–11). The disabled individual does not live in a vacuum. If people with disabilities are to become fully integrated into society, most authorities agree that *both* intrinsic and environmental barriers must receive everyone's attention.

Although recreational professionals can and should help to reduce or eliminate intrinsic and environmental barriers, the *unique* contribution that recreators can make is with the third type of barrier—communication barriers. By eliminating communication barriers as their first priority, recreators can help to provide a vital link between individuals with disabilities and their social environments. Once this is accomplished, the job of overcoming other barriers will become much easier.

Facilitate Communication

Providing accessible programs is one way to facilitate communication between individuals with and without disabilities. Such programs bring people together and offer an opportunity for intepersonal communication. Recreation professionals must do more than just bring these people together, however. Recreators should set an example for their nondisabled constituents by interacting appropriately with people who have disabilities. Additionally, recreators should aid the communication process between people who have disabilities and society's policymakers.

People who lack experience interacting with visibly disabled individuals sometimes feel uncomfortable initiating conversation. Hesitancy and some discomfort are normal reactions to any unfamiliar situation, so recreators should expect to feel uneasy at first. It is essential to overcome these initial feelings, however. Before long the person's disability will become less noticeable, and his or her "normalcy" will become apparent. The following tips for interacting with an individual who has a disability are modified from "When You Meet a Handicapped Person," by an unknown author. They provide an excellent guideline for community recreators.

- Remember, a person with a disability is a *person*. He or she is like anyone else, except for specific physical or mental limitations.
- Just be yourself, and show friendly personal interest in him or her.
- Learn basic signs and finger spelling for talking with individuals who are deaf.
- Talk about the same things you would with anyone else.
- Give physical assistance only if requested by the individual.
- Independence is important to everyone. If the situation dictates, perhaps ask, "Do you need assistance?"
- Be patient and let the person with a disability set the pace in walking or talking.
- Don't be afraid to laugh with him or her.

- Don't be overprotective or shower the individual with kindness. Don't offer pity or charity.
- Avoid making up your mind in advance about the capabilities of the person. You may be surprised how wrong you can be in making judgments about the individual's interests and abilities.

Facilitating interpersonal communication is extremely important. It is equally important, however, for recreators to facilitate communication between individuals with disabilities and leaders in the community. Miller (1979), Hutchison and Lord (1979), Owen (1981), and many others have stressed the necessity for special population members to express their own needs to policymakers. Hutchison (1980) noted, "As with many other change movements, greatest progress will be made when those oppressed by negative attitudes and poor services take an active role in changing attitudes and practices which block community involvement" (p. 7). Recreation professionals should search for ways to assist with this process. The following are some possibilities:

- Assist in the development of consumer groups, which bring together special population members with similar needs, interests, and goals.
- Analyze the community's power structure (Jewell, 1983), identify decision makers, and assist efforts to increase their awareness of barriers to participation.
- Keep abreast of meetings, hearings, and so on, that offer opportunities for people with disabilities to express their views.
- Provide to consumers information and resources that may be useful in discussions with policymakers.
- Offer seminars on interpersonal communication for people with disabilities to include ways to improve both expressive and receptive communication.
- If necessary, serve as an "advocate" to speak for people with disabilities who are unable to articulate their own needs.

Recreation professionals are in a unique position. Their jobs offer the chance to provide an ideal atmosphere for eliminating communication barriers, and effective communication between individuals with disabilities and the rest of society is the key to reducing or eliminating most barriers to participation. Careful planning and a great deal of energy are required, but it is well worth the effort. As Bowe (1978) emphasized, "We are talking about retrofitting an entire society, renovating buildings and subways, altering entrenched bureaucracies, and, perhaps most difficult of all, changing people themselves. But it must be done" (p. 225).

──────────────── **SUMMARY** ────────────────

Barriers to participation in recreation and leisure activities are experienced by everyone, but people who have disabilities face more and greater barriers than their nondisabled peers. Some of these barriers are *intrinsic;* thus, they result from the individual's own limitations. Other barriers are *environmental;* they are caused by external forces that impose limits on the individual. Finally, some are *communication* barriers, which block interaction between the individual and his or her social environment. Although recreation professionals can assist with overcoming all types of barriers, they should establish the elimination of communication barriers as their first priority. By reducing or eliminating communication barriers, recreators can help to establish a vital link between people with disabilities and their social environments. Once this is accomplished, the task of overcoming other barriers becomes much easier.

Suggested Learning Activities

1. Make a list of ten items regarding elimination of barriers to recreation participation that you would address if asked to testify before your city council.

2. Explain how an individual's perception of his or her own skill can act as a barrier to recreation participation.

3. Simulate a disability (blindness, paraplegia, etc.) and attend an organized recreational program. Identify each barrier encountered according to the types listed in the chapter.

4. Interview the director of a community recreation program and determine what actions are being taken to eliminate barriers to participation in that program. Discuss the strengths and weaknesses of these actions.

5. Of the three types of barriers outlined in the chapter, which is the key to reducing or eliminating most other barriers to participation? Explain why.

6. Interview an individual with a disability and determine (a) his or her recreational needs, interests, and desires, and (b) intrinsic,

environmental, and communication barriers that limit his or her participation.

References

American Bar Association. *Eliminating Environmental Barriers.* Washington, DC: ABA Commission on the Mentally Disabled, 1979.

Bowe, F. *Handicapping America: Barriers to Disabled People.* New York: Harper and Row, 1978.

Bregha, F. J. Leisure and freedom re-examined. In Goodale, T. L. and P. A. Witt, eds. *Recreation and Leisure and Issues in an Era of Change.* State College, PA: Venture Publishing, 1980, pp. 30–37.

Bruck, L. *Access: The Guide to a Better Life for Disabled Americans.* New York: Random House, 1978.

Carpenter, R. Integration, self–concept and recreation. In Witt, P. *Community Leisure Services and Disabled Individuals.* Washington, DC: Hawkins and Associates, 1977, 109–114.

Csikszentmihalyi, M. *Beyond Boredom and Anxiety.* San Francisco: Jossey-Bass, 1975.

Gunn, S. L. Structural analysis of play behavior: Pathological implications. In Hitzhusen, G., ed. *Expanding Horizons in Therapeutic Recreation V.* Columbia, MO: University of Missouri, 1978, 98–113.

Hutchison, P. Perceptions of disabled persons regarding barriers to community involvement. *Journal of Leisurability,* 7(3) 4–16, 1980.

Hutchison, P., and J. Lord. *Recreation Integration.* Ontario, Canada: Leisurability Publications, 1979.

Illich, I., I. K. Zola, J. McKnight, J. Caplan, and H. Shaiken. *Disabling Professions.* London: Marion Boyers, 1977.

Jewell, D. C. Comprehending concepts of community power structure: Prerequisite for recreation-integration. *Journal of Leisurability,* 10(1) 24–30, 1983.

Labanowich, S. *Transportation Counseling for Handicapped Individuals: A Manual for Rehabilitation Professionals.* Washington, DC: George Washington University, 1979.

Langer, E. J., S. Fiske, S. E. Taylor, and B. Chanowitz. Stigma, staring, and discomfort: A novel-stimulus hypothesis. *Journal of Experimental Social Psychology,* 12(5), 451–463, 1976.

Matthews, P. R. Why the mentally retarded to not participate in certain types of recreational activities. *Therapeutic Recreation Journal,* 14(1), 44–50, 1980.

Miller, J. Barriers to participation. *Australian Journal for Health, Physical Education and Recreation,* 84, 25–27, 1979.

Murphy, J. F. An enabling approach to leisure service delivery. In Goodale, T. L. and P. A. Witt, eds. *Recreation and Leisure: Issues in an Era of Change.* State College, PA: Venture Publishing, 1980, 197–210.

Owen, J. Advocacy 'with' instead of 'for' consumers. *Journal of Leisurability,* 8(3), 19–20, 1981.

Park, D. Recreation. In the White House Conference on Handicapped
    Individuals. *Volume One: Awareness Papers.* Washington, D.C.: The White
    House Conference on Handicapped Individuals, 1977, 119–131.

Richler, D. Access to community resources: The invisible barriers to
    integration. *Journal of Leisurability*, *11*(2), 4–11, 1984.

Socio–Techological Instrumental Modules Project. *Accessibility for the
    Handicapped.* Stony Brook, NY: State University of New York at Stony
    Brook, 1978.

Witt, P. *Community Leisure Services and Disabled Individuals.* Washington,
    DC: Hawkins and Associates, 1977.

Wright, B. A. Developing constructive views of life with a disability.
    Rehabilitation Literature, *41*(11–12), 274–279, 1980.

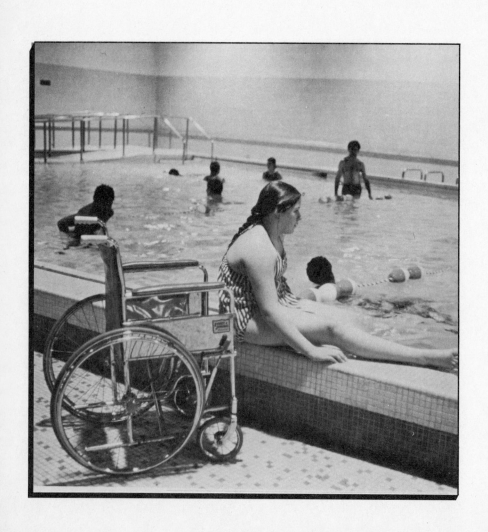

5

Design of Accessible and Usable Recreation Environments

Most recreation and leisure service professionals would probably agree with the principle that America's parks, playgrounds, and recreation centers should be totally accessible to and usable by all people. Yet in the past a vast number of recreation facilities in the United States have been usable only by persons who do not have visual, audial, mental, or mobility impairments. Today, however, there is a growing public consciousness regarding environmental design for persons with disabilities. For example, one cannot visit most large cities in the United States without noticing curb ramps in sidewalks and ramps into public buildings. This heightened public awareness has been felt in recreation and park facility design.

This chapter deals with the design of appropriate recreation environments for all people, including disabled persons. Initial coverage is given to common terms and pertinent legislation. The major portion of the chapter is devoted to a discussion of guidelines and recommendations for creating usable public recreation facilities, with special attention directed to playgrounds.

TERMINOLOGY

For the purpose of this chapter, it is necessary to define particular terms often found in the literature concerning recreation environments designed to meet the needs of persons with disabilities. Terms are provided for the following definitions: accessibility, usability, mobility impairments, visual impairments, audial impairments, and mental impairments, mental retardation, and mental health problems.

- *Accessibility* refers to the elments in the manmade environment (site or building) that allow approach, entrance, and use of facilities by persons with disabling conditions. The term is often used to indicate that a facility complies with specified standards to permit use by those whose sensory or physical impairments might otherwise limit their use of the facility.
- *Usability* refers to a manmade environment providing the opportunity for maximum use by those with sensory or mobility impairments. Occasionally, the word is used with the term accessibility to indicate that a facility not only meets minimum accessibility standards but is actually usable by individuals with disabling conditions.
- *Mobility Impairments* restrict or curtail movement or ambulation. Semi-ambulatory persons may use crutches, canes, or walkers for assistance in walking.
- *Visual Impairments* involve partial or total loss of vision. Most visually impaired persons have some vision, so they can distinguish light and large objects, and often can read large print.
- *Audial Impairments* involve partial or total loss in hearing, thus preventing the perception of normally audible sounds.
- *Mental Impairments* refer to any sort of limitations that restrict mental functioning. The term is generally used to refer to individuals with mental retardation or persons experiencing problems in mental health. Because of the broad nature of this term, it is more appropriate to use the terms "mental retardation" and "mental health problems."
- *Mental Retardation* is a developmental disability in which subaverage intellectual functioning results in impairment of learning and adaptive behavior.
- *Mental Health Problems* are psychological and emotional difficulties that lead to maladaptive behavior deterimental to the individual or group's well-being.

LEGISLATION

Growing public awareness of the problems of disabled persons has led to several pieces of federal legislation that have impact upon the design of recreation facilities. Chief among these are the Architectual Barriers Act of 1968 (P.L. 90–480) and Section 504 of the Rehabilitation Act of 1973 (P.L. 93–112).

The language of these federal statutes dictates that the needs of persons with handicapping conditions be considered by those recreation agencies that utilize federal funds. The Architectual Barriers Act specifies, "Any building, or facility, constructed in whole or in part by federal funds must be made accessible to and usable by the physically handicapped." Section 504 of the Rehabilitation Act states, " . . . no otherwise qualified handicapped individual in the U.S. . . . shall solely, by reason of his handicap, be excluded from participation in, be denied the benefits of, or be subjected to discrimination under any program or activity receiving federal assistance." Thus it is clearly the mandate of the government of the United States that public recreation facilities supported by the federal government be accessible to all people. In addition, many state and local laws stipulate barrier-free architectual design for public facilities.

GENERAL GUIDELINES FOR PLANNING RECREATION FACILITIES

Dimensions—Space Requirements

A basic point of departure in thinking about design components for persons with disabling conditions is to deal with dimensional requirements. In order to do this, space requirements for an average adult wheelchair user are considered since designs to accomodate this individual should ensure spaces large enough for other persons.

Wheelchair Dimensions. Dimensions for an average, manual, adult-sized wheelchair are provided in Figure 5–1. These dimensions are highlighted below.

- The length of the chair itself will be 42″ to 48″. With another 6″ required for toe space, the total length required for wheelchair users is 48″ to 54″.
- The width of the average wheelchair is 24″ to 26″. When collapsed, the most commonly used wheelchairs are 11″ wide.
- The height of the seat from the floor is approximately 19″.
- It is 27″ from the floor to the user's lap and 30″ from the floor to the armrests.
- The height of the pusher handles is 36″ from the floor.

There are some specially equipped adult-sized wheelchairs that may exceed these dimensions. Of course, children's wheelchairs will

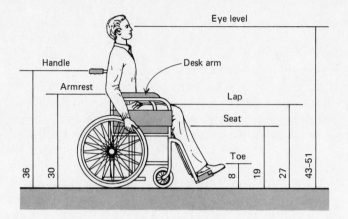

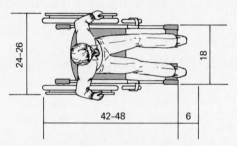

Figure 5–1. Dimensions of adult–sized wheelchairs.

be smaller than those designed for adults. The junior-sized chair has a seat 16″ wide and 18″ from the floor. Thus space requirements, such as the turning radius, will necessarily be reduced for children.

Space Requirements for Maneuvering Wheelchairs. The following are space requirements for those using standard, adult-sized wheelchairs:

- A turning radius of 64″ × 64″ is required in order to make a full 360-degree turn.
- A minimum width for a corridor or path that allows a pedestrian and a wheelchair user to pass is 48″, although a wider width to accomodate two wheelchairs to pass would be recommended.
- The minimum width for a corridor or path that allows two wheelchairs to pass is 60″, although a space of 72″ would be recommended.

- A minimum door opening width of 32″ is needed by a person in a wheelchair.
- The width of a corridor or path with a door or gate should exceed the width of the door or gate by 18″ to 24″ in order to allow the space needed to maneuver the chair while opening the door or gate.

Reaching From a Wheelchair. Each wheelchair user is unique in his or her range of reach because of differences in size, strength, range of motion, and degree of involvement. The reach dimensions presented here are averages. Devices should therefore be placed well within the figures presented so they may be accessible to all.

- The reach for a wheelchair user facing a wall and reaching diagonally is approximately 48″ from the floor. Thus switches, telephones, and other such devices should be placed less than 48″ from the floor. Minimum height is 15″ from the floor.
- An upward side reach can be made to the height of 54″ from the floor. A downward side reach can be made down to 9″ from the floor. Thus shelves and cabinets should be placed within the range of 9″ to 54″ from the floor.
- An average person in a wheelchair can reach a maximum of 25″ across a table when seated at the table. A comfortable reach would of course be less. Thus relatively narrow shelves and work spaces are dictated.

Special Considerations for Other Persons

General concepts to consider when planning areas and facilities for other populations are as follow:

- Some persons experience difficulty in operating devices that call for grasping or twisting because of chronic impairments that affect the skills required to manipulate objects (such as door knobs). Therefore, devices should be chosen that make it possible to manipulate the objects without the need to grasp or twist.
- Persons may lack the strength and stamina needed to be successful in completing tasks such as opening heavy doors or using revolving doors. Decreased strength and stamina may particularly be a problem for old people. Doors should not be heavy to open and rest areas should be considered in all recreation facilities, especially along paths.
- For those with visual impairments, raised letters should be used on signs.

- The use of different textures on walks or paths may be used to provide visually impaired persons with location cues. Textured borders on the edge of paths would be an example of providing such a cueing aid.
- Audible cues may be provided such as bells signaling once for an up elevator, twice for a down elevator, or verbal announcements of each floor on the elevator.
- For those with severe auditory impairments, signage is particularly important. Signs with precise and clear messages should be placed at a height within the range of vision of both children and adults.
- Simplicity should be a keynote in design for persons possessing mental impairments. For example, signs should be as simple as possible (i.e., use short words or easily understood symbols), and in the design of buildings and other facilities ambiguity should be avoided so as to minimize uncertainty and confusion.

PARKS AND OUTDOOR RECREATION AREAS

Numerous design elements are found within park and outdoor recreation areas. Although in the section that follows a number of these elements will be treated as separate entities, it is critical to remember the importance of the physical relationship between these design elements. This point is made clear in *Barrier Free Site Design* (1975), published by the U.S. Department of Housing and Urban Development with the American Society of Landscape Architects Foundation. Within this document it is stated:

> Unless there is a relationship of continuous accessibility between forms of transportation, site elements, and building entries, the value of making any one of these components more accessible is lost. Consequently, it is imperative that *all* elements of circulation be made as easily accessible as possible. (p. 20)

Signage. Identification, directional, and information signs are helpful to all users of park and recreation facilities. Proper signage is particularly beneficial for persons with hearing and speech impairments since they may not be able to communicate with others to obtain information.

The international symbol of accessibility (see Figure 5–2) should be displayed at the entrance and at various points within the park or recreation area to inform people that it provides for persons with disabilities. Facilities within the park or recreation area that should be appro-

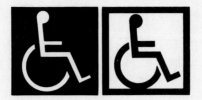

Figure 5–2. International symbol of accessibility.

priately marked with the symbol include rest rooms, entrances to buildings, trails, and picnic areas. In addition, all parking spaces designated for use by disabled individuals should be clearly marked with the symbol of accessibility, and where diagrams or maps are provided the symbol should be used to indicate accessible buildings or areas.

Signs should be placed at a height of within the range of vision and reach for both children and adults. Preferably signs should be located at eye level (between 43″ and 51″) for wheelchair users. Consistency should be employed in height and location when mounting signs so that they may be easily found.

For ease in reading, signs should be made with light-colored characters or symbols on a dark background and have a nonglare surface. Identification signs for rooms (including rest rooms) should have raised characters, using the standard alphabet and Arabic numbers since the vast majority of persons with severe visual impairments do not read Braille. The characters should be at least $\frac{5}{8}$″ in height but no higher than 2″. They should be raised a minimum of $\frac{1}{32}$″ and have clearly defined edges. Signs with raised letters can also be used to identify and interpret points of interest. Most authorities would probably agree, however, that sighted guides or audio tape devices are more effective means of presenting information.

Parking. Special parking accomodations are required for some persons with disabling conditions: Passenger loading zones permit disabled persons to gain access to automobiles; special parking spaces are required by disabled drivers who need extra space to transfer safely, as well as by those with stamina limitations and by visually impaired individuals who must have safe access to and from parking areas. Both loading zones and parking spaces need to be located as close as possible to the shortest accessible route to the building or area being utilized.

The loading zone parallel to the auto must be a minimum of 4′6″ wide to allow the car door to fully open. The surface of this area should contrast in color and texture with the portion of the area occupied by the auto. Should the loading zone be on the same level as the walk, bollards or similar objects should be used to separate the loading zone from the walk. If there is a grade difference, a curb ramp may be constructed. The overall dimensions of the area should be approximately 12′6″ wide (including the 4′6″ loading zone) and 25′ to 50′ long, depending on whether it accomodates one or two cars. Finally, gradual access to the main road must be provided, and proper signage, utilizing the symbol of accessibility, should be posted to identify its use as a passenger loading zone.

Angled or 90-degree parking spaces provided for disabled people need to be at least 12′6″ in width (including an access aisle at least 4′6″ wide) and 20′6″ in length. The front of the space should have a precast car stop (i.e., wheel stop) to keep cars from overhanging the walk. An alternative is to provide a 3′ strip to the walk to allow for the overhang of the front of the cars. Of course, a curb ramp will be necessary if there is a difference in level between the parking area and walk.

Parallel parking spaces should be approximately 12′6″ in width and 24′ long. If the walk parallel to the space is at road level, bollards or similar objects should be used to separate the areas. A curb ramp may be installed if there is a grade difference between the road and walk.

Curb ramps should have a maximum grade of 1:12 (8.33%). Two common types of curb ramps are the ramp with a returned curb (Figure 5–3) and the flared ramp (Figure 5–4). If there is a flare on the sides of the ramp, it should be no steeper than 1:8 (12.5%). No matter the type, all curb ramps should be a minimum of 3′ wide and should blend smoothly with the street or parking lot and the walk. Ramps should be constructed to blend at a common level with the street or parking lot and the walk. It is recommended that the entire curb ramp be made to

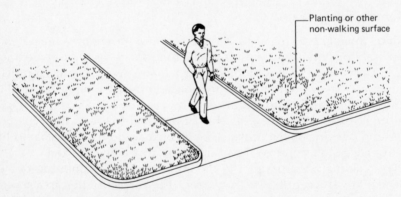

Planting or other non-walking surface

Figure 5–3. Returned curb.

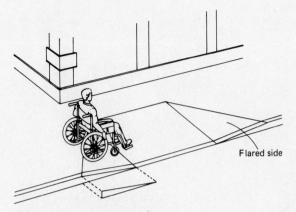

Figure 5–4. Flared sides.

contrast in both color and texture with the walk surface so that it is not a hazard for those who have visual impairments.

How many parking spaces need to be designated for the use of disabled persons? This is a difficult question and will probably require some amount of judgment on the part of designers and park and recreation administrators. Accessibility standards published by the Illinois Department of Conservation in *Mainstreaming Handicapped Individuals: Parks and Recreation Design Standards Manual* (1978) stipulate 2 spaces be designated for disabled persons where parking facilities have 1–20 spaces, 3 spaces where 21–65 spaces are found, and 4 spaces where 66–95 spaces exist. No matter how many spaces are supplied, each should be marked that it is reserved for the use of persons with disabilities, and the international symbol for accessibility should be posted on a sign or painted on the parking surface of each space.

Walks and Trails. Parks and outdoor recreation areas commonly provide walks to connect major buildings with other areas. Trails are also common features in parks and outdoor recreation areas.

When walks join parking lots and streets they must be made to meet the level of the other surfaces. In many instances curbs are not constructed in park and recreation areas so that there is a natural blending of walks with parking lots and streets. Illustrations presented in the previous section cover the design features when curb ramps are necessary in parking facilities. These same principles may be employed when a walk meets a street or driveway. Design features become far more complex, however, when walks meet the intersection of two curbed streets. It is recommended that information be sought from

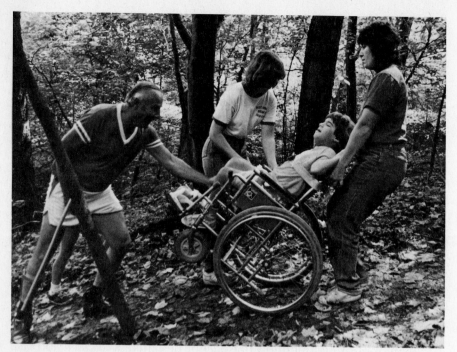

Figure 5–5. Ecological barriers, such as hills and rough terrains, may limit independent participation by wheelchair users. Accessible walks and trails enable most people with disabilities to enjoy nature without depending on others for assistance. (Courtesy of the League for the Handicapped, Baltimore, MD.)

experts or illustrated literature on accessibility be reviewed to obtain alternatives for designing acceptable curb ramps at intersections.

Walks should be a minimum of 48″ wide. However, a width of 60″–72″ is preferable so that wheelchairs may easily pass. Walk gradients should not exceed 5 percent and preferably should be less. If a walk does approach the maximum grade or is unusually long, rest areas with benches and room for wheelchairs should be provided. Surfaces in front of rest stops should be textured differently than the walk in order to provide location cues for visually impaired persons. Nonslip surfaces such as brushed concrete or asphalt are recommended for the overall walk surface. Minimum use of expansion joints is also recommended, and where joints are used they should not exceed $\frac{1}{2}″$.

Most authorities object to the designation of "handicapped trails." An alternative to designating trails for the use of persons with disabilities is to provide several different types of recreational trails within a park or outdoor recreation area. The trail system can then reflect a wide range of user preferences and abilities. *A Guide to Designing Accessible Outdoor Recreation Facilities* (1980), published by the U.S. Department of Interior, suggests five classifications for trails. A brief description of each follows.

- Class I trails are short ($0'-\frac{1}{4}$ mi), hard surface (concrete or asphalt) trails with very little grade (a maximum of 1:50 or 2 percent slope). The recommended width is 48″ (one way) to 72″ (two ways). Rest areas with benches, shelters, and interpretation stations are placed every 100′ to 150′.
- Class II trails are $\frac{1}{4}$–1 mi, surfaced with asphalt, wooden planking, or solidly packed crushed stone, and may have a slope of 1:20 (5%). The width for Class II trails is 36″–48″ (one way) to 48″–60″ (two ways). Rest areas with benches, shelters, and interpretation stations are placed every 200′–300′.
- Class III trails are 1–3 mi long, are surfaced with a firm, well compacted material (such as pea-gravel), and may have a slope of 1:12 (8.33%). The width of the trail is 36″–48″. Rest areas consist of occasional natural benches and interpretation stations where needed (using 500′–600′ as a guideline).
- Class IV trails are 3–10 mi in length, are surfaced with bound wood chips or class 5 gravel mixed coarse, and may have a slope of 1:8 (12.5%). The trail width is 24″–36″. A rest area or interpretation station is located every mile.
- Class V trails are over 10 mi, have surfaces that are sandy or made of rocks or rough, unbound wood chips, and that follow the slope of the land or use steps. The width of the trail is not defined and rest areas are not developed unless there is a particularly unique feature that requires interpretation.

By employing this five-level classification system, or a similar system, park and recreation professionals can provide appropriate levels of experiences to suit persons with a variety of interests and abilities. Of course, proper signage is important to the successful utilization of such a trail system since users must be informed of the length and difficulty of each trail. Also important is that consideration be given to the needs of the visually impaired. Overhanging tree branches should be cut back and textural changes should be used on hard surface trails to indicate interpretations or rest areas.

Before closing this segment on trails, it should be mentioned that a particularly interesting approach to trail design is displayed by the "All People's Trail," located in the Shaker Lakes Regional Nature Center in Cleveland, Ohio. The "All People's Trail" is a completely accessible trail constructed of wood and concrete. The use of wood allowed the designers to elevate parts of the trail so that all can enjoy being in the middle of a marsh area, overlooking a small waterfall, looking down into a creek, and, in general, having a new perspective from which to view nature. The trail truly provides a unique outdoor experience in which all may participate.

Picnic Areas. Picnic tables need to be designed to accomodate wheelchair users. Usually this is accomplished by designing picnic tables so that a wheelchair user can sit comfortably at one end of the table. Paths should lead to at least some of the tables in any picnic area and grills should be usable by wheelchair users. Specific dimensions for tables and grills are provided in the following section on furnishings.

Furnishings. Site furniture includes tables, grills, benches, drinking fountains, and telephones. Most sources agree that *tables* should be a minimum of 30″ from the underside of the table to the ground and should allow 24″ clearance from the end of the table to the undersupport. This allows the wheelchair user to sit at either end of the table. *Grills* 30″ in height and located adjacent to hard surfacing can be most easily utilized by wheelchair users. While not all grills in any picnic area need to accommodate persons in wheelchairs, a number should be provided adequate to the needs of the population using the facility. *Benches* with setting heights of 18″ to 20″ and widths of no more than 18″ are most ideal. Backrests and arm supports should be included. Benches should be set back so that they do not obstruct walkways, and adequate space should be provided around them so that a wheelchair user may sit in his or her wheelchair beside someone seated on the bench. *Drinking fountains* should be surrounded with paved areas to provide easy access and avoid mud puddles. Hand-operated levers allow the greatest ease in turning on the water. For adults, the spout should preferably be 34″ to 36″ from the paved area. For children the height should be approximately 30″. A push-button public *telephone* should be located on a hard surface for use by disabled persons. The entrance to the phone should be at least 30″ wide in order to allow wheelchair users access to the coin slot, receiver, and push buttons. Normally it is best to plan for the highest operable part of the telephone to be no more than 4′ from the surface.

Water-Related Areas

Some of the most popular recreational activities take place in water-related areas. The section that follows discusses swimming, fishing, and boating facilities.

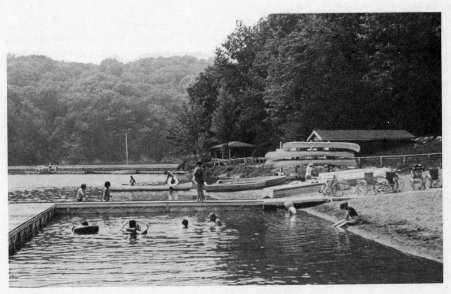

Figure 5–6. A walk leads through the sand to the water.

Beaches. Sand—a highly desirable element at the beach—can create difficulties for wheelchair users and those who may have mobility problems. Designers must therefore make certain there are walks or pathways through the sand to the water. Concrete walks can be constructed. An alternative is to build a stabilized sand path to the water. No matter what particular method is used, the walk or path should not be steep (a maximum slope of 8.33 percent is recommended) and it should lead to the water's edge or to swimming platforms or docks. Where platforms or docks do not extend into the lake, a concrete pad may be constructed so that there is a hard surface under the water to aid the entry of disabled persons. Sometimes handrails are constructed to follow (placed at about 32″ in height) the walk and entry into the water.

Pools. The best pool design is that which allows disabled people to choose from several options to enter the water. One means to aid entry is to construct a ramp. Such ramps should have a slip-resistant surface, 32″ handrails, and a slope of no more than 8.33 percent. A second means is to provide steps. Steps should be deep enough to allow an adult to sit on them. Handrails can be provided along the steps. A third means for people to enter the pool is for them to sit on the pool deck and swing their legs over the side into the water. A portable device with steps can be placed on the deck so that wheelchair users may transfer to it and then move down its steps to deck level. A final means of helping disabled persons into a pool is a hydraulic lift. Such a lift will normally not be required. However in instances when large persons must be assisted into the pool, the hydraulic lift can be very useful.

Fishing Piers. Fishing piers can be constructed to meet the needs of persons with disabilities. Of course, fishing piers should be made accessible by the provision of a walk or hard surface pathway. It is important that the walk or path blend with the pier so there no difference in level between the two. The surface of the pier should have spaces of less than $\frac{1}{2}''$ between the planks. Around the bottom edge of the pier there should be a kick plate to keep foot pedals of wheelchairs from slipping off the pier. Handrails or armrests and bait shelves should be provided. Probably the best design is to build an armrest about 36″ high with a slope of approximately 30 degrees. This board can be used by those fishing to rest their arms and fishing poles. An 8″ to 12″ bait shelf about 30″ from the surface of the pier offers a place for fishing gear. If children are the principal users of the pier, then slightly reduced heights would be appropriate for the armrest and bait shelf. Benches and some type of shaded seating area are other features that may enhance fishing piers.

Boat Docks. As with fishing piers, access to boat docks should be over hard surface walks or paths and there should be no difference in level between the dock and the walk or path. Again, as in the case of the fishing pier, spaces between planks should be no wider than $\frac{1}{2}''$. Handrails may be constructed around the edge of the dock where they do not restrict access to boats.

Recreation Buildings

This section covers accessibility information regarding recreation buildings. Both exterior and interior design elements are discussed.

Exterior Circulation and Entrances. Designated parking spaces need to be located as near as is practical to the accessible entrance of each recreation facility. The guidelines on parking provided earlier in the chapter provide more exact information on design features for parking areas.

Ideally the approach to the entrance of the building will not be on a slope, or any slope will be minimum. The suggested guidelines for walks presented earlier in this chapter may be applied when designing walks leading to buildings. Chief among design considerations for walks are their grade, width, and surface.

All major entrances of recreation buildings should be made accessible in order to avoid having persons with disabilities use the "back door," "service entrance," or other similar entrance. Involved in this principle is not only respect for individuals with disabilities but the need for all persons to have access to major exits in cases of emergency.

The surface directly in front of entrances should be level or have only a very slight slope (of no more than 2 percent). When an automatic door is not provided, adequate space should be allowed on either side of the door to permit wheelchair users to easily open the door. Manual doors should be equipped with handles that do not require grasping or a twisting motion of the wrist. The door should have a width of at least 32" and should have a threshold of no more than $\frac{1}{2}$" in order to allow wheelchair access. The pressure required to open the door should never exceed 15 lb for exterior doors and will hopefully be much less than this maximum. Revolving doors are not practical since they cannot be used by people in wheelchairs.

Ramps. Both exterior and interior ramps may be utilized in recreation buildings. Any walk or path may be designated a ramp if it has a slope 5 percent or greater. While curb ramps may be slightly steeper, other ramps should not exceed a slope of 8.33 percent (1:12 ratio) with a slope of 5 percent preferred (1:20 ratio). Handrails on both sides are a necessity on practically all ramps (except curb ramps) in order to protect people or to provide support. Normally handrails on ramps are placed around 32" in height. However, if the building is often used by children, a second set of handrails 24" in height should be added. Handrails should extend 12" beyond the top and bottom of the ramp.

The minimum width for ramps is 36", with 60" being needed for ramps over which wheelchairs often pass. A level space at least 5' in length and as wide as the ramp should be provided at the approach and at the top of the ramp. Long ramps or ramps with turns should have level platforms to allow users to rest or to easily negotiate the turn. On long straight run ramps a rest platform of 3' in length is recommended. Turning platforms are larger. The platform for a ramp with one 90-degree turn should be 4' deep by 5' long. For a switchback type of ramp the turning platform needs to be at least 8' deep and 5' wide.

Stairs. Stairs and elevators should be provided in addition to ramps since some persons have difficulty using ramps. Because persons wearing leg braces and others may trip if the nosing on stair steps is squared, a smooth nosing on steps is generally recommended. As with ramps, handrails should be installed on both sides of the stairs. The handrails should be placed about 32" from the surface (i.e., tread) of each step and should extend 12" beyond both the top step and the bottom step. A second set of handrails should be provided in recreation facilities that serve children. These should be placed 24″ above the surface of the steps.

Tactile warning devices can be utilized as cueing aids for visually impaired persons to alert them of stairs. For example, in buidings with carpeting or vinyl tiles, rubber tiles can be laid at the top of stairs to offer a surface tactile warning signal. It is important that tactile warning signals remain consistent throughout the entire building. Finally, adequate lighting on stairs is necessary to allow users to detect the step nosing.

Elevators. Elevators should be placed in an area close to the main entrance of the building and the normal path of travel of building users. The elevator call buttons should be located so wheelchair users can reach them. It is recommended that the center of button panel be 40″ from the floor. Raised numbers may be placed on the button panel in order to identify the floor. These numbers should be raised a minimum of $\frac{1}{32}$″ from the surface and be at least $\frac{1}{2}$″ high. They should have clearly defined edges. To be easily seen, the numbers should contrast in color with the background on which they are placed.

Visual and audible cueing devices should be used to indicate the direction of an approaching elevator car. Visual signals can be given by installing arrow shaped direction indicators. The "up" indicator arrow should be white and the "down" arrow red. Audible cues can be given by signals that sound once for "up" cars and twice for "down" cars.

The inside of the elevator car must be large enough to accomodate at least one person in a wheelchair and allow this individual to move to a position from which he or she can operate the elevator controls. The controls need to be so located that the highest button is no more than 54″ from the floor of the elevator. Emergency controls should be located below the standard controls so that they are accessible to wheelchair users. Also inside the car should be handrails mounted on the side walls (and preferably rear wall) at a height of 30″ to 32″ from the floor of the elevator.

It is of course necessary that all elevators be adjusted so that, when stopped, the floor of the car will be level with the building floor. Elevator doors should have safety edges and door opening sensing devices to prevent the door from closing and injuring someone entering or leaving the car.

Lodges and Cabins with Bedrooms. Every effort should be made to make certain that newly constructed or remodeled lodges and cabins with bedrooms provide for the needs of physically disabled people. While ideally all lodge or cabin bedrooms will be made accessible to, and usable by, physically disabled persons, this may not be possible. In

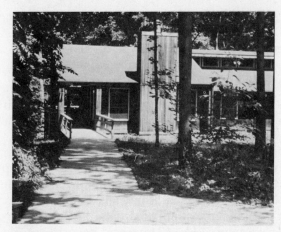

Figure 5–7. Cabin at Bradford Woods, home of Camp Riley for campers with disabilities.

this case a certain percentage of bedrooms should accomodate disabled individuals. The Illinois Department of Conservation (*Mainstreaming Handicapped Individuals*, 1978) recommends a minimum ratio of two bedrooms per twenty bedroom units be usable by persons with physical disabilities.

Hallways and corridors should be at least 42″ wide and all doors should have a minimum width of 32″. Within the rooms the floor space should be large enough to permit the furniture to be placed with adequate space (approximately $4\frac{1}{2}'$ to 5′) for wheelchair users to move about. The floor should be unwaxed. If carpeting is used it should be a low-pile, wall-to-wall carpet so that wheelchairs may move easily on it.

It is important that essential elements are of the proper height. The top of the mattress on the beds should be approximately the same height as the seat of the wheelchair to allow for ease in transferring. Controls such as light switches and thermostats should be placed within reach of wheelchair users, at a maximum of 4′ from the floor. Windows should be easily opened and closed by those in wheelchairs. Ideally, windows will be placed low enough so wheelchair users may be able to see the out-of-doors from them.

Closets and other clothing storage facilities should be designed with wheelchair users in mind. Closets should allow ease in entry and should have hanging rods within comfortable reach. Spring closed or self closing drawers should be avoided.

Many of the suggestions in the next section on rest rooms can be applied to bathrooms for bedroom units. Of course, the floor space of individual bathrooms for bedroom units will be much smaller than for public restrooms. Therefore it will be important to design individual bathrooms so that those in wheelchairs may close the door for privacy and have sufficient room to move about.

Rest rooms. Within any given park and recreation area it is important to have at least one public restroom for each sex that accomodates disabled persons. It is recommended that a minimum of 5' by 5' of clear floor space be provided so that wheelchair users may have sufficient turning space in public rest rooms.

At least one accessible toilet stall should exist in each rest room. This stall needs to be a minimum of 36" wide and 66" to 69" deep (66" if wall-hung stall, 69" if floor-hung stall). Doors should be a minimum of 32" wide and should open outward. Handrails should be placed on either side of the stall at a height of approximately 32"–33". These handrails should be approximately 54"–55" long and have an outside diameter of $1\frac{1}{2}$". The toilet seat should be 20" from the floor to allow for ease in transferring. Standard 18" water closets may be used if a 2" filler ring is installed so that the seat is raised to the proper 20" height. Wall-hung water closets are preferred over floor-mounted ones since the wall-hung type provides additional space for wheelchair footrests.

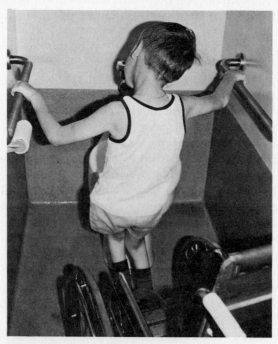

Figure 5–8. Accessible toilet stall.

Men's rest rooms should also have at least one wall-mounted urinal. This urinal should be placed with the basin lip not more than 19″ from the floor for adults and 14″ for children.

The lavatory should be mounted to provide a 29″ clearance from the floor, with a maximum height to the top of the rim of 34″. All pipes under the lavatory should be covered or insulated in order to protect wheelchair users from burning themselves. This is particularly important to protect those without sensation in their legs.

Towel racks, towel dispensers, hand dryers, and other such devices should be placed so that they are easily accessible to wheelchair users. These should be placed no higher than 40″ from the floor.

Showers are sometimes found in rest rooms or locker rooms in recreation facilities. If showers are provided, they should accomodate disabled persons. Shower stalls equipped for disabled individuals should not have thresholds (or only slight thresholds) and nonslip surfaces. On each shower stall a hinged seat should be mounted 19″ from the floor so that it may be folded out during the use of the shower. Grab rails are a necessity and should be placed at a height of approximately 32″. Water control levers should allow for ease in gripping and, like the soap tray, should be placed less than 40″ from the floor. The provision of a hand-held diversionary shower head with a flexible hose will allow those seated to shower more easily.

Concluding Statement on the Design of Parks and Outdoor Recreation Areas

Many sources of information on design consideration for handicapped people are available to the park and recreation profession. Chief among those used as references for this chapter were *American National Standard Specifications for Making Buildings and Facilities Accessible to and Usable by Physically Handicapped People, An Illustrated Handbook of the Handicapped Section of the North Carolina State Building Code, Barrier Free Site Design, Accessibility Standards Illustrated, Design Standards to Accomodate People with Physical Disabilities in Park and Open Space Planning, Mainstreaming Handicapped Individuals*, and *A Guide to Designing Accessible Outdoor Recreation Facilities*. These are listed in the references for the chapter.

No matter what the source of information, it is important to remember the warning issued earlier in the chapter by the American Society of Landscape Architects. That is, the planner must consider *all* parts of the facility since these must flow together in order to assure the area is truly accessible. Table 5–1 provides a checklist that may be used to determine the accessibility of park and recreation facilities.

Table 5–1
Checklist for Accessibility of Park and Recreation Facilities

Signage

1. Is the international symbol of accessibility displayed at the entrance?
2. Is the international symbol of accessibility displayed at various points within the facility to inform persons of accessibility?
3. Are parking spaces designated for use by persons with disabilities marked with the symbol of accessibility?
4. Do diagrams or maps provide the symbol of accessibility to indicate accessible buildings or areas?
5. Are signs located at eye level (43″ to 51″) for wheelchair users?
6. Are signs made with light-colored characters or symbols on dark backgrounds?
7. Do identification signs for rooms (including rest rooms) have raised characters at least $\frac{5}{8}$″ but no greater than 2″?
8 Are signs placed near the closest approach?
9. Are signs well lighted, if used at night?
10. If used, are exhibit labels large enough to read?

Parking

1. Is a loading zone available 12′6″ wide and 25′ long, with an area parallel to the auto of 4′6″ to allow the car door to open fully?
2. Is the loading zone separated from the walk by a curb, bollards, or similar objects?
3. Is there a curb ramp if a curb is next to the loading area?
4. Are angled or 90-degree parking spaces 12′6″ wide and 20′6″ long?
5. Are parallel spaces 12′6″ wide and 24′ long?
6. Do spaces have provisions to keep cars from overhanging walks?
7. Is there a curb ramp, if a curb exists?
8. Are curb ramps no more than 8.33 percent grade?
9. Are curb ramps made to contrast both in color and texture with the walk surface?
10. Are adequate numbers of spaces provided for persons with disabilities?

Walks and Trails

1. Are walks joining parking lots and streets made to meet the level of the other surfaces?
2. Are walks at least 48″ wide?
3. Are walk gradients 5 percent or less?
4. Do walks approaching the maximum grade, or those unusually long, have rest areas? Are surfaces in front of the rest areas textured differently than the walks?
5. Do walks have nonslip surfaces?
6. Do trails reflect a wide range of user preferences and abilities?
7. Are trails clearly marked for length and degree of difficulty?
8. Are overhanging tree branches on trails cut?
9. Are textural changes used on hard surface trails to indicate interpretations or rest areas?

Picnic Areas

1. Are picnic tables designed to accommodate wheelchair users (with a minimum of 30″ to the ground and 24″ to the undersupport from the end of the table)?
2. Do paths lead to some of the picnic tables? Grills?

Table 5-1 (Continued)

Picnic Areas

3. Are grills approximately 30″ in height?
4. Do benches have sitting heights of 18″ to 20″ and widths of no more than 18″? Are backrests and arm supports included?
5. Is there adequate space around benches so that wheelchair users may sit beside someone seated on the bench?
6. Are drinking fountains set in paved areas? Do they stand 34″ to 36″ from the ground for adults? 30″ for children?

Telephones

1. Is a push-button public telephone available? Is it located on a hard surface?
2. Is the entrance to the phone at least 30″ wide?
3. Is the highest operable part of the telephone no more than 4′ from the surface?
4. Are telephones equipped for persons with hearing impairments?

Water-Related Areas

1. Are pathways provided on beaches through the sand to the water?
2. Are paths sloped no more than 8.33 percent?
3. Is the pool designed to allow disabled persons to enter the water by means of a ramp? Steps? Portable device with steps placed on the deck? Hydraulic lift?
4. Are fishing piers made accessible by providing a path to them?
5. Do the surfaces of docks and piers have spaces of less than $\frac{1}{2}$″ between planks?
6. Is there a kick plate at the bottom edge of fishing piers? Are handrails provided?

Buildings and Ramps

1. Are designated parking spaces for persons with disabilities located near the entrance?
2. Are all major entrances accessible?
3. Are surfaces in front of entrances level or have only a very small slope?
4. Are entry doors at least 32″ wide with a threshold of no more than $\frac{1}{2}$″?
5. Are any manual doors equipped with proper handles?
6. Are doors relatively easy to pull open?
7. Are ramps on a slope of 8.33 percent or less?
8. Are proper handrails on ramps?
9. Are ramps at least 36″ wide? Do they have nonslip surfaces?
10. Are level spaces (5′ in length or more) provided at the approach and at the top of the ramps?

Stairs and Elevators

1. Are stairs and elevators provided in addition to ramps?
2. Do stair steps have smooth nosing?
3. Are handrails on both sides of the stairs?
4. Are handrails about 32″ from the surface of each step? Do they extend 12″ beyond both the top step and the bottom step?
5. Are tactile warning cues provided to alert persons with visual impairments to stairs?
6. If the building serves children, are handrails provided 24″ from the surface of each step?
7. Are stairs adequately lighted?

111

Table 5–1   (*Continued*)

Stairs and Elevators

8. Are elevators placed near the main entrance?
9. Are elevator cars large enough to accommodate at least one person in a wheelchair and to allow that person to move to a position to operate the controls?
10. Are elevator buttons easily accessible to wheelchair users?
11. Are raised numbers placed on the button panel?
12. Are visual and audial cueing devices used to indicate the direction of approaching elevator cars?

Lodges and Cabins with Bedrooms

1. Do doors have a clear opening of at least 32″?
2. Are hallways and corridors at least 42″ wide?
3. Does floor space in rooms permit wheelchair users to move freely around furniture?
4. Do floors have nonslip surfaces? If carpeting is used, is it low-pile, wall-to-wall carpet?
5. Are light switches and other controls within reach of wheelchair users (a maximum of 4′ from the floor)?
6. Are bed mattresses approximately the same height as the seats of the wheelchair users who usually occupy the room (i.e., children or adults)?
7. Do closets allow use by wheelchair users?

Rest Rooms

1. Is there at least one rest room for each sex that accommodates physically disabled persons?
2. Can wheelchair users easily enter the rest rooms?
3. Is there a minimum of 5′ × 5′ of clear floor space to provide turning space for wheelchair users?
4. Are toilet stalls at least 36″ wide? At least 66″ deep? Equipped with doors at least 32″ wide that open outward? Equipped with handrails on either side approximately 33″ high and 55″ long with an outside diameter of 1½″?
5. Is the seat in toilet stalls 20″ from the floor—designed for persons with disabilities?
6. Does the men's rest room have at least one wall-mounted urinal place with a basin lip of not more than 19″ for adults? 14″ for children?
7. Is the lavatory mounted to provide 29″ clearance from the floor with a maximum height to the top of the rim of 34″?
8. Are drain pipes and hot water pipes covered or insulated?
9. Are mirrors, towel racks, dispensers, hand dryers, and other such equipment placed so they are easily accessible to wheelchair users, no more than 40″ from the floor?
10. Do showers, if provided, accommodate persons with physical disabilities by having no thresholds (or very slight thresholds)? No slip surfaces? A hinged seat, mounted 19″ from the floor? Grab rails at approximately 32″? Control levers less than 40″ from the floor?

Although the design of facilities to meet the needs of children has been mentioned several times, the central point of focus of this chapter has been with adults. If children are the primary users of a facility, their needs should be given a great amount of consideration. Those planning facilities for children should remain ever conscious of the need to accomodate children with disabling conditions. One of the primary play areas of children is the playground. The final portion of this chapter deals with the design of playgrounds with the disabled child in mind.

PLAYGROUNDS

Through play children develop intellectually, emotionally, and motorically. As Frost and Klein (1979) have stated, "Play is the chief vehicle for the development of imagination and intelligence, language, sex role behavior, and perceptual-motor development in infants and young children" (p. 50). As with any child, play is a necessary experience in the development of the child who has a disabling condition.

Gordon (1972) has observed a tendency for many infants and children with disabling conditions to be passive and to display a superficiality in relating to people and objects. Frost and Klein (1979) have suggested that children who are disabled may have difficulties in the following skills: "extent of exploration; initiation of activities; response and approach to others; attention to people, materials, and tasks; acceptance of limits and routines; respect for rights of others; seeing self as able to do and achieve" (p. 219). Obviously, infants and children displaying such behaviors have not had the experiences required to allow them to develop the competencies to interact with confidence with other persons or with the physical environment. Sadly, because of the inadequately designed playgrounds that too often exist in our communities, many of the more than seven million disabled children in the United States (Bowers, 1979) have been deprived of the opportunity to experience play environments that encourage the realization of natural developmental outcomes.

This is not to say, however, that special playgrounds must be designed for the exclusive use of children with disabling conditions. One of the most important concepts to remember about children with disabilities is that they are first and foremost children. Most special children have one or perhaps two disabilities and are average or above average in most areas of ability. The special child is a normal child who typically deviates from the average only on one or two characteristics (Moore et al., 1979). Also, by constructing playgrounds to serve all children, children both with and without disabling conditions can gain experiences playing with children possessing different characteristics. Such exposures have the potential to broaden the understanding of all children regarding individual differences (Austin, 1978). Finally, fundamental economic reasoning dictates that a single playground would be less expensive than two playgrounds. From all perspectives, it seems to make little sense to build community playgrounds for the use of any single group. Therefore, as a general principle, playgrounds should be designed so they are usable by *all* children.

The Inadequacy of Traditional American Playgrounds.
Traditional American playgrounds were seemingly designed to serve two primary purposes. Apparently the major reason for the establishment of playgrounds was to provide gross motor activities. The slides, swings, merry-go-rounds, seesaws, and monkey bars of the traditional playground certainly do not encourage types of play other than motor behaviors. The second major purpose of the design was evidently to allow ease of maintenance. This was commonly done by having all apparatus made of steel and usually placing this equipment in a sea of asphalt. Traditional American playgrounds, to say the least, were unimaginative in design and built with the needs of the maintenance crews ever in mind.

What Should Playgrounds Be Like?
Unquestionably those responsible for traditional American playgrounds failed to provide well-designed play areas for our children. But what should playgrounds be like? In recent years a number of authors have attempted to answer this question (e.g., Dattner 1969, Bengtsson 1970, Hagan 1974, and Frost & Klein 1979). Most of these authors have given consideration to the needs of disabled children in their writings. Still other authors (e.g., Gordon, 1972; Austin, 1978; Bowers, 1979; Moore et al., 1979; and Grosse, 1980) have published works that have focused specifically upon designing playgrounds that meet the needs of children with disabilities.

In reviewing this body of literature, four broad areas of concern emerge. These are: (1) accessibility, (2) health and safety considerations, (3) the provision of an interesting and challenging environment, and (4) the need for variety. The sections that follow review these four areas.

Accessibility.
Wheelchair users, children using crutches, and children with braces are regularly denied play experiences because play areas have not been

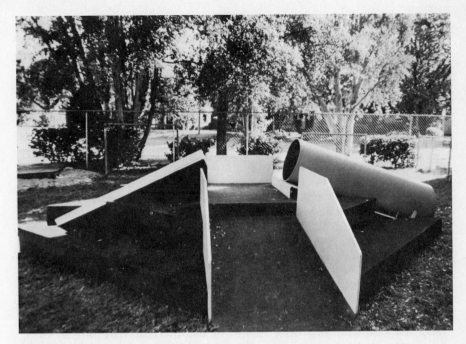

Figure 5–9. Note the use of the ramp and railing in a playground designed by Dr. Lou Bowers.

made accessible (Grosse, 1980). To be sure, accessibility is a primary issue in the design of community playgrounds.

A number of design features can be employed to make an outside play area accessible. The following recommendations for increasing accessibility have been drawn from Gordon (1972), Austin (1978), Bowers (1979), Frost & Klein (1979), Grosse (1980), and Beckwith (1985).

Hard Surface Paths. Hard surface paths or trails should allow entry to the play area and then wind their way throughout the playground so that a child may reach any piece of apparatus by use of the path. The paths should be wide enough to permit two wheelchairs to pass. Sharp angles should be avoided in laying out the path system in favor of gentle curves. Also to be avoided are steep slopes. Paths should not exceed a grade of 5 percent, with slopes of 3 or 4 percent preferred. Finally, space close to each piece of apparatus should be provided so that children may park their wheelchairs or leave crutches or walkers in order to give them the freedom to crawl or use the apparatus for support while exploring the play environment.

Ramps. Ramps can make playgrounds accessible by first permitting access to the play area and then by allowing children access to play apparatus. A slope of not more than 8.33 percent is recommended for all ramps. Preferably the slope will be much less than this suggested maximum. Ramps are well suited to replace stairs or ladders. For example, a ramp can provide access to a slide. Free standing ramps should be so designed as to prevent the child from accidently slipping off the edge. This may be done by means of two railings—one at the bottom edge of the ramp and a second higher one that may be used as a handrail. Or walls may be constructed on the ramps and handrails attached to the walls. Two sets of handrails at two different heights will enable children of various sizes to negotiate the ramp. The highest handrail should be 24″ from the floor of the ramp.

Railings. Railings can be used to enable children to move about the playground more easily. Children with balance problems can use the equipment by supporting themselves with the railings. Children who have visual impairments can employ the railings to guide their movements. The use of bright paint on the rails can serve as visual cues for those children who are partially sighted. Of course it is important to make the railings the proper height to accomodate the children using them. The size of the diameter of the railing is also important. For children with mobility problems, the average handrail with a diameter of $2\frac{1}{2}″$ is of little use. A smaller railing of $\frac{3}{4}″$ to $1\frac{1}{2}″$ has been recommended by the Pittsburgh Architects Workshop (1979). Another source (A Playground for all Children, 1978) has suggested handrails have a diameter of no more than $\frac{3}{4}″$ to allow ease in use by amputees with hooks.

Elevated Areas. Elevated areas may be constructed to allow children in wheelchairs to engage in sand and water play or complete gardening projects. Freestanding sand and water tables, which accomodate wheelchairs, may be purchased or constructed. For sand play, a mound of dirt can be cut out to accomodate a wheelchair and then the mound can be covered with sand. A small wall can be constructed to surround the cutout area. It is important that the cutout area is designed so it is of the correct height (approximately 32″) and allows the child to easily reach the sand. Garden boxes can be built with railroad ties, which can be stacked to form boxes and filled with soil. Here again proper height is important. The wheelchair user should be able to reach the soil from his or her wheelchair or by transfering from the wheelchair to sit on the top rail. Most designers believe that children should be afforded the option to leave their wheelchairs whenever they desire. Therefore, it is probably best not to "over design" playgrounds by building too many elevated areas since this may discourage children from leaving their wheelchairs.

Health and Safety Considerations.

A few common-sense measures can help assure a safe and healthy play environment that challenges children without posing undue risks. Several recommendations follow under the headings of general considerations, surfacing, and apparatus. Primary sources for this section are Gordon (1972), Frost and Klein (1979) and *A Guide to Designing Accessible Outdoor Recreation Facilities* (1980) produced by the U.S. Department of Interior.

General Considerations. One often neglected element on playgrounds is seating for adults who accompany children to the play area and who wish to have a comfortable vantage point from which to view the child at play. Benches should, if possible, be in a shaded area. Protection from the sun should also be provided for the children. Trees and/or shelters may be used for this purpose. For some, a shaded area is a desirable convenience. For others it is essential. Children taking certain medications may need to avoid exposure to the sun in order to prevent nausea, severe sun burns, or other harmful reactions. Those who may not perspire normally must have shade to avoid becoming overheated. Other children who lack skin sensitivity may be burned by contact with metal parts on apparatus that have become hot due to exposure to the sun (Pittsburgh Architects Workshop 1979). Another general consideration is that of providing accessible rest rooms and drinking fountains a relatively short distance from the playground. Easy access to water is imperative for some disabled persons who require regular fluid intake (Smith, 1981). Finally, a fence with gates (3'–4' wide) that can be locked should be provided around playgrounds adjacent to a street or those used primarily by young children.

Surfacing. Children will occasionally fall from apparatus. Therefore falls should be anticipated and prepared for when installing surfaces. While hard surfaces such as asphalt and cement are desirable from a maintenance perspective, these surfaces are not desirable from a safety standpoint. Grass is a most desirable surface for open areas of the playground, but resiliant surfaces are needed under all equipment. A protective surface must be installed under equipment where falls would be anticipated. Materials such as rubber mats, sand, pea gravel, and tanbark can be used to form a protective surface.

Apparatus. One basic playground safety principle is that all apparatus should have rounded edges. All rough or jagged edges need to be smoothed off when equipment is put in place and regular maintenance checks need to be made to assure that the edges remain safe.

Another basic principle is to normally avoid the use of hard, wooden seats on swings. Flexible rubber seats provide a better alternative for traditional swings. Safety belts may be installed for swings adapted for use by children with disabilities. For children with strength limitations, those who are amputees or paraplegics, and others who can benefit from the stabilization provided, safety belts (along with back supports and leg supports) are useful additions to swings. In fact, safety belts can be used not only on swings but on seesaws and other pieces of apparatus where children are seated (Pittsburgh Architects Workshop, 1979).

Stabilization is a critical factor to consider in designing equipment for disabled children. There is a noticeable absence of support devices on many traditional pieces of playground equipment. Swings, seesaws, spring animals, and similar pieces require a great deal of balance and control; the lack of some type of devices to provide back and leg support makes their use quite difficult for many children who have conditions. Therefore, to allow these children safe access to this equipment, alterations need to be made (Pittsburgh Architects Workshop, 1979). Specific guidelines for making adaptations for swings, seesaws, and merry-go-rounds are provided later in this chapter.

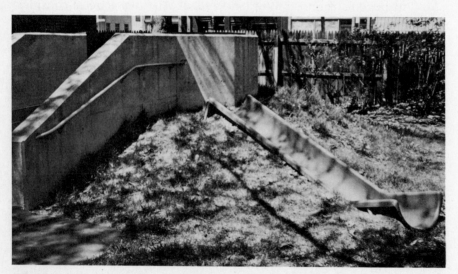

Figure 5–10. A slide built into a hillside in a playground designed by Richard Dattner.

To enable children with strength or mobility limitations to safely move about, handholds and handrails should be installed where appropriate. Of course, handrails are essential to ramped areas and steps. Here it may be desirable to provide two sets of handrails to accomodate children of various sizes.

A final area of concern is that of height. A great deal of analysis should go into the selection of equipment and its installation to be sure it is of a safe height for the user. Smaller children naturally need smaller apparatus. Other design concepts, such as building slides into hillsides or using climbing ropes or platforms set on one another to allow children access to a slide, not only eliminate the need for a ladder but reduce the danger of having a child fall from a high place.

The Provision of an Interesting and Challenging Environment.
Several design principles have been brought forth on how to make a playground interesting and challenging for children. The concepts that follow are based largely on the work of Frost and Klein (1979) and Moore and the University of Wisconsin-Milwaukee group (Moore et al., 1979).

Multiple Skill Level. The play environment should provide for multiple levels of skill so that the child is challenged without unreasonable demands being made on his or her abilities. Ideally, there is just enough challenge to stimulate the child to try the next skill level. Therefore, it is important to provide graded levels of complexity on the playground. For example, there may be several ways to reach the top of a slide, each of which may be slightly more challenging to the child. These might range from a ramp to platforms to climbing a cargo net. Such alternatives also provide clear points of accomplishment so the child will realize he or she has succeeded at the task. All children, and particularly disabled children, need successes in order to build positive self-concepts.

Opportunities for Sensory Stimulation. Children need opportunities for all sorts of sensory stimulation. Playgrounds should offer a wide variety of sensory experiences including things to feel, smell, see, and hear. For example, surfaces can be made to have different textures so that children with visual impairments may learn to discriminate between types of surfaces. Flowers and other plants may be grown to offer visual beauty as well as pleasing aromas. A variety of colors can be used on the playground, and some equipment may be designed so that children can manipulate it to produce sounds.

Soft Play Things Offer Emotional Release and a Sense of Control. Not all equipment must be of steel or wood. A soft play environment made of foam rubber covered with a variety of colored fabrics can offer new experiences to children. In such an environment children may release tensions and emotions without harming themselves. Designers of the New York University Medical Center playground (Gordon, 1972) used pits made of covered foam rubber so that children with severely limited mobliity could express themselves through motion by moving their bodies on the soft and giving surface. An alternative to foam rubber is the use of air-filled apparatus.

Equipment Placement to Facilitate Continuous Play. Play should be allowed to naturally flow from one activity to another. In the placement of equipment, consideration should be given to possible alternative play behaviors once a particular activity ends. The child should be given several alternatives from which to choose his or her next play activity. For example, are opportunities other than returning for more sliding available at the bottom of the slide? Play patterns can grow and expand if adequate environmental cues are provided the child. On the other hand, overstimulation at decision points must be avoided for those children not yet ready to tolerate dealing with too many stimuli.

The Need for Variety.

Closely related to the need for an interesting and challenging environment is the necessity for variety in play environments. The content for this section, like the one that preceded it, has been drawn primarily from the works of Frost and Klein (1979) and Moore and his colleagues (Moore et al., 1979).

Broad Range of Areas and Equipment. The playground should provide for almost any imaginable type of play in which children normally engage. Children certainly need equipment that allows for gross motor activity. But children also require places for play involving organized games, drama, building things, growing plants, and other activities. Defined boundaries should set apart the more active areas from other areas of the playground. One means of zoning the playground is by building waist-high railings throughout the play area. Such a railing system would also serve as a guide for visually impaired children and would enable those children with braces, crutches, canes, and walkers to stabilize themselves as they move about the playground (Pittsburgh Architects Workshop, 1979).

Equipment Offering a Variety of Uses. Some equipment pretty much defines its own use since it has a singular purpose. Swings are for

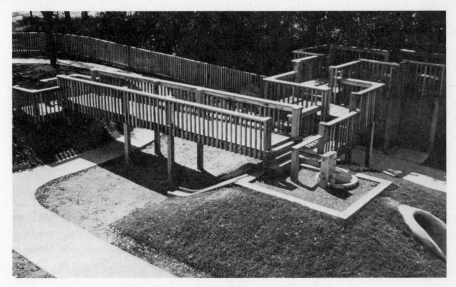

Figure 5–11. An interesting preschool playground at Flower Mound, New Town, in Texas.

swinging and slides are built for sliding. This equipment is generally not as useful as equipment that serves multiple functions. The playground designer should analyze each piece of apparatus to see if it provides for a variety of uses. For example, a variety of spatial experiences might be gained by a piece of apparatus that allows the child to crawl or climb under it, on it, through it, beside it, across it, above it, and around it. Ambiguous objects such as wooden climbing structures or rocks allow children to be creative and to use their imaginations.

Manipulation of Loose Parts. Closely related to the principle of offering a variety of uses is the idea of providing loose parts that the child can manipulate in a number of ways. Moore and his colleagues (Moore et al., 1979) classify loose parts into three categories. These are manufactured objects that are to be made into a specific end product (e.g., a puzzle), things that are manufactured but have a variable finished form (e.g., Tinker Toys), and thirdly, things found in the natural environment (e.g., old tires, boards, sand) that can be used in any variety of ways. The use of loose parts allows the child to have some amount of control over his or her environment—to change it or to manipulate it. Adventure playgrounds are made up entirely of loose parts such as lumber, bricks, cardboard boxes, and old tires from which the children build whatever they desire. Moore and his colleagues (Moore et al., 1979) state that the use of loose parts (including adventure playgrounds) has been successfully employed with mentally and physically disabled children. They mention, however, that some children will need to be shown an example of a finished product before actually attempting to construct something for themselves.

Places and Spaces. Children need a variety of places to accommodate different types of play. Open spaces are required for group play and games. Other places should be provided for play by a single child or a small group of children. While children require opportunities for group play, they also need places where they can gain privacy on the playground. Some small spaces need to be provided for the child for solitary play or for just escaping to be by himself or herself. Small group play may be facilitated by designing areas where two to four children may play together. Sand and water areas or playhouses may be designed for this purpose.

Adapting Existing Equipment

One means to begin assuring adequate play areas for children with disabilities is to modify equipment on existing playgrounds. Specific suggestions have been offered by the Pittsburgh Architects Workshop (1979) on how to adapt traditional playground apparatus to make them usable by children with disabling conditions. The material that follows is based on the work of the Pittsburgh Architects Workshop.

Slides
A soft ground surface may limit access to both conventional and timber slides. An initial improvement would be to provide a hard surface path to a hard surface pad (with a 6' diameter) at the base of the steps or ramp leading to the top of the slide.

Conventional Slides. Steps on conventional metal slides are too steep and too narrow for the use of children who are semi-ambulatory. The original steps may be replaced by ones adjusted to 45 degrees or less. These new steps should be 2'6" to 3' wide with a depth of 4" to 6". The space between steps should preferably be 4" and no more than 6". In replacing existing handrails on steps, ones approximately $\frac{3}{4}$" in diameter should be used. At the top of the steps a platform 2' long (from front to back) and approximately 3' wide should be constructed to allow needed space for the child to prepare to go down the slide. The sliding board should be 2'6" to 3'6" in width in order to accommodate disabled children, rather than the standard 1'6" to 2'6" size. A soft landing surface (6' in diameter) should be provided at the bottom of the sliding board. Outside of this landing area, a hard surface circulation path should be located for the use of semi-ambulatory children. Within the landing area, a short railing extending from either side of the bottom of the sliding board may be constructed to aid physically disabled children in getting up after coming off the end of the slide into the landing area. Finally, trees may be planted near the slide in order to provide shade to keep the sliding surface relatively cool on hot summer days.

Timber Slides. Pipes are often placed on timber slides to be used as climbers to reach the platform. Since this access would be difficult for many children with disabilities, alternatives may need to be employed to allow access to this apparatus. One means is to use either telephone poles or railroad ties cut at various lengths and placed on end to form stairs up the platform. Handholds may be placed on the support posts of the apparatus for use by children in gaining stability and pulling themselves up the stairs. Another alternative is to construct a ramp at least 4′ wide. As with any ramp, handrails should be placed on either side to facilitate movement by the children. Rubber coverings can be used on handrails and on the tops of support posts to cushion falls. On the platform, an elevated box may be constructed to allow children a more gradual transfer to the surface of the sliding board. It is recommended that the box be 2′ long, 3′ wide, and 1′ to 1′6″ high. As in the case of the conventional metal slide, the sliding board and landing areas should be made to accommodate the needs of children with disabilities. (See the prior section on conventional slides for details.)

Seesaws

Another piece of traditional apparatus discussed by the Pittsburgh Architects Workshop (1979) is the seesaw. A basic improvement, as with the slides, is to allow access to the seesaw by means of a hard surface path.

To provide stability when the child is mounting the seesaw, a pipe or post device may be constructed on which the end of the seesaw can rest. A permanent installation of this device would require a seesaw that could be swung to the side so it could be placed on the stationary post for mounting and then be returned to its original position. An alternative to having a seesaw that rotates would be to build a stabilizer post that could be moved once the child had mounted the seesaw.

Two things can be done to lessen the impact of the seesaw when it hits the ground. One is to provide a soft surface beneath the seesaw. The second is to add shock-absorbent padding at the ends of the seesaw. Various types of rubber padding (e.g., a piece of auto tire) may be attached to the bottom of the seesaw to absorb the shock.

Several adaptations can be made to the seat in order to better accommodate children with disabilities. The first is to make the seat wider (10″–12″) so it is easier to straddle. A second is to add a back support to provide stability for children with balance problems. Another is to attach leg supports from 1′6″ to 2′ from the front of the seat. These supports, which extend about 8″ from each side, should be curved up on their ends to keep the legs from falling off. Finally, the addition of safety belts allows a margin of safety for those children who experience difficulty with balance and stability.

Handles on conventional seesaws are 1″ to $1\frac{1}{2}″$ in diameter. As indicated earlier, this size is too large from many disabled children. To accommodate these children, a $\frac{3}{4}″$ piece of pipe can be bolted into the existing handle.

Swings

A hard surface path leading to a 6′-diameter concrete pad directly under the swing offers the wheelchair user the opportunity to transfer to the seat of the swing. The path should come into the pad at a 45-degree angle so that there is a soft landing area directly in front of the swing. The placement of an inverted U-shaped metal pipe (1″–$1\frac{1}{2}″$ in diameter and 2′–2′6″ in height) in the concrete pad would enable users to stabilize themselves while getting seated. This railing should be set in the pad 10″ to 12″ from the path of the swing. (Even though this clearance is recommended by the Pittsburgh Architects Workshop, it would seem highly important to make certain that the swing could not strike the railing.)

Other modifications for an adapted swing include the addition of a back support, leg support, and safety belts. The back support should be at least 1′6″ in height. The leg support should fold back under the wooden or metal seat when it is not needed by the child who has the ability to operate the swing without the device. When extended, the leg support should clear the ground by at least 6″ to 8″. The safety belts help assure that the child with stability problems will not fall from the swing. They are easily attached to the seat.

It is recommended by the Pittsburgh Architects Workship (1979) that in each set of four swings, one swing should be adapted in the fashion indicated in this section. For those agencies that do not wish to modify existing swings, commercial playground equipment manufacturers now offer molded plastic seats for purchase.

Merry-Go-Round

As with other adapted equipment, it is important that a hard surface path lead to the merry-go-round. It is not desirable, however, to have hard surfacing surrounding the merry-go-round; a soft ground surface should be provided around the merry-go-round in order to minimize injuries resulting from falling from the apparatus.

Handrails on merry-go-rounds are usually made of metal pipe $1\frac{1}{4}''$ to $1\frac{1}{2}''$ in diameter. At the minimum, one set of handrails should be replaced with smaller pipe (i.e., $\frac{3}{4}''-1''$). Other adaptations that can be made are to stretch wire mesh or a rope net between the posts for the handrails to form a back support and to attach safety belts to the base of the pipes.

Railings Around Equipment

A waist-high railing around an area, such as the merry-go-round or see-saw, will zone it off to protect children with visual or perceptual impairments from getting hurt by moving into the equipment when it is in use. Such railings also serve to guide visually impaired children around the playground. An optional refinement would be the attachment of a sound-producing device to the merry-go-round, seesaws, or other apparatus to indicate to the visually impaired that it is in use.

The interested reader is referred to *Access to Play* by the Pittsburgh Architects Workshop (1979) for further details on the adaptations covered in this section, as well as for adaptations for climbers. *Access to Play* contains many excellent diagrams that illustrate suggested adaptations.

A Final Word on Playgrounds

As previously stated, it is not normally necessary or desirable to provide separate playgrounds for children with disabilities. Playgrounds can be designed with all children in mind. If play environments are well designed, the great majority of disabled children can join their nondisabled peers in healthful play experiences in our city parks, on our school grounds, or wherever playgrounds are provided.

SUMMARY

This chapter dealt with concerns in designing appropriate recreation environments for all people, including those with disabilities. The chapter began with a discussion of terminology and legislation related to designing environments to meet the needs of individuals with disabilities. Following this introduction, the major portion of the chapter was devoted to guidelines and recommendations for creating usable recreation facilities. The final segment of the chapter covered the topic

of designing playgrounds so that they will accommodate children who
have disabilities.

Suggested Learning Activities

1. Using Table 5–1 (p. 110), access a local park or campus recreation
    facility. Several students may join together to access a state,
    regional, or national park.

2. Drawing upon the information from the section on playgrounds,
    access a local playground for design criteria.

3. Using an actual playground, report how you would adapt existing
    equipment to meet the needs of all children, including those with
    disabilities.

4. Prepare a slide show on proper design of either parks or
    playgrounds.

5. Participate in a telephone lecture given by an authority on
    playground design for children with disabilities.

6. View an audio-visual presentation on facility or playground design
    for persons with disabilities. Several films and slide shows are
    available through Indiana University, University of Missouri, and
    University of South Florida.

References

A Guide to Designing Accessible Outdoor Recreation Facilities. Ann Arbor,
    Michigan: Heritage Conservation and Recreation Service, U.S. Department
    of Interior, 1980.

American National Standards Institute. *American National Standard
    Specifications for Making Buildings and Facilities Accessible to and Usable
    by Physically Handicapped People.* New York, NY: American National
    Standards Institute, Inc., 1980.

A Playground for All Children: Resource Book. Washington, DC: U.S.
    Government Printing Office, 1978.

Austin, D. R. Playgrounds for the handicapped. In D. J. Bradamus, ed., *New
    Thoughts on Leisure.* Champaign, IL: Office of Recreation and Park
    Resources, University of Illinois, 1978.

Beckwith, J. Play environments for all children. *Leisure Today.* In *Journal of
    Physical Education, Recreation and Dance,* 56(5):32–35, 1985.

Bengtsson, A. *Environmental Planning for Children's Play.* New York: Praeger
    Publishers, 1970.

Bowers, L. Toward a science of playground design: Principles of design for play centers for all children. *Leisure Today*, In *Journal of Physical Education, Recreation and Dance.* 50(8):51–54, 1979.

Dattner, R. *Design for Play.* New York: Van Nostrand Reinhold Company, 1969.

Frost, J. L., and B. L. Klein. *Children's Play and Playgrounds.* Boston: Allyn and Bacon, Inc., 1979.

Gordon, R. *The Design of a Pre-School Therapeutic Playground: An Outdoor "Learning Laboratory."* New York, NY: Institute of Rehabilitation Medicine, New York University Medical Center, 1972.

Grosse, S. J. Making outdoor play areas usable for all children. *Practical Pointers.* Reston, VA: American Alliance for Health, Physical Education, Recreation and Dance, 1980.

Hagan, P. *Playgrounds for Free.* Cambridge, MA: The MIT Press, 1974.

Jones, M. A. *Accessibility Standards Illustrated.* Springfield, IL: Illinois Capital Development Board, 1978.

Mace, R. L., and B. Lasett, eds. *An Illustrated Handbook of the Handicapped Section of the North Carolina State Building Code.* Raleigh, NC: North Carolina Department of Insurance Engineering Division, 1977.

Mainstreaming Handicapped Individuals: Parks and Recreation Design Standards Manual. Springfield, IL: Department of Conservation. 1978.

Moore, G. T., U. Cohen, J. Oerbel, and L. van Ryzin. *Designing Environments for Handicapped Children: A Design Guide and Case Study.* New York: Educational Facilities Laboratories, 1979.

Pittsburgh Architects Workshop. *Access to Play: Design Criteria for Adaptation of Existing Playground Equipment for Use by Handicapped Children.* Pittsburgh: Pittsburgh Architects Workshop, Inc., 1979.

Ries, M. L. *Design Standards to Accommodate People with Physical Disabilities in Park and Open Space Planning.* Madison, WI: University of Wisconsin Recreation Resource Center, 1973.

Smith, R. W. Personal Communication. November 11, 1981.

U.S. Department of Housing and Urban Development with the American Society of Landscape Architects Foundation. *Barrier Free Site Design.* Washington, DC: U.S. Government Printing Office, 1975.

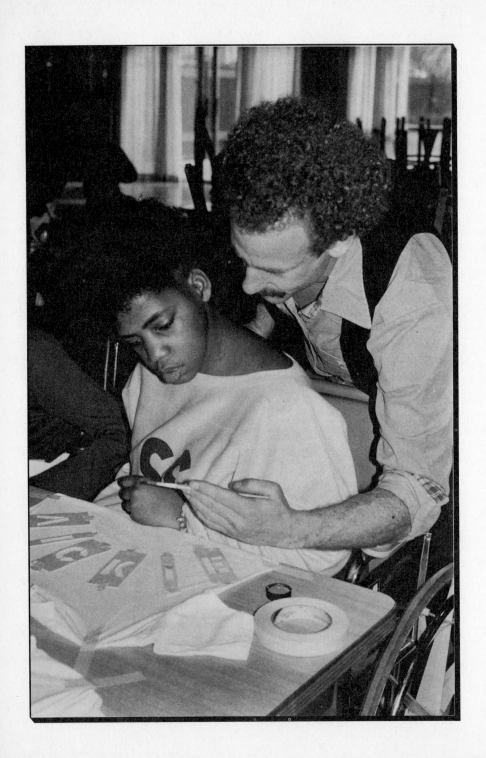

6

Program Planning Processes

A student majoring in recreation was asked to conduct a three-day camp program for a group of children who were mentally retarded. The student promptly began planning activities such as crafts, a campfire program, and hiking. This is actually the reversal of the procedure that should take place. The student should have first assessed the needs of the participants.

The first step in program planning must include needs assessment. Recreators should find out what their clients want to do and determine their abilities. Next, recreators should develop program goals and write objectives that correspond with the interests and abilities of the participants. The participants should be included in this process if at all possible. In most instances, persons who are disabled should define their own program goals and objectives. Stating goals and objectives can enhance the evaluation of leisure services since the recreation specialist may compare pre-stated goals and objectives with actual outcomes in order to make informed decisions about changes in programs and services.

Selecting and modifying (if necessary) activities is the last step in the planning process. This selection process should be based on the relationship between needs and those leisure services that have the potential to meet goals and objectives. Again, persons with disabilities should be encouraged to play an active role in this stage of the program planning process.

NEEDS ASSESSMENT

The first step in the program planning process is needs assessment. The goal of needs assessment is to facilitate effective program planning (Farrell and Lundegren, 1978). This step can take two forms. One form deals with determining the need for recreation services for persons with disabiilties, and the other form concerns the needs, interests, and abilities of the participants.

The Need for Recreation Services

The number of persons with disabilities in the community or geographic area where programming is to take place should be identified. The fact that persons who have disabilities reside in your community will, in part, help justify leisure services. Some communities have conducted surveys in order to establish such information. The kind of information that might be useful includes age, sex, disabling condition, and special considerations. Special considerations could entail transportation barriers, architectural barriers such as steps and curbs, the need for medication, and special kinds of assistance such as transferring persons from their wheelchairs to the swimming pool.

Although persons with disabilities within many communities tend to make up six to eight percent of the population, it is wise to conduct a survey to obtain more detailed information, as well as to verify numbers and types of disabilities. The process of identification is not an easy one. O'Morrow (1980) suggests several reasons why it is difficult to collect information on the prevalence of special populations. Among these reasons include "the fact that the line of demarcation between the 'normal' or 'average' and the individuals most often considered to be a special population member cannot always be agreed upon" (p. 9). O'Morrow notes further that definitions change and laws differ from state to state. Another difficulty is the way in which information is reported. Agencies do not seem to have any standard reporting procedure. In addition, due to confidentiality, obtaining names, addresses, and other pertinent information is often difficult. In addition to going to the schools and social agencies or conducting a survey, some communities have tried other techniques to identify persons with disabilities. For example, communities have advertised their programs on television and in local newspapers to get individuals with disabilities to come forward and, ultimately, take part in community programs. In other instances, the recreation department or agency has tried to contact and publicize programs through water bills sent to residents in the community.

In summary, in order to establish the need for programs, the recreator has to verify the fact that there are persons who are disabled who live in the community and who lack leisure opportunities. Information concerning individuals with disabilities and the lack of leisure opportunities must be delineated. Consideration must also be given to questions concerning the extent of need for specialized or separate programs for persons with disabilities, and the degree to which they can be integrated into general community recreation patterns (Frye and Peters, 1972). Advertising and marketing special recreation services seems to be one way to determine the need for such services.

Determining Individual Needs, Interests, and Skills

The fact that human beings have certain needs that are essential to their survival and other needs that add to the quality of their life is well documented. These needs are physical, social, and psychological in nature. As Frye and Peters (1972) suggest, all people, including individuals who are disabled, have needs. O'Morrow (1980) points out that persons with disabilities have the same needs, interests, and aspirations as their non-disabled counterparts. Most professionals in the recreation and leisure field are in agreement that individuals can satisfy some of their needs through participation in recreational experiences. Frye and Peters (1972) note that:

> The fundamental rationale both for strengthening links between treatment-centered and community leisure services and for developing community-based recreation services for ill or disabled people stems from the concept of recreation as a life-continuous force. (p. 116)

Many writers suggest that despite illness or disability, and regardless of where individuals reside, they are entitled to recreative experiences. Thus, not only is recreation and leisure viewed as meeting needs, it is also seen by many as a legal right. For instance, the Kennedy Foundation has fought for the legal rights of mentally retarded persons by using the "pursuit of happiness" clause from the Bill of Rights.

There is much evidence in the literature suggesting that activities leading to leisure outcomes can benefit individuals by contributing to their mental, emotional, physical, and social development. Research, for example, on sociodramatic play demonstrates that such opportunities contribute to the development of problem solving skills by enhancing such qualities as concentration and cognitive spontaneity (Compton and Witt, 1981). Many writers have indicated that mental health is related to the fantasy and make-believe aspect of play. Menninger (1960) has commented that the individual can find satisfaction through the emotional release of pent-up energies by participating in active, competitive situations, although research has not always been supportive of this notion. We do know, however, that adequate leisure participation can provide the individual with such benefits as positive self-concept, fitness, enjoyment, and overall well-being. It is also important to recognize that the lack of opportunity and, in fact, deficits in leisure functioning may curtail individual growth and development and, in some cases, create undesirable behaviors such as depression and feelings of inadequacy.

How Needs, Interests, and Abilities Are Identified

Needs, interests, and abilities are identified in various ways. The following is a brief listing with some examples, to illustrate:

- Some needs and interests are identified by the consumer of the leisure service. For example, an individual might say: "I feel inadequate because I can't seem to meet anyone," or participants in some activities may help restructure those activities because of their needs. A good example of this phenomena would be the rule changes that have occurred in wheelchair sports, particularly in wheelchair basketball wherein the participants vote on rule changes.
- Interests and skills can be determined from direct observation. For instance, the autistic child does not respond to social cues (smiling) in the environment and this lack of response is observed by the recreation worker. The recreation worker may observe that a child with cerebral palsy is having difficulty holding a fishing rod or crayon. This observation may prompt the adaptation of a device to facilitate the fishing or coloring skills of the child.
- Interviewing the parents or the spouse of an individual who is disabled may help the recreator ascertain needs that leisure participation can help satisfy. For example, parents might tell you that their child would like to learn to swim or to play the guitar.
- Needs, interests, and abilities may be identified through formal testing. The Leisure Diagnostic Battery (LDB), developed by Compton and Witt (1981), is an innovative approach to the assessment of leisure functioning. It covers a wide range of components inherent in leisure functioning including social

skills and leisure attitudes, and looks at the ability of an individual to satisfy needs via leisure involvement. Several leisure inventories and leisure counseling tools have been developed to assess participation patterns as well as preferences and interests (Hubert, 1969; Overs, 1970; Mirenda, 1973: McKechnie, 1974; and McDowell, 1974).

Once needs, interests, and skills are identified through testing, direct observation, interviewing, and listening to the consumers, the next step is developing goals and objectives. The achievement of these goals and objectives would mean the satisfaction of needs and interests of participants.

GOALS AND OBJECTIVES

Once needs assessment is completed, the establishment of program goals and the writing of program objectives should take place. Recreators seek to accomplish their goals and objectives by means of leisure services for persons with disabilities conducted in a variety of settings. These goals and objectives can be stated in many different ways. In this section, the focus will be on writing goals and objectives as outcomes for groups of participants. It should be noted that the principles and techniques of writing goals and behavioral objectives can be applied to individuals as well as groups.

It is important to distinguish between goals and objectives. Goals are general statements of intent while objectives are more specific outcomes described in terms that are measurable (Mager and Pipe, 1970). Both goals and objectives answer the question: "Where are we going?"

In the recreation field, the formulation of goals should be based on the strengths, interests, and skills of the individuals participating. Here are some examples:

Goal 1: Improve socialization skills with peers.
Goal 2: Facilitate enjoyment during leisure.
Goal 3: Increase physical fitness.
Goal 4: Improve ability to cooperate with others.

Sometimes, goals are stated as evaluative questions. The same goals stated in the question format become:

Goal 1: Is there improvement of socialization skills with peers?
Goal 2: Are participants enjoying themselves during leisure?

Goal 3: Is physical fitness better now?
Goal 4: Do they cooperate better with others?

Reducing Goals into Objectives

Having determined program goals, the next step is to translate these goal statements into behavioral objectives. Gronlund (1970) and others (Mager, 1962, and Mager and Pipe, 1970) have discussed the process of reducing a goal to behavioral terms. Table 6–1 outlines this process.

This procedure gives you an operational definition of your goal, which is referred to as a behavioral objective. You will find that some behaviors seem essential to attainment of the goal while others are not essential but serve to add weight or strength to the evidence. For instance, you would probably state some essential cognitive (intellectual) skills if your goal is to "Appreciate the art work of Picasso," arguing that some foundation of information is needed for appreciation. On the other hand, one of your performance or behavioral statements might read, "During a discussion of art, the children talk voluntarily about Picasso's art." While this latter behavior might well be indicative of interest in Picasso's work, you would not say the goal was not met simply because you did not observe that particular behavior.

Table 6–1
Example of Reducing a Goal to Behavioral Terms

Steps	Example
1. Write down the goal.	1. Improve socialization skills.
2. Ask: How shall I know success when I see it? What will the individuals be doing?	2. The individuals will be doing such things as sharing, helping and/or talking with others.
3. List the behaviors which, taken together, would tell you that the goal had been achieved.	3. • Sharing (person shares crayons). • Helping (person helps another child put the crayons away). • Talking (person talks with another child while they are coloring).
4. Eliminate from the list any items that are redundant or trivial.	4. None.
5. Remove from the list any items that prove to be goals.	5. None.
6. Ask: Would I be willing to say that they had achieved the goals?	6. Yes.
7. If "yes," you're done. If "no," continue steps 2–6.	7. _____

Writing Behavioral Objectives

A behavioral objective describes the outcome of the leisure experience in terms of the performance or behavior desired of the individuals who are engaging in the recreation activity. It describes your leadership intent in unambiguous terms. A behavioral objective:

1. provides direction for the leader
2. conveys intent to others, including the participant
3. provides a guideline for selecting activities, equipment, etc.
4. provides a guide for evaluating the program.

Behavioral objectives usually contain a *behavior, condition(s)*, and/or *criteria*. These elements are outlined in the following points.

1. Identify the behavior. In effect, complete the sentence: "I will know the individual is demonstrating the desired behavior when the person can . . ." State *only* the action or *behavior.*
2. If necessary, identify the *conditions* under which the behavior will take place—the "givens," or restrictions that will help individuals as they perform.
3. If necessary, identify the *criteria* of successful performance— the minimum standards of correctness, time, or other measures that you consider important. Many times successful performance is based upon past behaviors of the individual as compared to a standard and/or group. (Mager and Pipe, 1970)

EXAMPLES of behavioral objectives that include these elements are listed below.

1. Given all the basic shapes—cone, cylinder, prism, and sphere *(conditions)*, the participants will identify orally *(behavior)* each one of the four shapes *(criteria)*.
2. Within three months *(condition)* the participants will follow the rules of the game *(behavior)* 90 percent of the time *(criteria)*.
3. After two months of lessons *(condition)*, the participants will swim *(behavior)* one length of the pool *(criteria)*.

It is important to discriminate *outcome objectives* from process objectives. Be careful to keep separate the objectives you define that describe outcomes (that is, measurable end-products of the recreation program) and those that define processes (that is, the means for accomplishing them).

Let's look at two *Incorrect* examples.

Example #1: The leader will demonstrate how to use the book cradle.

Example #2: The children will use the book cradle for 15 minutes

In the first example, good practice is violated by the error of specifying a response that is to be made by the leader instead of the person. For the second example, the objective contains a more common error. It describes the children's behavior, but it does not describe the desired outcome. Rather, if you read it carefully, you will note that it prescribes a means by which children can use a device to help them do something, such as read or color.

A *corrected* version of this same objective might be:

After being shown how to use the book cradle properly *(condition)*, the children will use it to read, color, or paint *(behavior)* during their leisure at least twice per week *(criteria)*.

Taxonomy

The objectives for a program should reflect the different levels of skill attainment it intends to produce. Participation in recreation programs may help individuals develop skills and attitudes at several levels depending on their needs, interests, and capacities. Objectives can be stated in one of three domains: cognitive, affective, and psychomotor. However, it is understood that participating in activities usually involves all three domains. This means that we are thinking, feeling, and acting when we are participating in recreational activities.

One way to help yourself include objectives at varied levels is to consult the taxonomies of educational objectives written by Bloom (1956) and others (Krathwohl et al., 1964; Harrow, 1972). Bloom developed a cognitive domain taxonomy, while Krathwohl and associates developed an affective domain, and Harrow, a psychomotor domain. Below are operational definitions of these domains with examples of behavioral objectives.

1. *Cognitive domain* includes those objectives that emphasize intellectual outcomes such as knowledge, understanding, and thinking skills.

Cognitive objective: State the rules of checkers.

2. *Affective domain* includes those objectives that emphasize feeling and emotion such as interests, attitudes, appreciation, and methods of adjustment.

> Affective objective: Demonstrate good sportsmanship by not cheating during the game.

3. *Psychomotor domain* includes those objectives that emphasize motor skills such as swimming, running, grasping, and so on.

> Psychomotor objective: Place the marble into the container.

Another helpful hint in writing objectives includes writing single rather than compound objectives. An example of a compound objective would be:

> *Identify* and *match* five pieces of material with corresponding colors.

In the above example, the children are asked to perform two behaviors or actions: (1) identify and (2) match. One way to correct a compound objective is to write two separate objectives. Thus, the previous example might look like this:

> 1. *Identify* five pieces of different colored material.
> 2. *Match* five pieces of material with corresponding colors.

The following are some examples of potential program objectives that are based upon strengths, interests, or needs.

SELF-HELP
1. Drink from cup without assistance.
2. Eat unaided.
3. Walk to bathroom by self.
4. Use toilet without help.
5. Brush teeth.

COMMUNICATION
1. Listen to music.
2. Respond correctly to request (e.g., "Give me the brush").
3. Initiate conversation with peers.

SOCIALIZATION
1. Reach for toys.
2. Show interest in game by watching it.

3. Wait his or her turn in the game.
4. Share crayons with others.
5. Enjoy activity as demonstrated by smiling and laughing.
6. Throw the ball to playmate.
7. Kick ball without falling.
8. Obey directions ("Go stand by the door.")
9. Draw shapes (circle, triangle, etc.)
10. Clap hands when music is played.

SELECTION AND MODIFICATION OF ACTIVITIES

As you will recall, the first step in program planning is to assess the needs and interests of individuals. The second step is to determine goals and objectives. Once the objectives are stated, the leader and the participants should decide what recreational experience will be best. It is important that the participants are capable of meeting the requirements necessary to take part in the activity and that the particular activity has the potential to contribute to the attainment of the goals and objectives. This brings us to the topic of activity analysis.

Activity Analysis

Activity analysis has been primarily viewed in two ways. The first is from the vantage point of assessing an individual's leisure behavior patterns and, second, as a procedure for evaluating the inherent quality of activities. The material presented here concerns the latter perspective. Gunn and Peterson (1978) give us the following definition: "Activity analysis is a procedure for breaking down and examining an activity to find inherent characteristics that contribute to program objectives" (p. 156). Gunn and Peterson go on to emphasize that activity analysis occurs independently of the individual and "the goal is simply to understand the activity and its inherent characteristics" (p. 157). Their view of activity analysis is similar in the revised edition of this earlier text (Peterson and Gunn, 1984).

What to Look at When Doing an Activity Analysis
Usually, an individual who is participating in an activity is involved in three behavioral domains: psychomotor, affective, and cognitive. For instance, in a game of racquetball, the motor responses include running, grasping the racquet, and hand–eye coordination. Affectively, racquetball requires control of emotions during the game. Cognitive skills

such as remembering rules and thinking about strategy are also important considerations.

In addition to the three behavioral domains, it is important to look at social interaction patterns. Avedon (1974) identifies eight interactive patterns. These include:

1. *Intra-individual.* Action taking place within the mind of a person, or action involving the mind and a part of the body, but requiring no contact with another person or external object. Day-dreaming would be an example of this interactive process.
2. *Extra-individual.* Action directed by a person toward an object in the environment, requiring no contact with another person. Examples of this interaction pattern would include playing a pinball machine alone, walking by one's self or working on a solitary art project.
3. *Aggregate.* Action directed by a person toward an object in the environment while in the company of other persons who are also directing action toward objects in the environment. What has been termed "parallel play" is an example of aggregate. Activities such as watching a movie and playing bingo would be examples of this interaction pattern.
4. *Inter-individual.* Action of a competitive nature directed by one person toward another. It is inherent in backgammon, checkers, singles tennis, and a variety of other one-on-one encounters.
5. *Unilateral.* Action of competitive nature among three or more persons, one of whom is an antagonist or "it." Any number of "it" games like "hide and seek" would be examples of this process.
6. *Multilateral.* Action of a competitive nature among three or more persons, with no one person as an antagonist. This process is exemplified in many card games such as poker and hearts.
7. *Intragroup.* Action of a cooperative nature by two or more persons intent upon reaching a mutual goal. Singing in a group or playing a video game with a partner would be examples of intragroup patterns.
8. *Intergroup.* Action of a competitive nature between two or more intragroups. A variety of team sports such as basketball and football exemplify this interactive process.

Other factors for analysis might include the amount of leadership, whether or not equipment is required, duration of the activity, and the number of participants needed for the activity. The following Activity Analysis Form is a modified and shortened version of the Activity Analysis Rating Form presented by Peterson and Gunn (1984).

ACTIVITY ANALYSIS FORM

Name of Activity _____
Brief Description _____

Physical Aspects

1. Strength   Little or no 1 2 3 4 5 Much strength
                   strength

2. Speed   Little or no 1 2 3 4 5 Much speed
                   speed

3. Endurance   Little or no 1 2 3 4 5 Much endurance
                   endurance

4. Flexibility   Little or no 1 2 3 4 5 Much flexibility
                   flexibility

5. Agility   Little or no 1 2 3 4 5 Much agility
                   agility

6. Other; please specify:

   _____Little or no 1 2 3 4 5 Much _____
   _____Little or no 1 2 3 4 5 Much _____

Social Aspects

1. Interaction Patterns
   • intra-individual
   • extra-individual
   • aggregate
   • inter-individual
   • unilateral
   • multilateral
   • intragroup
   • intergroup

2. How much physical contact does the activity demand?
   little 1 2 3 4 5 much

3. How structured is the activity?
   unstructured 1 2 3 4 5 structured

4. What type of interaction is required?
   nonverbal 1 2 3 4 5 verbal

5. How noisy is the activity?

little or no noise 1 2 3 4 5 much noise

Cognitive Aspects

1. How complex are the rules that must be adhered to?

simple 1 2 3 4 5 complex

2. How much strategy does the activity require?

little strategy 1 2 3 4 5 much strategy

3. How much concentration is required?

little concentration 1 2 3 4 5 much concentration

Affective Aspects

1. Rate the opportunities for the expression of the following emotions during the activity.

	never				often
joy	1	2	3	4	5
guilt	1	2	3	4	5
fear	1	2	3	4	5
pain	1	2	3	4	5

2. Rate the likely responses.

failure	1	2	3	4	5	success
dissatisfaction	1	2	3	4	5	satisfaction
rejection	1	2	3	4	5	acceptance

Administrative Aspects

1. Leadership   minimum   1 2 3 4 5 maximum

2. Equipment   none   1 2 3 4 5 much equipment

3. Participants   _____ fixed numbers
_____ multiple
_____ any number

The skill to analyze activities makes it possible for the recreator to select appropriate activities for the predetermined goals and objectives. As suggested by Gunn and Peterson, "It is obviously valuable to use activities that have inherent in their structure the qualities that relate most directly to the objectives. This information is only ascertained by activity analysis. The process also allows several activities to be compared so that the best ones can be selected and used" (p. 179).

It is impractical to do a formal activity analysis on every activity experience planned and conducted by the recreator. However, the recreator should be cognizant of inherent qualities of activities and periodically use a formal system in order to keep his or her activity selection skills finely tuned.

Modification of Activities

Occasionally, it will be necessary to modify activities in order to meet the needs of those being served. Changes in structure and activity rules may be more apparent with persons with disabilities than with their nondisabled peers. Certainly the literature in the recreation field includes numerous references to "adapted" activities. A point that Labanowich (1978) makes in his article about wheelchair sports is that we need to be careful not to slant recreational activities to give them (activities) an air of "temporariness," particularly for children and youth. According to Labanowich, such activities may "fail to convey a sense of realism for the participant projected against their utility as later life pastimes" (p. 12). While this is a valid statement, it could be argued that play experiences may serve many purposes relative to skill development, socialization, and overall adjustment, yet have little carryover value. Perhaps the main idea here is that activities performed by persons who are disabled are meaningful and/or beneficial to these persons either from a developmental point of view or from a carryover perspective.

Keeping the thought that activities should be beneficial or meaningful to the individual, the leader should ask the question: "Will modifying or adapting the activity be unfair and/or detract from the meaningfulness of the activity for the individual?" The following are some guidelines that should be considered when selecting and modifying activities for persons who have disabilities.

1. Change as little as necessary. For example, try to keep the structure and the rules of a game as close as possible to the existing

game. It is better to undermodify so as to challenge the individual and to provide normalized experiences.

2. Where possible, involve the person in the selection and activity modification process. Many times the user is a good source of information. The rules for wheelchair basketball are based on this phenomenon. All of the modifications have historically needed the approval of the participants.

3. There may be elements of competition to consider when working with groups of children and adults. For instance, in the Special Olympics, past performance, age, and sex of the participant are usually taken into consideration when pitting one person against another.

4. Try to offer activities that are characteristic of those individuals who are in the mainstream of society. That is, offer to persons with disabilities the same leisure opportunities that exist in society. The normalization principle should be emphasized and the idea of inventing activities should be de-emphasized.

5. Where possible, activities should have common denominators, especially if they are modified. For example, in wheelchair basketball everyone plays in a wheelchair and follows the same rules. The wheelchair and the fact that everyone follows the same rules are the common denominators for equality in participation.

6. In many instances the person with a disability is cast in the role of spectator. The authors of this text strongly feel that individuals should be provided opportunities to participate in, and in some cases be "nudged" into, participant-based activities.

7. Although the authors do *not* devalue cooperative and other noncompetitive leisure experiences, the person who is disabled should have ample opportunities to participate in equitable competitive situations.

8. Start at the level where the participants are currently functioning. This does *not* mean starting at the lowest level.

9. Individuals should be given opportunities for free choice. This may enhance the feeling of control and reduce feelings of "learned helplessness."

Peterson (1976) presented what she termed a "Selection of Activity and Modification Model" (SAMM). The important feature stressed in the SAMM is answering questions and making the appropriate decision. If the answer is "no" for the question "Do clients have the physical skills necessary for participation?" then another question is posed: "Can the

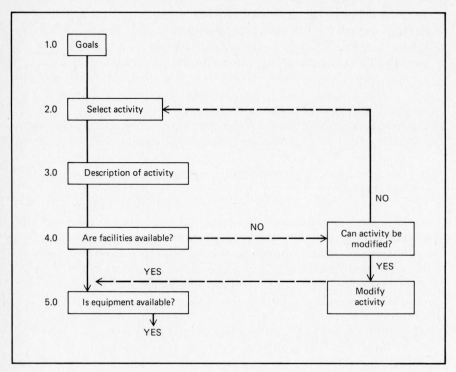

Figure 6–1. Modified version of the Selection of Activities and Modification Model (Peterson, 1976).

activity be modified for the existing skill level?" If "yes," then follow the guidelines for selecting and modifying activities. Figure 6–1 is a modified version of the Selection of Activity and Modification Model (Peterson and Gunn, 1984).

──────────────── **SUMMARY** ────────────────

This chapter has dealt with the program planning process. Discussion focused on needs assessment, the formulation of goals and the writing of behavioral objectives, and the selection and modification of activities. It was stressed that needs assessment is the first step in the program planning process. The main point is to establish that there are persons who are disabled who live in your community and who lack leisure opportunities.

Once needs assessment is completed, the establishment of group goals and the writing of behavioral objectives should take place. The recreation practitioner is encouraged to write group goals and objectives to convey intent to others, to provide a guideline for selecting activities, and as a guide for evaluating the program.

The final section of the chapter covers the selection and modification of activities. This section highlighted activity analysis and presented guidelines for selecting and modifying activities for persons who have disabilities.

Suggested Learning Activities

1. Develop a one-page survey that could be used as an instrument to identify individuals in the community who are disabled.

2. Within the context of a recreation program for children who are disabled, list three goals. For each goal write one behavioral objective and include conditions and criteria for acceptable performance.

3. Observe a group of special population members engaged in a leisure activity. Then, design a plan for implementing individual objectives within the group process.

4. Write two behavioral objectives and include conditions and criteria for mentally retarded teenagers who are learning how to swim.

5. Specify one objective in each of the three domains (cognitive, affective, and psychomotor) for disabled persons who want to improve their basketball skills.

6. Using the activity analysis form in this chapter, analyze one of the activities listed below or some other leisure activity with which you are familiar.
   a. checkers
   b. bowling

7. Take an activity and adapt it to a particular special population group. For example,

   ■ What kind of adaptations might you make in volleyball for a group of elderly persons who have difficulty in mobility?

   or

   ■ What kind of changes might you make in a painting activity for quadriplegic individuals?

References

Avedon, E. M. *Therapeutic Recreation Service: An Applied Behavioral Science Approach.* Englewood Cliffs, NJ: Prentice-Hall, Inc., 1974.

Bloom, B. S., ed. *Taxonomy of Educational Objectives Handbook I: Cognitive Domain.* New York: David McKay Co., Inc., 1956.

Compton, D., and P. A. Witt. *The Leisure Diagnostic Battery: Background, Conceptualization and Structure.* Denton, TX; North Texas State University, June 1981.

Farrell, P., and H. M. Lundegren. *The Process of Recreation Programming Theory and Techniques.* New York: John Wiley & Sons, 1978.

Frye, V., and M. Peters. *Therapeutic Recreation: Its Theory, Philosophy, and Practice.* Harrisburg, PA: The Stackpole Co., 1972.

Gronlund, N. E. *Stating Behavioral Objectives for Classroom Instruction.* London: The Macmillan Co., 1970.

Gunn, S. L., and C. A. Peterson. *Therapeutic Recreation Program Design Principles and Procedures.* Englewood Cliffs, NJ: Prentice-Hall, Inc., 1978.

Harrow, A. J. *A Taxonomy of the Psychomotor Domain.* New York: David McKay Co., Inc., 1972.

Hubert, E. "Leisure Interest Inventory." Masters Thesis, University of North Carolina, Chapel Hill, 1969.

Krathwohl, D. R., B. S. Bloom, and B. B. Maria. *Taxonomy of Educational Objectives, Handbook II: Affective Domain.* New York: David McKay, 1964.

Labanowich, S. "The Psychology of Wheelchair Sports," *Therapeutic Recreation Journal* 12(1), 11–77, 1978.

Mager, R. F. *Preparing Instructional Objectives.* Palo Alto, CA: Fearon Publishers, 1962.

Mager, R. F., and P. Pipe, *Analyzing Performance Problems* or '*You Really Oughta Wanna'.* Palo Alto, CA: Fearon Publishers, 1970.

McDowell, F., Jr. "Toward a Healthy Leisure Mode: Leisure Counseling," *Therapeutic Recreation Journal* 8(3), 96–104, 1974.

McKechnie, G. E. "Psychological Foundations of Leisure Counseling: An Empirical Strategy," *Therapeutic Recreation Journal* 8(1), 4–16, 1974.

Menninger, W. C. "Recreation and Mental Health," in *Recreation and Psychiatry.* New York: National Recreation Association, 1960.

Mirenda, J. *Mirenda Leisure Interest Finder.* Milwaukee, WI: Milwaukee Public Schools, Dept. of Municipal Recreation and Adult Education, 1973.

O'Morrow, G. S. *Therapeutic Recreation: A Helping Profession,* 2nd ed. Reston, VA: Reston Publishing Co., Inc., 1980.

Overs, R. P. "A Model for Avocational Counseling," *Journal of Health, Physical Education and Recreation* 41(2), 36–38, 1970.

Peterson, C. A. "State of the Art Activity Analysis," *Leisure Activity Participation and Handicapped Populations: Assessment of Research*

Needs. Arlington, VA: National Recreation and Park Association and Bureau of Education for the Handicapped, U.S. Office of Education, April 1976.

Peterson, C. A. and S. L. Gunn. Therapeutic Recreation Program Design: Principles and Procedures, 2nd ed. Englewood Cliffs, NJ: Prentice–Hall, Inc., 1984.

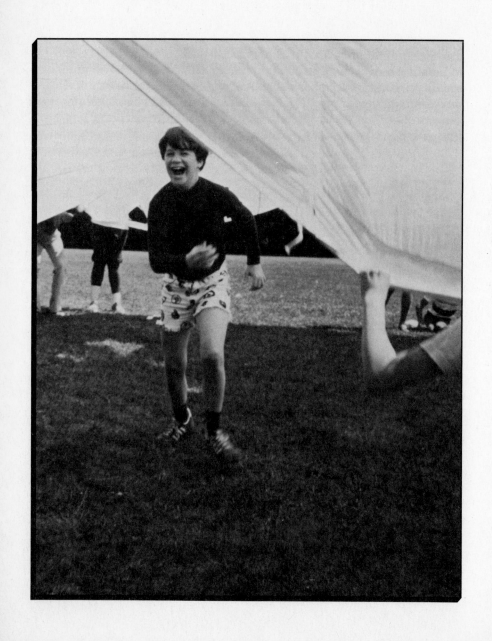

7

Special Recreation Programs— Exemplaries and Standards

This chapter presents seven programs as examples of special recreation programs offering leisure services to individuals who are disabled. The programs, selected because of their positive features, represent a variety of services and structures. They were chosen from seven different states across the country, primarily larger cities. It is hoped that by learning what kinds of programs and services exist in different areas of the United States readers will be better prepared to organize their own programs.

In addition to modeling new programs after examplary programs, such as those discussed in this chapter, professional standards may be useful in the establishment of special recreation services. The final segment of the chapter deals with guidelines for the development of special recreation services.

ADAPTIVE PROGRAMS, AUSTIN PARKS AND RECREATION DEPARTMENT*

The "Special Populations Program" was established in June, 1974, as a city-funded operation within the Community Recreation Division of the

---

*Information in this section was taken from materials furnished by the Austin Parks and Recreation Department.

149

City of Austin Parks and Recreation Department. The program name changed to Adaptive Programs in January, 1978. From the onset, the focus of the Adaptive Programs has been toward an integrated program with mainstreaming of disabled individuals into existing programs. Adaptive Programs stresses choice, involvement, and self-direction while offering recreational experiences, new challenges, and friendships. Those served by Adaptive Programs include persons three years old and older with the following disabling conditions: physical disabilities including visual and hearing impairment, mental retardation, emotional disturbance, learning disabilities, and those eliciting delinquent behaviors.

The recreation staff attempts to parallel recreation programs so that when skills are learned in the Adaptive Programs, they will carry over into existing general recreation programs. Adaptive Programs are divided into three phases: integrated, transitional, and adaptive (segregated). The integrated phase provides assistance in getting the disabled person into regular existing programs and classes. The transitional phase is a "one-shot" experience to introduce the individual to recreational programs and to orient the person to the philosophy of recreation while encouraging participation in regular recreation activities. The third phase is for the person who has little recreational experience and needs encouragement or skill development to participate and interact with nondisabled individuals. Within the Austin Parks and Recreation Department, transitional activities have typically included theater productions, hayrides, canoeing and backpacking trips, ice cream socials, and bowling. Special adaptive classes offered have included sewing for individuals with visual impairments, developmental gymnastics, T-ball, cooking, dance, soccer, camping, aquatics, and adaptive pre-school.

The Adaptive Programs Section has entered into several cooperative agreements with other agencies in an effort to (1) reduce duplication, (2) enhance the quality of programs, (3) provide additional facilities, and (4) provide more services to more persons with disabilities in the Austin area. For example, cooperative arrangements have been made with Criss Cole Rehabilitation Center for the Blind, the Austin Independent School District, and the Austin–Travis County Mental Health–Mental Retardation Center. The Criss Cole Center shares facilities and programs while the Austin–Travis County MH–MR Center and the Austin Parks and Recreation Department cooperatively operate a day camp for emotionally disturbed youngsters.

Since 1977, the Adaptive Programs section has had three full-time staff members, allowing expanded programming. A neighborhood community program was started in 1979 to complement existing city-wide programs. Volunteers have been utilized extensively in an effort to maintain a lower participant/leader ratio and to offer more variety in programming and quality of supervision. The following are some activity highlights that reflect the Adaptive Programs offerings.

ADAPTIVE PROGRAMS SUMMER HIGHLIGHTS

■ *At Your Leisure*—A learning-through-leisure program that emphasizes socialization and development of recreational activity skills and attitudes, and promotes independent, self-directed use of leisure. Meets Mondays, 6:30–9 P.M. at Mayfield Park. *Fee:* Annual registration fee.

■ *Cooking Basics*—A basic introduction that will focus on menu planning, food preparation, and table etiquette. Two 6-week classes for teens and adults will be held at the following locations:

1. Jordan Recreation Center: Wed 7–8:30 P.M.
2. Bedichek Community School: Thur 6:30–8 P.M.

Fee: The participants will prepare a meal for a guest of their choice on the last class night.

■ *Creative Movement*—This program emphasizes body awareness, gross motor skills, fitness, and self-expression, and will introduce some basic dance movements designed for youth 6–12 years of age. Two 3-week sessions will meet on Tuesdays and Thursdays from 3–4 P.M. at Cook Community School.

■ Session I: June 9–June 25
■ Session II: June 30–July 16

■ *Kaleidoscope*—This program will be held Monday through Friday at Mayfield Park for youth 6–12 years old. Activities for each 2-week session will include: crafts, nature study, creative dramatics, group sports and games, "special" days and water play at Bailey Park, and one overnight in the building at Mayfield Park. Session times and dates are listed below.

■ Session I: June 8–June 19   8:30 A.M.–12 noon
■ Session II: June 22–July 2   8:30 A.M.–12 noon
■ Session III: July 13–July 24   8:30 A.M.–12 noon
■ Session IV: July 27–August 7   8:30 A.M.–12 noon

■ *Kid Kapers*—A wide variety of activities for youth 6–12 years old. Activities will include: crafts, creative dramatics, group sports and games, puppetry, storytelling, and others.

■ *Leisure Lunchbox*—Bring a sack lunch to eat, and afterward enjoy leisure activities for adults led by an Adaptive Programs staff member. Socialization and fun are the main emphasis of this program. Meets for 6 weeks on Tuesdays (June 9–July 14) 11:30 A.M.–1:00 P.M. at Maplewood Community School.

■ *Pottery*—A basic introduction to handbuilding pottery techniques for teens and adults.

■ *Swimming*—Specially trained instruction in a small class setting, working on basic skills for the more involved handicapped individual, or those who need some special skill development before moving into the integrated "Learn-to-Swim" program. There are three 3-week sessions for youth (6–16 years). *Adult Swimming* is still to be arranged in regard to time and location. Sessions will be 3 weeks in length, 2 nights per week.

■ *Teen Trek*—This program will be held Monday through Friday from 10:00 A.M.–2:00 P.M. at Bailey Park for teens 13–19 years old. Activities for each 3-week session will include a wide variety of leisure programs, with the main emphasis on leisure education, career exploration, and socialization. Session dates are listed below.

■ Session I: June 8–June 26
■ Session II: July 6–July 24

■ *Walking for Fitness*—The emphasis of this 6-week program for disabled teens, adults, and family is on fitness, conditioning, and socialization. A warm-up exercise program will be developed for each participant. Meets on Thursdays (June 11–July 16) from 7–8:30 P.M. at Cook Community School.

■ *Weight Conditioning*—Use of a universal gym for teens and adults, specifically designed to meet the needs of the disabled. Meets Tuesdays and Thursdays (Session I: June 9–July 2; Session II: July 7–July 30) from 6–7 P.M. at Northwest Recreation Center. *Fee:* Annual registration fee.

ADAPTIVE PROGRAMS SUMMER SPECIAL EVENTS

■ *Tubing on the San Marcos River*—This family outing will take place on Saturday, June 6. Transportation, inner tubes, and life jackets will be provided. We will meet at the Parks & Recreation Department Office Annex on Dawson Road, south of the City Coliseum barns, at 12:30 p.m., and will return at approximately 5:30 p.m. Bring your bathing suit, towel, sun lotion, any snacks

you may desire, and enough money for an ice cream cone on the way home. *Fee: Register by June 4th!!*
- *Balloon Day and Water Play*—A *lot* of fun with activities using balloons, and refreshing water play in the afternoon. For youth (6–12 years). Meets Tuesday, July 7, from 10:00 A.M.–2:00 P.M. at Bailey Park. Bring a sack lunch and your swimsuit. *Fee:* Free.

DIVISION OF THERAPEUTIC RECREATION, CINCINNATI RECREATION COMMISSION*

In 1968, the Cincinnati Recreation Commission established the Division of Therapeutic Recreation to offer a variety of community recreation programs to children, teens, and adults who were disabled. The overall goal of the Division is to provide recreation services for persons who are ill or disabled living in the Greater Cincinnati Area. The purposes of the program are to aid in individual growth and development, to contribute to the quality of life, and to enhance a leisure lifestyle. The budget is made up of city tax dollars and has grown from less than $3,000 in 1968 to more than $200,000. Over 100 unique and varied recreational programs are offered on a yearly basis. Nominal fees are assessed for the Division's programs, in addition to a yearly membership fee. The Division of Therapeutic Recreation works with ages six and up and employs a supervisor and four full-time program coordinators who initiate and organize the programs, as well as train and supervise staff and volunteers.

Program formats vary according to the seasons, disabilities, and participants' ages and functional levels. The unique and varied program formats currently being implemented by the Division include:

1. *Activity Programs:* May incorporate music and dance, movement exploration, arts and crafts, nature lore, creative dramatics, games, physical fitness activities, field trips, and swim instruction.
2. *Sports and Athletics:* Seasonal clinics teach tennis, golf, soccer, floor hockey, basketball, flag football, racquetball, and neighborhood games. Fall/winter bowling leagues and spring/summer softball teams are also offered annually.

---

*Information in this section was taken from materials furnished by the Cincinnati Recreation Commission, Division of Therapeutic Recreation.

3. *Adapted Aquatics:* Programs consist of swim instruction, water games, swim and diving meets, and aquatic shows. A week-night "post therapy swim" is offered for teens and adults with physical disabilities. In the summer, swim instruction is an integral part of the eight-week day camp program.
4. *Outdoor Adventures:* Consists of high-skill-level nature activities that may include canoeing, camping, backpacking, rappelling, horseback riding, cross-country skiing, and orienteering.
5. *Socials and Special Events:* Include dances, clubs, banquets, parties, holiday events, and experiences in the community such as movie-going or restaurant dining.
6. *Specialized Skill Programs:* A sample of these leisure life skills offered on a seasonal basis may include ceramics, dance instruction, carpentry, and trimnastics.

Program Skill Level Continuum

Concern for meeting the individual needs of program participants prompted the development of a program skills-level continuum (see Table 7–1). The skill levels are used by the staff in developing goals and objectives, planning programs, and assessing individuals.

The first skill level described by the Therapeutic Recreation Program Skill Level Continuum is Level I. Level I activities are geared to persons with developmental disabilities who need a 1:1 or 1:2 staff-to-participant ratio in order to learn basic sensory motor and self-help skills. Lists of appropriate skills for each level are used by staff for goal setting and assessment. These listings have been termed *skill sheets* by the staff. Level I skill sheets are used as a guide for planning program objectives and activities and for assessing the skills of severely or profoundly disabled children, teens, or adults and young physically disabled children. An individual who is severely mentally retarded may need to work on Level I skills his or her entire lifetime, whereas a young child who is mildly mentally retarded or is physically disabled may use skills learned in Level I as a bridge to grow and to develop skills presented in Levels II through IV. Specific skills included in the Level I skill sheets involve body awareness, sensory stimulation and discrimination, and basic visual perception activities. Sequential self-help skills are also presented on the Level I skill sheets in the areas of eating, toileting, personal hygiene, and dressing.

Level II activities are geared to persons who possess sensory motor skills and who are able to begin functioning in a group situation. Individuals at skill Level II are ready to learn basic fine and gross motor skills that are prerequisite to learning high-level recreation activities. An adult who is severely mentally retarded may work on refining the

Table 7–1
Cincinnati Recreation Commission
Division of Therapeutic Recreation
Program Skill Level Continuum

Level 1	Level II	Level III	Level IV
Programs for persons exhibiting basic needs who need a 1:1 or 1:2 staff ratio, working on the development of basic socialization, sensory-motor, self-help, and motor coordination skills.	Programs for persons possessing sensory motor skills, able to function in group situations and begin refining basic fine and gross motor and self-help skills for high-level recreation activities.	Programs for persons possessing skills necessary to learn high-level recreation activities.	Integration
Evaluation Requirements:	Evaluation Requirements:	Evaluation Requirements:	
■ Sensory motor skill assessment	■ Sequential motor development skill assessment	■ Sports/leisure activity skill assessments	
■ Sequential motor development skill assessment	■ Self-help skill assessment	■ Outdoor Adventure skill assessment	
■ Self-help skill assessment	■ Socialization skill assessment	■ Self-help skill assessment	
■ Socialization skill assessment	■ Attitudes, values, and emotional development skill assessment	■ Socialization skill assessment	
■ Attitudes, values, and emotional development skill assessment	■ Mobility assessment (for physically disabled individuals only)	■ Attitudes, values, and emotional development skill assessment	
■ Mobility assessment (for physically disabled individuals only)	■ Cognitive development skill assessment (for individuals with learning disabilities only)	■ Mobility assessment (for physically disabled individuals only)	
■ Body awareness and sensory-motor (for physically disabled)	■ Self-help (for physically disabled)	■ Cognitive development skill assessment (for individuals with learning disabilities only)	
■ Self-help (for physically disabled)	■ Sequential Motor Resource Sheet	■ Self-help (for physically disabled)	
■ Sequential Motor Resource Sheet			

skills presented in Level II indefinitely, whereas a young mildly retarded teen may use fine and gross motor skills learned in Level II to play a team sport that is classified by the continuum as a Level III activity. Specific skills included on the Level II skill sheets involve individual socialization skill assessment as well as fine and gross motor and basic activity skills.

Level III programs are geared to children, teens, and adults who possess skills necessary to learn high-level recreation activities. Activities included on the Level III skill sheets involve team sports, specific leisure skills, and outdoor adventure skills. A teenager who is mentally retarded may participate in a softball league sponsored by the Division of Therapeutic Recreation to refine his skills and learn the rules necessary to eventually compete on a public team in his community. For some individuals involved in Level III programs, being integrated into a community softball league (Level IV on the continuum) is a challenge and a true possibility. For other individuals, integration would not be the most appropriate, least restrictive environment. Their individual needs would best be met by continuing in Level III activities sponsored by the Division.

Integration is the fourth and final skill level on the Division of Therapeutic Recreation's program level continuum. Integration is attained by individuals with disabilities when they leave a program sponsored by the Division of Therapeutic Recreation to become a participant in a community recreation program. Such a program has specially trained staff or volunteers who program for, or work with, special populations. During the various stages of integration, the involvement of the Division staff becomes that of facilitator, trainer, consultant, and advocate. It is the philosophy of the Division that once an individual is successfully integrated into a community center program he or she is no longer at a disadvantage (handicapped) in relation to the specific skill he or she is performing.

The continuum is unique because many individuals who are learning skills presented in Levels II and III of the continuum may, at the same time, be working on basic self-help skills presented in Level I. For example, an individual who is in an Outdoor Adventure (Skill Level III) program, may also be working on his or her personal hygiene and toileting skills, which are classified as Level I. General recreation programs group individuals into the most appropriate skill levels in order to meet individual needs. A day camp program, therefore, may divide into specific skill level groups to work on the competencies listed on the assessment sheets. However, the entire group will get together to eat lunch and participate in scheduled group socialization activities.

As different programs use the continuum as a guideline for planning program objectives and activities, the flexibility of the continuum becomes apparent. In some general activity programs, for example, children benefit from skills listed in more than one level. For those in the process of moving from Level I to Level II, the most appropriate activities for them might be a mixture of skills listed in both levels. An individual could be learning the gross motor skills presented in Level II and at the same time benefit from the tactile stimulation activities presented in Level I. A teen with a severe physical disability who due to his or her physical involvement is in Skill Level I may become involved in a Level III program because it best fulfills his or her cognitive, social, and emotional needs. For example, a teenager with a degenerative disease and severe physical involvement, may no longer benefit from Skill Level I and II activities. Therefore, he or she may become part of the Level III Outdoor Adventure Program for physically disabled teens because it gives the opportunity to learn more about the community and to socialize with peers.

Final Comment

The philosophy of the Cincinnati program involves elements of the continuum method, employs principles of normalization, and cooperates with parents and agencies serving special populations. The program has been nicely summed up in the following quotation from Barbara ("Sam") Browne (1984). Browne is Supervisor of the Division of Therapeutic Recreation.

> In the final analysis, life is a continuum of experiences. Quality programming for special populations is the life of the Division of Therapeutic Recreation. Through constant evaluation by staff, participants and the general public, the Division is constantly striving to improve the quality of its programs. The staff has learned and experienced a great deal in the years that the Division has been in existence. The Division has grown from its experiences and has dedicated itself to making Cincinnatians realize that, even though individuals may be handicapped in certain situations, *recreation* does not have to be one of them.

CITY OF MIAMI DEPARTMENT OF RECREATION, PROGRAMS FOR THE HANDICAPPED*

With the thought that it is the responsibility of municipal government to provide services to citizens who are disabled, the City of Miami has

---

*Information in this section was taken from materials furnished by the City of Miami, Department of Recreation, Programs for the Handicapped.

developed a comprehensive system to serve persons with disabilities. The Handicapped Division of the Department of Recreation was formed in 1973. The following goals exemplify the interests of this Division.

1. Monitor and assure the City's compliance with the Rehabilitative Act of 1973, as amended, and other state, federal, and local legislation that impacts the City's services.
2. Give impetus to the City of Miami Advisory Committee for the Handicapped as per Resolution #78–127.
3. Coordinate City Services that relate to the community's disabled.
4. Monitor compliance with City building and housing codes and the sensitivity of these to the needs of the disabled.
5. Serve as a communication link between the City of Miami government and disabled citizens.
6. Establish a link with the government in Central and South America to create and exchange information and training in the area of community services to the handicapped.
7. Secure State, Federal, Foundation, and private funding for the provision of existing and additional services.

The following are seven types of services provided by the Handicapped Division:

1. *Training for Independent Living*—Classroom and on the job training for mentally retarded adults aimed at providing permanent vocational placement for participants, eliminating these individuals from state aid or other programs.
2. *Barrier-Free Design*—Develop plans for the removal of architectural barriers from the community's park facilities. Acquire funds to complete this work.
3. *Leisure Services*—Provision of leisure time services to disabled citizens who are not able to become involved in programs with the general population.
4. *Non–Work Oriented Activity Center*—Activities in self-help skills, pre-vocational aptitude, and academics to improve the independence of previously institutionalized citizens.
5. *Community Relations*—Information source for community members in areas related to various special populations.
6. *Education*—Classes in cooperation with Miami-Dade Community College, the Association for Retarded Citizens, and area Community Schools in money and banking, community adjustment, cooking, travel training, basic speech and language, and other lifetime skills courses for previously institutionalized citizens.

7. *Staff Training for Adapted Recreation (STAR)*—The in-service training of general recreation staff to recognize the attitudinal and architectural barriers that prohibit the delivery of equal services to the disabled in a recreational setting.

Funded Projects

The City of Miami has been a national leader in obtaining funding from outside sources to support special recreation services. Monies were obtained, for example, from the U.S. Department of Education Office of Special Education and Rehabilitation Services for Project STAR (Staff Training for Adapted Recreation). The purpose of Project STAR was to develop an in-service training model to be utilized by public park and recreation departments to prepare their staff to include citizens with disabilities as participants in their programs. City of Miami recreation staff members, of course, were able to benefit from training provided through Project STAR.

Another example of a project funded by an outside source was Project CARE (Continuum of Adapted Recreation Education). Project CARE was designed to address leisure education needs of citizens with disabilities who live in the Greater Miami area. This project, too, was funded by a grant from the U.S. Department of Education Office of Special Education and Rehabilitation Services.

Project CARE was based on a full spectrum participation philosophy. According to this philosophical position, no member of society, including the estimated 60,000 citizens with disabilities residing in Miami, should be denied the right to participate in and benefit from a full range of leisure education experiences.

In order to fulfill this philosophy, the City of Miami developed a continuum flow pattern for appropriate placement in leisure and education programs. The level of advancement begins with the Leisure on Wheels program in the homes of individuals who are homebound. Leisure on Wheels focuses on participants who are not in an organized program due to behavioral problems or functional level. This homebound program serves the individual for two hours per day, two days per week. A parent or guardian of the homebound individual is encouraged to become involved with the program on a regular basis.

The next phase of the flow pattern is termed the Transitional Training Program. This segment is designed to transfer the homebound participant into a more involved community skills program designed to expand the participant's successful inclusion into the general community. The final phase in the flow pattern, prior to total integration into the mainstream of the community, is the general recreation program offered by Programs for the Handicapped. Components of this program include, but are not limited to, activities such as creative arts, sports and fitness, outdoor education, aquatics, and special events.

Final Comment

As can be readily surmised, the City of Miami program for individuals who are disabled has many thrusts. The primary focus, however, remains that of providing disabled citizens in the Miami area with equal access to recreation services. As Kevin Smith, Program Coordinator for the Handicapped, states:

> There is oftentimes a rehabilitation plan developed for [disabled individuals] when they are going through the required therapies which prepare them for the community. A major flaw in this plan is that the community has not been prepared for them. Community-based recreation is one of the best possible modes for eliminating the barriers which exist for both concerns. It offers the disabled an opportunity to participate in a non-threatening activity with a high potential for success while it offers the general community the opportunity to observe and participate with the disabled, eliminating the lack of awareness as to capabilities, stimulating community education toward the disabled, and increasing the entire community integration process. (Smith, 1984)

DISTRICT OF COLUMBIA DEPARTMENT OF RECREATION, SPECIAL PROGRAMS DIVISION, PROGRAM FOR THE MENTALLY RETARDED & PHYSICALLY HANDICAPPED*

The Program for the Mentally Retarded & Physically Handicapped (MRPH) recently changed to Therapeutic Recreation Services, was initiated in 1954 by the D.C. Department of Recreation. A three-week summer day camp was established for thirty elementary age children with orthopedic impairments on a budget of $2,161 donated by United Cerebral Palsy. The development of services evolved in four major phases: the initial years, 1954–1961, which depicted the growing pains of the program; the developmental years, 1962–1965, where potential and actual growth in services occurred; the expansion years, 1966–1969, which saw major financial aid to the Program; and the reorganization years, 1970–1974, that provided cohesive management and administra-

---

*Information in this section was taken from materials furnished by the D.C. Department of Recreation, Special Programs Division.

tion of the program. Today, the program provides comprehensive therapeutic recreation services involving a continuum of care to an enrollment of over 3000 with a year–round staff of 40—both certified therapeutic recreation specialists and assistants—and an additional summer staff of 70—mostly high school and college students. Service components offered by the program include: programming, counseling, job placement, referrals, transportation, outreach, training and technical assistance, media/material services, and consultation. Geographically, the Program operates six centers and four day camps which are school, park, and recreation-based settings located throughout the city in wards I, II, III, IV and VI of the District of Columbia's 630 square miles in area (Mitchell, 1975).

The MRPH Program Managers/Directors meet yearly in April with organizations, agencies, and various other groups to advise, to exchange information with colleagues, to pool community resources, and to initiate plans to encompass Recreation Services to the disabled. The centers also maintain communication in working with parent clubs, allied disciplines, and community advisers; confronts them personally on areas of specific concerns, presents program data results of individuals/groups achievements in conferences, and together discuss and suggest methods needed to achieve program effectiveness.

Various sheltered programs are available for the severely/profoundly involved. The program provides a wide range of activities/programs which are centered around the following areas of development: basic independent functioning, perceptual motor skills, socialization and communication (which are exclusively in therapeutic recreation settings with programmed interaction with other levels of services), and participation in prescribed, closely supervised activities.

Transitional programs are designed specifically to assist the clients who are ready to move towards more independent recreation and leisure pursuits. The Community Awareness Program (CAP) and Mainstream Project are the major vehicle for client transition. Intermural sport teams, D.C. Special Olympics, high risk activities, wheelchair sports, and Boy/Girl Scout Clubs are also highly utilized.

In concert with the D.C. Public School's special education criteria, namely behavioral levels and functional abilities, the Program for the Mentally Retarded and Physically Handicapped provides the following levels of services to children, youth and adults:

Level I. Assessment of leisure function; recreation/leisure services in community recreation centers; leisure counseling/guidance (facilitation); recreation/leisure in nonpublic sector; limited use of special recreator or therapeutic recreation services when needed, e.g: travel, special events. Fifty percent of their recreation services in regular recreation programs.

Level II. Twenty-five percent of their recreation services in regular recreation programs.

Level III. Participants in closely supervised activities such as special events, sports, etc.

Level IV. Close supervision in settings; attention to fundamental motor/movement skills development.

A significant step toward meeting the recreation and leisure interests of persons with disabilities in the District of Columbia has been the opening of the D.C. Center for Therapeutic Recreation. This municipal recreation center, opened in 1977, was specifically planned, designed, and publicly funded for use by individuals with disabilities with the ultimate goal of fostering the mainstreaming of participants into regular programs.

From the Center's beginning, the major disability groups enrolled in the program have been persons who are mentally retarded or orthopedically and health-impaired. Over the last few years, the participants at the Center have also included persons with hearing impairments, visual, emotional, and health problems.

Architectural barriers were taken into account in the design of the D.C. Center for Therapeutic Recreation. There are no steps except to mechanical areas. Even in shower areas and outside doors, all sills are flush. Parking spaces for persons with physical disabilities are close to building entrances. All outdoor sport areas were designed for wheelchair users—including a unique miniature golf course with access slots along the curbs allowing wheelchairs free mobility on and off the course. All sinks and drinking fountains are designed and located for use by persons who are disabled. In areas where counters are required, at least a portion of these have been placed at wheelchair height. This includes kitchen counters, washroom areas, arts and crafts counters, and shop counters. The specifically designed swimming pool includes many features that make it accessible:

■ A ramp was provided for the deck into the pool for easy direct access by wheelchairs.

■ The floor of the pool was designed with a minimum slope from 2'6" to 3' so that the wheelchair users with additional muscular disabilities in hands and arms would not by gravity roll into water over their heads.

■ A deep water alcove was provided for special training. This was protected from shallow areas by under-water railings. It is protected from stubles on the deck by a continuous bench that also serves as a wheelchair transfer point into deeper water.

■ Removable guide rails were provided at one end of the pool to assist in therapy and swimming instruction.

■ The pool deck was sloped back toward the pool (contrary to usual practices) to reduce water collection and slipping on the deck.

Programs Provided by the Special Programs Division

A variety of programs are conducted by the Special Programs Division. Included in the program offerings are programs developed through federally funded projects (PREP and "I CAN") and the Joseph P. Kennedy, Jr. Foundation (Let's Play to Grow).

PREP and "I CAN." A children's project, referred to as the Preschool Recreation Enrichment Program (PREP)* and the "I CAN"† system, has been employed by the staff within the Special Program Division. The purposes of PREP are to foster the development and utilization of the child's fine and gross motor, social, self-help, cognitive, and language skills. Essentially, the program is structured so the child can both learn and practice new skills through everyday life experiences—particularly play activities. The "I CAN" program is an individualized instructional management system with resource materials for teaching physical recreation and associated skills, to preschool children through youth, with special needs. As a system, "I CAN" is built around a set of objectives correlated to diagnostic assessment instruments, prescription instruction through diagnosis, evaluation, and planning individualized instruction. The child is guided through a continuum of skills that are needed for health and fitness.

Let's Play to Grow. In 1979, the D.C. Department of Recreation was one of ten sites in the United States to be selected and funded by the Joseph P. Kennedy, Jr., Foundation to conduct a Model Program of "Let's Play to Grow." This program is designed to bring the positive aspects of play to families with children who are disabled. It is a program of activities

---

*Designed and developed by Karen Littman of the Maryland National Capital Park and Planning Commission through a grant from the Bureau of Education for the Handicapped, Office of Education, U.S. Department of Health, Education, and Welfare.

†The "I CAN" system was developed by Dr. Janet Wessel of Michigan State University through a grant from the Bureau of Education for the Handicapped, Office of Education, U.S. Department of Health, Education, and Welfare.

designed to provide each family with an opportunity for physical participation, interaction, and sharing. "Let's Play to Grow" was developed through the actual life experiences of parents of children with disabilities and the focus is on the child's physical and recreational development. Within the D.C. Recreation Program, families participate once a week in the "Let's Play to Grow" curriculum, which includes basic throwing and catching skills, water activities, camping, dance, and infant stimulation.

Other programs include an aquatics infant stimulation program and a senior citizens aquatics program, both of which were initiated in 1979 at the D.C. Center for Therapeutic Recreation. Youngsters who are mentally retarded participate in the Special Olympics, giving these children and youth an opportunity to compete in track and field events, swimming, bowling, frisbee, and gymnastics. An example of a program schedule of activities follows.

AN EXAMPLE OF A PROGRAM SCHEDULE OF ACTIVITIES PROVIDED BY THE D.C. DEPARTMENT OF RECREATION FOR HANDICAPPED PERSONS

Mamie D. Lee Therapeutic Recreation Center

Monday thru Friday 11:30 A.M.–3:00 P.M.	Inschool Program (SMR)	4 to 13 years
3:30 P.M.–5:30 P.M.	DC Special Olympics (MR)	ALL AGES
Monday & Wednesday 6:00 P.M.–8:00 P.M.	Let's Play to Grow Program (Autistic)	9 to 15 years
Tuesday 6:00 P.M.–8:00 P.M.	Activity/Swim Program (Nat'l Children Center)	9 to 15 years
Thursday 6:00 P.M.–8:00 P.M.	Activity/Swim Program (Learning Disabled)	9 to 15 years

Sharpe Health Therapeutic Recreation Center

Monday, Tuesday & Friday 11:30 A.M.–3:00 P.M.	Inschool Clubs	9 to 20 years
Monday 3:30 P.M–5:30 P.M.	Bowling (Physically Handicapped)	9 to 13 years
Monday, Tuesday 3:30 P.M.–5:30 P.M.	Kennedy Institute	13 years & above
4:30 P.M.–6:30 P.M.	Activity Program (Jones Treatment Center)	13 years & above

Wednesday 4:30 P.M.–6:00 P.M.	Swim Program (Kennedy Institute)	13 to 20 years
6:00 P.M.–8:00 P.M.	After 5 Social Club (PH)	20 years & above
	Activity/Swim Program (St. Elizabeth's)	Senior Citizens
Wednesday & Thursday 11:30 A.M.–3:00 P.M	Inschool Programs	4 to 20 years
4:30 P.M.–6:00 P.M.	Activity/Swim Program (Kennedy Institute)	13 to 20 years
Thursday	Activity/Swim Program (Area B Community Mental Health Center)	10 to 14 years
6:00 P.M.–8:00 P.M.	Explorer's Club (MR)	20 years & above
	Activity/Swim Program (St. Elizabeth's)	Adults/Sr. Citizens
Friday 4:30 P.M.–7:30 P.M.	Open/Family Swim	ALL AGES
AS SCHEDULED	DC Special Olympics	ALL AGES

D.C. Center for Therapeutic Recreation

Monday thru Friday 8:30 A.M.–2:30 P.M.	Preschool	$2\frac{1}{2}$ to 5 years
8:30 A.M.–6:00 P.M.	Day Care	3 to 5 years
9:00 A.M.–10:00 A.M.	Infant Stimulation	6 mos to 2 years
10:00 A.M.–11:00 A.M.	Activity/Swimming (St. Elizabeth's)	ADULTS
2:00 P.M.–4:00 P.M.	Life Skills (St. Elizabeth's)	20 years & above
6:00 P.M.–8:00 P.M.	Community (Gym)	20 years & above
Monday thru Wednesday 9:30 A.M.–11:30 A.M. 1:30 P.M.–3:30 P.M.	Activity/Swimming (St. Elizabeth's)	20 years & above
6:00 P.M.–8:00 P.M. (Feb–Apr)	Workshop/Auto/ Mechanics/Disabled & Able-bodied)	20 years & above
Monday and Thursday 11:00 A.M.–12 noon	Preschool	$2\frac{1}{2}$ to 5 years
9:30 A.M.–12:15 P.M.	Swimming Program (MR)	20 years & above
5:00 P.M.–6:00 P.M.	Basketball Practice (CYO)	9 to 16 years

Tuesday 8:30 A.M.–2:30 P.M.	Infant Stimulation	6 mos to 3 years
Tuesday and Thursday 9:30 A.M.–12:15 P.M.	Adult Activity	20 years & above
11:30 A.M.–12:30	Activity/Swim Community	ADULTS
12:00–1:00 P.M.	Activity/Swim Hope Village	ADULTS
1:00 P.M.–2:00 P.M.	Infant Swim	6 mos to 2 years
1:30 P.M.–3:30 P.M.	Activity/Swim Community	ADULTS
5:00 P.M.–6:00 P.M.	Activity/Swim Area B Community Mental Health	ADULTS
6:00 P.M.–8:00 P.M.	Activity/Swim	ADULTS
	Open Swim	ALL AGES
	Walk-in Swim (handicapped Hospital for Sick Children)	
Tues., Wed., & Thursday 6:00 P.M.–8:30 P.M.	Basketball Practice (wheelchair)	20 years & above
Thursday 9:30 A.M.–3:30 P.M.	Community/Activity	20 years & above
Tuesday & Thursday 3:30 P.M.–4:45 P.M.	Community (non-handicapped)	9 to 16 years
Wednesday 1:30 P.M.–3:30 P.M.	Activity/Swim (St. Elizabeth's)	ADULTS
5:00 P.M.–6:00 P.M.	Activity/Swim (Mamie D. Lee)	ADULTS
6:00 P.M.–8:00 P.M.	Walk-in Swim	ADULTS

During the seventies the Program achievements included the supervision of over 40 Universities' field placement students, the addition of wheelchair-accessible buses to the fleet, recipient of national awards for excellence from the American Association on Mental Deficiency and National Therapeutic Recreation Society; a unique barrier free recreation facility was opened (DC Center for Therapeutic Recreation) attracting national and international acclaim as a Program Model and an Architectural Showcase, participation in nationally organized events, i.e. Special Olympics, Very Special Arts Festivals, Let's Play to Grow, and utilization of such recreation curricula as I CAN, PREP, and Project Explore.

The most important growth aspects in the eighties have included the following: establishment of a Beep Ball League (visually impaired), opening a new center devoted mainly to the performing arts and most importantly named in memory of a young woman with mental retardation, Joy Evans, designing and implementing a Therapeutic Infant Play Program (TIP), and the adoption of the new Classification Standards—the 638 Series, Recreation Therapist.

MAINE-NILES ASSOCIATION OF SPECIAL RECREATION (ILLINOIS)*

A number of Special Recreation Associations have been established in Illinois since the early 1970s. The Maine-Niles Association of Special Recreation (M-NASR) is one of several such associations established because member park districts recognized that the leisure needs of individuals who were disabled were not being met. Committed to the idea that individuals have the *need* and *right* to make productive and enjoyable use of their leisure time within their own communities, in 1972, seven park districts became supportive members of Maine-Niles Association of Special Recreation. M-NASR was formed under special legislation in the State of Illinois that permits two or more park districts or municipalities to join together to form a special recreation association to serve persons with disabilities.

M-NASR is dedicated to providing comprehensive leisure services for children and adults having diverse disabling conditions. Persons with various levels of mental retardation, physical disability, emotional disturbance, hearing impairments, visual impairments, and multiple disabilities are provided opportunities for quality leisure activities specifically oriented toward individual ability levels and limitations.

It must be realized that not every individual who is disabled is in need of specialized recreation services. M-NASR has taken the position of selecting and evaluating the programs of the member Park Districts on their appropriateness for individuals who are disabled. Integrated programs have been designed for those participants able to participate in some of the ongoing Park District programs. In those cases, consultation and professional input from the M-NASR staff is provided. By offering recreation programs within the mainstream of the commu-

---

*Information in this section was taken from materials furnished by the Maine-Niles Association of Special Recreation (M-NASR).

nity, and by providing opportunities for involvement in new situations and environments, individuals with limiting conditions can learn and become comfortable with leisure opportunities that they will later be able to pursue independently.

Lynn Parfitt, Executive Director of M-NASR, has stated that:

> We have found that many of the people served with appropriate training and experiences, will eventually be involved in the mainstream of society. By providing them with opportunities to participate in quality leisure activities and an opportunity to develop a positive self-concept, the local park district will be providing a service that can upgrade the quality of life in the total community. M-NASR functions as a significant contributing factor to after-institutional care services and, more significantly, as a community preventative measure, an alternate to institutionalization. (Parfitt, 1984)

The staff at the Maine-Niles Association has developed these basic program philosophies:

1. *Programs may be leisure-oriented.* This will allow opportunities for relaxing, self-motivated leisure experiences that can eventually be pursued independently.
2. *Programs may be individualized and goal-oriented.* These programs can be structured to meet individual therapeutic or remedial needs.
3. *Programs may be an extension of the educational program in which the participant is involved.* Information can be obtained from classroom teachers and professional school staff members. A leisure program can then be structured to reinforce educational objectives.

Funding for M-NASR is primarily through special legislation that allows park districts to tax up to 2¢ per $100 of assessed valuation to fund programs for handicapped individuals. M-NASR operates on a budget of contributions from local member park districts and other sources. Sources such as foundation and corporate gifts, grants, fees, and charges make up approximately one quarter of the operating budget. M-NASR has received grants from the American Camping Association, the Illinois Department of Mental Health, and the Illinois Arts Council; such grants have kept program fees to a minimum.

Many of the children's programs stress *cooperation, skill development,* and *positive self-image.* Even with the tremendous amount of variety in programming, individual participants get plenty of attention. Parfitt indicates that "although program variety ranges from piano lessons to ice skating classes, an individualized ratio of one staff member to every four participants is usually maintained." A much needed volunteer core of community residents provides over 3000 hours a year of free service, making such a ratio possible. Nevertheless, Parfitt points out, M-NASR policy dictates that a trained recreation specialist be present to supervise every program.

M-NASR programs have been designed to meet the individual needs of every participant with age-appropriate activities. Recreation and leisure services are offered to all ages and disability groups year-round. In addition to over 250 programs and some 75 special events offered annually, M-NASR sponsors leisure education programs, several day camps, and overnight camping trips.

Over 200 children and some 100 adults enroll in camp programs each summer. A leisure education program takes place during the academic school day and includes nature activities, bowling, music, sports, and many other activities. Whenever possible, children are mainstreamed into affiliate park district programs. For example, seven children from one of M-NASR's ice skating classes were placed into the regular Park Ridge Recreation and Park District ice skating program for eight weeks. At the end of the session, three of these children performed in the Annual Ice Show.

The Maine-Niles Association of Special Recreation provides a cardiac exercise program for individuals with heart disease or those who have been identified as "high risk." The 48-week program provides medically supervised exercise three nights per week. This particular program is co-sponsored by the Chicago Heart Association for Northern Cook County with stress test information being provided by the Skokie Valley Hospital. In addition, Special Recreation Associations (SRA) work very closely with the special education districts, fostering a total interdisciplinary approach to integrating children who are disabled into the community as active participants.

The Maine-Niles Association of Special Recreation has received recognition from numerous sources as an outstanding program. The Association received awards from the Illinois Therapeutic Recreation Society (1978) and was named 1981 winner of the National Gold Medal Award for "Outstanding Community Achievement for Disabled Citizens" by the Medalist Industries.

RECREATION CENTER FOR THE HANDICAPPED, INC., SAN FRANCISCO, CALIFORNIA*

The Recreation Center for the Handicapped, established in 1952 by Janet Pomeroy, is recognized nationally as a pioneer program and a

---

*Information in this section was taken from materials furnished by the Recreation Center for the Handicapped, Inc.

model in developing community recreation for persons with disabilities. The Center was founded with private funds in one room of an old pool building owned by the San Francisco Recreation and Park Department, with six physically disabled teenagers enrolled and with only volunteer help. When the Center moved into a newly constructed facility in 1973, enrollment had increased to 650 children, teens, and adults with a wide range of disabilities, served by a paid professional staff of 80, and corps of 120 volunteers. Today, the Center is a major provider of services to disabled persons in the City and County of San Francisco, with an enrollment of more than 1600, and a professional staff over 100 workers strong.

From the beginning, the Center has changed and evolved to keep pace with changing conditions and community needs. The Center is a community-based facility that serves individuals of all ages and disabilities. The purposes of the Center are:

1. To stimulate the development of skills, attitudes, and knowledge necessary for successful participation in community life through recreation, habilitation, education, and socialization experiences.
2. To provide developmental leisure programs designed to assist individuals with disabilities to progress to programs that are in the least restrictive environment.
3. To educate participants and community members, to act as advocates for the rights of disabled individuals, to train new and existing professionals, and to develop innovative programs that meet the ever-changing leisure-related needs of people with disabilities.

In 1970, the Center initiated an Outreach Program to serve the needs of children, teens, and adults who could not participate in programs at the Center. Programs are now being offered to persons in their own homes, in board and care homes for mentally retarded individuals, and in senior citizen complexes and residential care homes for elderly persons.

Many disability groups are represented among those who participate at the Center or through the Outreach Program. The majority of participants are mentally retarded. Some are also partially sighted, deaf, hard of hearing, neurologically disabled, emotionally disturbed or have a combination of these conditions. Other individuals have disabilities as a result of accidents, arthritis, cerebral palsy, or multiple sclerosis. Some participants are in wheelchairs, on crutches, and even bedfast.

The Center itself encompasses 18,000 sq ft and includes day care rooms, an arts and crafts room, drama and music rooms, a multipurpose room with stage, a fireplace, an adjacent kitchen, staff offices, and related facilities. A large swimming pool complex is 12,000 sq ft in the interior with the pool measuring 25′ × 75′. The facility also has a gymnasium and outdoor play apparatus.

Programming is offered through five major program departments: (1) Children, (2) Day Care, (3) Adult, (4) Outreach, and (5) Aquatics and Physical Fitness. A new smaller division has recently been established to serve adults with a dual diagnosis of mental illness and mental retardation. A wide range of indoor and outdoor activities are offered in the Center and throughout the Community.

Activities include, but are *not* limited to:

- Arts and Crafts
- Drama
- Dancing
- Physical Fitness
- Table Games
- Education Classes
- Cooking
- Films
- Outdoor Environmental Education

- Singing
- Music Appreciation
- Sports
- Swimming
- Discussion Groups
- Skills Training
- Sewing
- Cookouts
- Special Events

The San Francisco Recreation and Park Department and the Department of Social Services subsidizes a portion of the Center's budget on a contractual basis. A large proportion of the operating budget is raised by the Board of Directors through personal solicitation of individuals, service clubs, and groups; by letter solicitation of individuals; and by working with groups who conduct benefits for the Center. Fund-raising events such as horse shows, luncheons, and bazaars are conducted annually by these groups. It should be noted that parents of participants as well as some disabled persons themselves assist the Board in all fund-raising events. For example, one major contribution made by parents is a yearly donation of a bus as a result of fund-raising activities.

Final Comment

The Recreation Center for the Handicapped, Inc., has many unique programs that have not been discussed. One such program, Theatre Unlimited—a special ensemble performing group, is discussed in considerable detail in Chapter 9. Also, it is important to point out that the Center has been dynamic and progressive throughout the years. In their 30th Anniversary Report (Forman, 1982), Janet Pomeroy suggested that "the future of recreation for persons with disabilities has never been brighter." She went on to say that:

> The philosophy of the Recreation Center for the Handicapped has evolved over the years from providing recreation and leisure services to the inclusion of education and training components that seek to improve the quality of life for persons with disabilities while enhancing the professional skills of those who work with them. What has remained constant is the goal that these services must be available to all persons, regardless of disability, and that these programs will be provided in the community in which he/she resides in the least restrictive environment. (p. 1)

The Recreation Center for the Handicapped has forged a 20-year plan to address identified and projected needs. For example, a day care for children and a multipurpose center for elderly persons is being planned. The demands upon the Center for its use as a model site for training professionals, students, and volunteers, have grown beyond expectations. In order to meet future demand in this area, the Center is planning to build an education training and conference facility with dormitories. The following quotation from the 30th Anniversary Report (Forman, 1982) about the future seems to be an appropriate way to conclude this section.

> The future of the Recreation Center for the Handicapped will be shaped by the same current that sculpted its present and carved its beginning—the need of disabled persons for recreation and leisure services in a community environment. (p. 24)

PARKS, RECREATION AND LIBRARY DEPARTMENT, PHOENIX, ARIZONA*

Regarding leisure services to individuals who are disabled, the Phoenix Parks, Recreation and Library Department operates under the philosophy of nondiscrimination, mainstreaming, integration, and partial segregation when necessary. *All* local citizens are welcomed into the recreation program. The Phoenix program staff supports the conceptual

---

*Information in this section was taken from materials furnished by the Phoenix Parks, Recreation and Library Department.

goal of integration but has found that many youngsters who have disabilities need partially segregated programs.

In 1973, a Recreation Specialist III position was authorized by the City Council for the Parks, Recreation and Library Department. The position is titled Recreation Coordinator for the Handicapped, rather than Therapeutic Specialist, because the Department sees a basic difference in goals between a community program and that in a clinical setting. Initially, programs were developed with other program staff in the Department who had a budget to deliver these services. In addition, volunteers were used extensively. Programs for persons with disabilities have included special events, summer day camps, Special Olympics, and swimming.

The Phoenix special recreation program is guided by an advisory council. This council comprises community representatives, both agencies and individuals, whose goal is to identify the unmet needs of persons with disabilities by developing a communication network.

In Phoenix, there are self-contained schools, agencies, and institutions that serve individuals with specific disabilities. Children and young adults are either bussed to or housed in these facilities for education and training, yet once their formal day is completed and they either return home or to their assigned quarters, it is extremely difficult to regroup them for recreation programs. The Phoenix staff offers leisure skill education programs during school hours to meet these needs. To accomplish this, the Department employs several part-time specialists who travel to the self-contained settings to teach special programs and skills. These programs include individual music lessons, group singing, creative movement, adaptive aquatics, and arts and crafts.

A number of sports programs for persons who are physically disabled or mentally retarded are conducted throughout Phoenix. For several years, the Department has acted as a promotion and referral agency for three local wheelchair basketball teams. In conjunction with Special Olympics, co-ed leagues have been developed in basketball, volleyball, and softball.

In many instances, community cooperation has been gained in order to develop accessible and usable park and recreation facilities. Both private organizations and public programs have been able partners with the Parks, Recreation and Library Department.

In the late 1970s, a local group interested in expanding recreation opportunities for youngsters with disabilities chose to donate funds to the Department for use at a nearby park, rather than at a self-contained school or hospital. They agreed to fund the construction of a concrete "spray pad." It was pointed out to the group by the Department's staff that this approach would enjoy far greater usage and integration if it was built with the "limited" child in mind, and provide an enjoyable alternative to swimming for any nondisabled child. The structure was designed and built by Department personnel. It consists of a winding cave, complete with stalactites and stalagmites leading up to a water slide, guarded by a sea serpent and crocodile spraying a fine water spray. Water is sprayed, by a pre-set timer, both inside and outside the cave and down the slide. An adjacent "half cave" with bench affords shade for watchful chaperones.

During the 1981 fiscal year, the Parks, Recreation and Library Department was allocated a small portion of the Community Development Block Grant for initial barrier removal in parks. The monies were allocated for installation of ramps for entry to parks, designated parking, drinking fountains, and restroom renovation in community, district, and regional parks. Adult, Senior, and Community Centers in Phoenix were put in compliance with accessibility standards.

In 1982, the Telephone Pioneers of America, a group representing the telephone system's employees, proposed to the Department that a small undeveloped City neighborhood park be used for a "beep" ballfield and other recreation facilities used by persons with disabilities. After many revisions of ideas and goals, the Parks and Recreation Board approved the park be used for the requested purpose. The Pioneers hired a landscape architect to design the entire park. The architect worked closely with Department staff, who reviewed the plan on an on-going basis. The adopted plan for this 7.5-acre park includes a multipurpose area, stage, picnic area, hand court game area, swimming pool, exercise area, and two ballfields. The Department's concerns were primarily related to maintenance, should the park ever revert back to the City in the future. This cooperative effort is one that is unprecedented in Phoenix, and one that will provide significant return in recreation benefits to the citizens of the community.

With increased demands, especially for basic accessibility and opportunities for outdoor activities, block grant funding was used to provide for new facilities. A community park was funded to have a one-mile exercise course constructed with stations for both nondisabled and wheelchair participants. This park, which already has a swimming pool, apparatus area, ballfields, and other recreation facilities, has a pool lift and an accessible bathroom building planned.

As a result of increased awareness, the Department has established a committee for monitoring accessibility for all new facilities and parks under its jurisdiction. In addition, as parks are being designed and redesigned, parking lots surfaced, and picnic facilities replaced, accessibility is being considered along with safety, durability, legality, and enjoyability.

SUMMARY OF SEVEN PROGRAMS

By briefly reviewing seven different special recreation programs, including two that have "centers" (Washington, D.C., and San Francisco), it should be apparent that similarities and differences exist in all programs. For example, philosopically all programs tend to aim toward integrating individuals with disabilities into the mainstream. Yet, some programs offer fewer segregated activities than others. The Cincinnati Recreation Program purports to offer a fairly structured program skill level continuum. The Austin and Miami Programs tend also to provide noteworthy continuums, ranging from adaptive recreation services to integrated programming. Others offer a range of programs even though they may not be organized along a formal continuum. Although programs tend to focus on individual growth and development, it should be noted that family programs are included in programming efforts such as the "Let's Play to Grow" program in Washington, D.C.

The emphasis on "therapeutic" effects also tends to vary from program to program. While some programs focus almost exclusively on the recreative experience, such as the one in Phoenix, others give more emphasis to "therapeutic" benefits.

In terms of activities, a full range is being offered. Programs range from infant stimulation and preschool recreation (PREP) to senior citizen aquatics. Reflective of the varied nature of recreation programming designed to meet the needs, interests, and abilities of the specific population, programs address self-help skills, athletics and fitness, health education, home economics, arts, music, and drama among other areas.

Inter-agency cooperation was specifically illustrated in most program descriptions. Such cooperation is important to the success of special recreation services in the community.

For individuals who desire further information, the agency addresses for the programs referenced in this chapter are as follows:

■ Adaptive Programs
Austin Parks and Recreation Department
Municipal Building, Eighth at Colorado
P.O. Box 1088
Austin, TX 78767

■ Division of Therapeutic Recreation
Cincinnati Recreation Commission
222 East Central Parkway
Cincinnati, OH 45202

■ Programs for the Handicapped
Department of Leisure Services
City of Miami
P.O. Box 330708
Miami, FL 33133

■ Therapeutic Recreation Services
D.C. Department of Recreation
3149 Sixteenth Street, N.W.
Washington, D.C. 20010

■ Maine-Niles Association of Special Recreation (M-NASR)
7640 Main Street
Niles, IL 60648

■ Recreation Center for the Handicapped, Inc.
207 Skyline Boulevard
San Francisco, CA 94132

■ Community Recreation Programs for the Handicapped
Parks, Recreation and Library Department
City of Phoenix
125 East Washington Street
Phoenix, AZ 85004

STANDARDS AND SPECIAL RECREATION SERVICES

Standards are prescribed criteria of acceptable, desirable qualities or performances. Van der Smissen (1972) has made the following statement regarding standards:

> A standard is a statement of desirable practice, a level of performance for a given situation. Standards are indirect measurements of effectiveness using the cause and effect approach so that if stated desirable practices are followed, the program should be effective. (p. 4)

Standards, or guidelines,* then provide a professional field, such as parks and recreation, with principles on which to base practice. If guidelines are followed, an acceptable level of service should result.

---

*The terms standards and guidelines are used interchangeably within this chapter.

Van Andel (1981) has suggested that there are several ways standards can be utilized by park and recreation professionals. Among these he states two that specifically pertain to special recreation services:

1. Standards can be used to identify and define the basic elements needed to provide *quality* programs and services.
2. Standards can be used as an evaluative tool to effectuate change and/or improvement in the service being delivered.

Guidelines for Special Recreation Programs

Following Van Andel's ideas, it seems clear that public park and recreation authorities could benefit from standards for special recreation services. These guidelines would stipulate basic necessary elements and provide a means to evaluate the delivery of services. Such was the sentiment of members of the Board of Directors of the National Therapeutic Recreation Society (NTRS) who, in 1976, endorsed a project to develop guidelines for community-based recreation programs for special populations.

The guidelines that were to ultimately be approved and published by NTRS were largely based on the research of Winslow (1977). As a part of his master's studies, Winslow sent a questionnaire to 264 community park and recreation agencies in the United States that had existing programs for special populations. A total of 113 (42%) agencies responded to the survey. Based upon this data and other information, such as other studies and expert opinion, a set of guidelines were approved by the NTRS Board of Directors for approval in 1978. Vaughan and Winslow distributed the final report entitled, *Guidelines for Community-Based Recreation Programs for Special Populations*, in 1979.

Winslow's survey helped identify five main problem areas most frequently encountered in the provision of community recreation and park services to special populations. These are

1. Transportation
2. Budget allocation
3. Identification of special populations
4. Lack of trained program personnel
5. Architectural barriers

Within their report, Vaughan and Winslow briefly discuss each of the five problem areas and offer suggestions to alleviate each problem. In addition, specific guidelines for community-based special recreation programs are outlined by population size.

Specifically, the *Guidelines for Community-Based Recreation Programs for Special Populations* have four major headings. These are human resources, program, finances/funding, and transportation. The *human resources* portion calls for certain staffing patterns and personnel qualifications, depending on the population size of the city or jurisdiction. For example, where the population is over one million, the guidelines require that an administrative division be established for special recreation services and that its chief administrator be given the title of Director of Special Populations. Qualifications are stipulated for the director, supervisor, and program personnel. As the population size declines, the guidelines for staff and staff qualifications are reduced. For instance, a jurisdiction with a population of 25,000 to 49,999 is required to have only one employee who devotes 50 percent of his or her time to special recreation programs.

Under the *program* section, guidelines cover philosophy, program needs, employee awareness, the establishment of an advisory committee, steps in program implementation, and three types of programs (regular, transitional, segregated) to be provided. The *finances/funding* segment provides guidelines for various population sizes ranging from those over 500,000 to those under 25,000. Among items of concern are budgeting, fees and charges, and cooperative agreements with other agencies. Guidelines for the final major area, *transportation*, also are provided according to population size. The reader is referred to Appendix A for details on the entire set of *Guidelines for Community-Based Recreation Programs for Special Populations* published by NTRS (National Therapeutic Recreation Society).

Camping Standards

Standards set forth by the American Camping Association (ACA) provide criteria for ACA accreditation of camps. The ACA *Camping Standards with Interpretations for the Accreditation of Organized Camps* (1984) integrates standards dealing with campers with physical disabilities or mental retardation into the body of the standards, rather than having a separate section as had been the case in the 1980 version of the *Camping Standards*. It is important to acknowledge that standards for campers with special needs apply to *all camps* that may have *any* campers with disabilities and are not for application solely in "specialized" camps that serve only campers who are disabled.

What are some examples of ACA standards that relate to serving campers with disabilities? One is that any camp serving any campers who are physically disabled or mentally retarded must maintain prescribed staff-camper ratios (Standard C–5). Another standard, C–3, establishes qualifications for administrators. Administrative personnel must hold the minimum of a bachelor's degree in an area related to special populations or have at least 24 weeks of experience in working with the special populations being served by the camp. Still another example deals with camp facilities. Standard A–10 calls for program, sleeping, dining, and toileting facilities to be accessible to campers with restricted mobility.

Accessibility Standards

Before concluding this segment on standards, brief mention should be made of the American National Standards Institute (ANSI) standards for making buildings accessible to persons with physical disabilities. The ANSI standards are the primary source used when dealing with issues of accessibility. There are several references in this textbook to the ANSI standards. While these standards are of obvious importance to special recreation services, they are covered in Chapter 5 and, therefore, are not given extensive coverage in the present chapter.

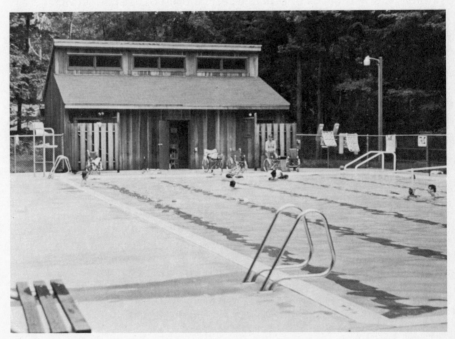

Figure 7–1. ACA standards for persons with special needs cover swimming pools.

—————————— SUMMARY ——————————

This chapter has presented information on exemplary special recreation programs in cities located throughout the United States. These exemplaries have been provided to help readers better understand actual programs in the hope that they will ultimately be better prepared to develop special recreation programs. The final segment of the chapter dealt with guidelines and standards for the provision of special recreation services. Included in this section were standards related to community-based programs, camping, and accessibility.

Suggested Learning Activities

1. Obtain information about community-based recreation programs for individuals with disabilities in your own community and present your findings orally or in written form.

2. Given specific demographic factors in your community, indicate how you would implement a special recreation program for persons with disabilities.

3. Tell how standards of practice can be used by leisure service professionals.

4. Discuss the Guidelines for Community-Based Recreation Programs for Special Populations.

5. Apply the Guidelines for Community-Based Recreation Programs for Special Populations to your own community (see Appendix A).

References

American Camping Association. *Camping Standards with Interpretations for the Accreditation of Organized Camps.* Martinsville, IN, 1984.

Browne, B. (Personal Communication). 1984.

Forman, T. P. *Outward Bound: A Statement for the '80's—30th Anniversary Report.* San Francisco: Recreation Center for the Handicapped, Inc., 1982.

Goldstein, J., and G. E. Van Andel. *Guidelines for Administration of Therapeutic Recreation Service in Clinical and Residential Facilities.* Arlington, VA: National Therapeutic Recreation Society, 1981.

Mitchell, Helen Jo. "The History of Recreation Services for the Mentally Retarded and Physically Handicapped in the District of Columbia Department of Recreation: 1954–1974," Unpublished Master's thesis, University of Maryland, 1975.

Parfitt, L. (Personal Communication). 1984.

Recommended Standards for Therapeutic Recreation Services in Clinical and Residential Facilities (unpublished paper, 1978).

Smith, K. (Personal Communication). 1984.

Van Andel, G. E. "Professional Standards: Improving the Quality of Services," *Therapeutic Recreation Journal* 15(2), 23–30, 1981.

Van der Smissen, B. *Evaluation and Self-Study of Public Recreation and Park Agencies*, rev. ed. Arlington, VA: National Recreation and Park Association, 1972.

Vaughan, J. L., and R. Winslow, eds. *Guidelines for Community-Based Recreation Programs for Special Populations.* Arlington, VA: National Therapeutic Recreation Society, 1979.

Winslow, R. "A Survey of Community Recreation Programs for Special Populations," Unpublished Master's Thesis, California State University, Northridge, 1977.

SPECIAL RECREATION PROGRAM AREAS

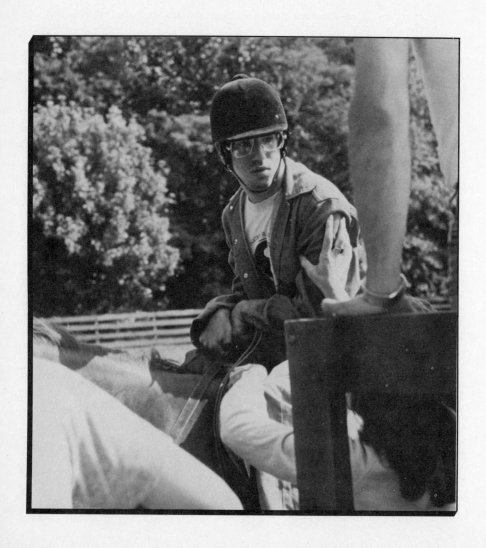

The following section highlights activities and successful programs that enable people with disabilities to pursue their recreational interests. Chapter 8, *Special Camping and Wilderness Experiences,* describes actual and potential contributions that organized camping and wilderness experiences offer to people who have disabilities. The importance of qualified and enthusiastic leadership is stressed, and a detailed presentation on wilderness-adventure programs is included. Chapter 9, *The Arts—For Everyone,* outlines the benefits of arts participation with everyone. Also, a special section features information on the National Committee, Arts with the Handicapped. The chapter concludes with two examples that emphasize the deep, personal meaning that comes from participation in the arts. Selected sports programs for people with disabilities are covered in Chapter 10, *Competitive Sports for Individuals with Disabilities.* The pros and cons of competitive sports programs are discussed, and detailed information on wheelchair sports and the Special Olympics is provided.

The emphasis of Section Three is on the benefits to people with disabilities of well-organized and professionally directed recreation activities. Most of the activities presented are easily incorporated into programs with disabled and nondisabled participants. Some of these activities, however, such as wheelchair sports and Special Olympics, are segregated experiences that restrict participation to people with disabilities. Including such examples in no way implies that the authors of this textbook advocate segregated programming for most people who have disabilities. To the contrary, we feel that each special population member should participate in the least restrictive recreational environment. We have highlighted some segregated recreation programs soley because they allow us to identify more clearly the benefits of a given recreational activity for all people with disabilities.

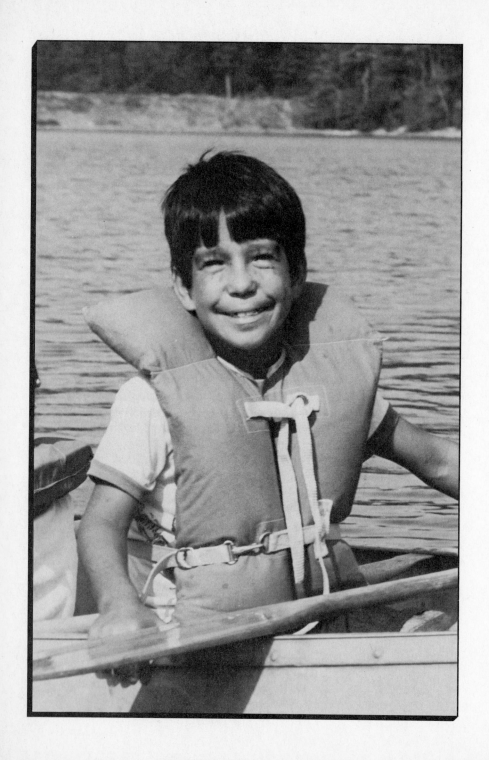

8

Special Camping and Wilderness Experiences

If you ask a group of people to define "camping," you might get as many definitions as there are people in the group. To one person camping might mean backpacking through California's High Sierras. To another it may bring back memories of childhood scouting trips to lakeside woods. Yet, another person may picture himself or herself sitting in an elaborate recreation vehicle (RV) parked in a neatly arranged campground. In truth, the word "camping" has come to refer to a wide variety of outdoor experiences. The equipment may range from simple to sophisticated; the surroundings, primitive to developed; and the activities, nature-based to indoor-oriented. Camping means many things to many people. This chapter, however, is concerned with *organized* camping programs and their potential for benefiting individuals with disabilities.

As the term implies, organized camping refers to outdoor living experiences that are carefully structured and supervised. The American Camping Association (ACA), a nationwide organization dedicated to organized camping, provides the following definition:

> [Camping is] a sustained experience which provides a creative, recreational and educational opportunity in group living in the out-of-doors. It utilizes trained leadership and the resources of natural surroundings to contribute to each camper's mental, physical, social, and spiritual growth. (ACA Standards, 1980, p. 8)

185

Clearly, then, camping as referred to in this textbook does not pertain to "escaping" urban living in recreation vehicles with all the comforts of home, nor does it apply to the solo backpacker who sets out on an extended hiking expedition. Each of these activities may meet the needs of its participants but neither contains all of the essential components of an organized camping experience. Betty Lyle (1947) wrote that five components are common to any definition of organized camping, including (1) out-of-doors, (2) recreation, (3) group living, (4) education, and (4) social adjustment. Despite the fact that her observation was made almost 40 years ago, the similarity between her remarks and the current ACA definition is striking. Adding one critical component to Lyle's list, trained leadership, provides an understanding of how organized camping differs from casual outdoor experiences. It is a *directed* experience that combines the unique properties of nature with the developmental potential of human group interaction. As an editorial in *Camping Magazines* (American Camping Association, 1985) stated:

> [Organized camping] is living in a community of people. It is face-to-face contact with the ebb and flow of human life—it is the civilizing, socializing, humanizing process of people working and playing and living together, closely, intimately. It is experimenting with hopes and aspirations, joys and sorrows, laughter and tears, successes and failures, moods and temperaments, and all humanity. It is *group* living—strong, virile, robust living together in the realm of people. Minus this human element, it is not organized camping. (p. 22)

Camping is fun, but equally as important, it offers unlimited opportunities for human interaction and personal growth. Each year thousands of campers go to summer camps expecting to become more comfortable with nature; most return more comfortable with themselves.

CAMPING FOR PEOPLE WITH DISABILITIES

Camping for special populations is traced to the 1880s, but it was not until the 1930s that a concerted effort was made to provide camping opportunities for large numbers of people with disabilities. At first, these programs focused upon therapy and treatment for children, but the camp environment's potential to aid personal growth of the *total* individual was eventually recognized by camp leaders. Since the 1960s, most camps for people with disabilities have closely paralleled camps for the general population. Their goals, objectives, activities, and organizational structures are similar. Although the camper to staff ratio may vary (camps for disabled individuals usually have fewer campers per counselor), the emphasis is the same—development of the total person through enjoyment of the out-of-doors.

The similarity between most special camps and so-called "regular" camps can be detected in the following general concepts listed by a National Easter Seal Society task force on special camping:

1. Persons with special needs should be afforded the same rewarding experiences that are available to the non-handicapped.
2. Special programs can play a major role in the rehabilitation or habilitation of persons with special needs.
3. The socio-recreational values to be derived from association with nature through camping are inherently therapeutic without regard to any concomitant medical or paramedical benefits that may accrue.
4. Group living and working or playing situations provide social and psychological opportunities not available in the clinical or educational setting. (Hardt, 1968, p. 2)

Clearly, the unique value of a camping experience is enhanced because the camp's leadership accepts an holistic view of the individual. All aspects of the person's life, from eating habits to activity selection, contribute to his or her personal fulfillment. Therefore, camps should provide quality opportunities in as many aspects of life as possible if the potential of a camping experience is to be fully realized. The girl who receives extensive physical therapy at camp undoubtedly benefits from the therapy. Does she, however, receive maximum benefit from all that camping has to offer? One long-time leader in the field of special camping, Jeanne Feeley from Pennsylvania, emphasized the importance of camping—not therapy—in her personal philosophy statement. Her words summarize the underlying theme of this chapter.

> I believe every person, handicapped, or not, should have at least one camp experience. . . . I believe in the intrinsic value of camping. We need to preserve these values for our children and our children's children. Let all people whether mildly, moderately, or severely handicapped know what good camping is. (Feeley, 1972, pp. 44–45)

Feeley did add one warning that should be kept in mind, however. Not everyone will enjoy camping. The once popular expression "different strokes for different folks" comes to mind. Some individuals will discover that outdoor activities and group living are perfectly suited to them; others will learn that the out-of-doors is not for them. The important thing is that everyone, whether disabled or nondisabled, has the *opportunity* to experience camping. Only through personal experience can one discover the potential benefits of a camp experience. As one teenaged camper remarked recently, "I can't believe it! I didn't even want to go on this (camping) trip; now I wish I could *live* in the woods!" Opportunity enables discovery. Unfortunately, only about 10 percent of youngsters who have disabilities in the United States receive the opportunity to discover camping (Hillman & Appel, 1978). The percentage of adults with disabilities who have experienced camping is probably even smaller.

Camp Objectives

Each camp should establish its own general objectives. These objectives are used to guide staff decision making in all aspects of the camp, including activity selection, food preparation, discipline techniques, personnel policies, administrative procedures, etc. The philosophy of the camp's governing body is usually reflected in the list of general objectives. It is important, therefore, that all objectives be clearly stated in writing. Wilkinson (1981) provided a list of six general objectives that reflect an holistic view of a camp's purpose. These general objectives, developed by the American Camping Association, are appropriate for most camps, no matter how many of their campers have special needs:

1. To provide each camper with the opportunity for wholesome fun and adventure in a safe and supervised outdoor program.
2. To help develop a concept of safe and healthful living by stressing wholesome daily health habits; by stressing safety in camp skills; by offering a change for increasing strength, vitality, and endurance; and by fostering freedom from mental tensions.
3. To contribute to the development of "at-home-ness" in the natural world by imparting an understanding of and appreciation for the world of nature, by fostering an understanding of man's dependency on nature and a sense of responsibility for conservation of natural resources, and by increasing the ability to use basic camping skills.
4. To increase a camper's concept of spiritual meaning and values through encouraging the development of a kinship with the security in an orderly universe, and through gaining an understanding of and appreciation for persons of other religions, cultures, nationalities and races.
5. To encourage the development of skills and knowledges that may contribute to wholesome recreation during later years.
6. To contribute to the development of the individual through adjustment to group living in a democratic setting by instilling

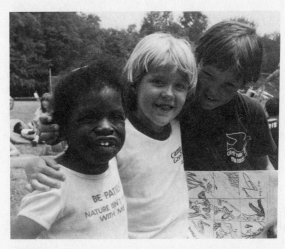

Figure 8–1. One goal of most organized camping programs is to provide group living experiences that enhance social understanding and responsibility. Camp is an ideal setting for cooperative activities that promote "togetherness" among disabled and nondisabled campers. (Courtesy of the League for the Handicapped, Baltimore, MD)

in him a sense of worth of each individual, by helping him to function effectively in a democratic society, and by helping him to develop a sense of social understanding and responsibility. (pp. 10–12)

Naturally, the preceding list of general objectives may not be ideal for all camps. Also, each camp should develop specific objectives that are more limited in scope and easier to measure than general objectives. Many camps are organized by sponsoring organizations to use the outdoor setting as a way of promoting specific special interests or outcomes. Religious camps, weight control camps, and computer camps are just a few examples of special interest camps. Therapeutic camps also fit into this category. Specific objectives are critical if a special interest camp is to achieve its purposes. Shea (1977) provides a few specific objectives that may be appropriate for special camps that emphasize therapy and (re)habilitation. Among these are:

■ To assess and diagnose the child's [disability] and to prescribe treatment and remediation to be implemented in another setting.

■ To serve as a temporary placement center before and/or after placement in an institution, foster home, or special class placement center. (p. 29)

General and specific objectives also may vary according to the type of camp. Day camps, resident camps, wilderness-adventure camps, trip camps, and family camps are examples of different camp types. Each type has its own advantages and these should be emphasized within the written objectives. Looking at Shea's specific objectives, we see that his first objective should be implemented in a variety of camp types, but his second objective most likely would be limited to a resident camp.

Properly written and publicized camp objectives are exceedingly important because they serve two main purposes. First, as stated earlier, they provide direction to all camp staff members. Thus, consistency and quality of services are more easily maintained. Secondly, written objectives provide essential information to parents and/or campers. If maximum enjoyment is to occur, the programs and operations of the camp must be well suited to the camper's individual interests. Written objectives help provide a basis for selecting the most appropriate camp. Vinton, et al., (1978) also stress the importance of objectives, and they provide five basic principles for camps serving children to follow. These principles should help any camp to create an appropriate atmosphere for achieving its objectives. They are:

■ Emphasize what the [child with a disability] can do rather than what he or she cannot do. Provide programs that are within range of abilities of the child.
■ Stress both the fun and the educational potential of each experience equally.
■ Provide a flexible program that is geared to the needs of each individual child.
■ Provide a situation that is as normal as possible, deviating or adapting only when necessary.
■ Stress participation in the democratic processes. Environmental education and camping should be a doing process, involving the child in all levels of planning and implementing the program. (p. 8)

Camp Leadership

Objectives provide direction in any camp program, but the camp's staff has responsibility for achieving these objectives. Anyone who has attended or worked in an organized camp can testify to the importance of a competent and enthusiastic staff. This is especially true in a camp that has campers with disabilities. It is easy for a counselor to become frustrated if the pace of camp is slowed by campers with physical disabilities, or if maintaining discipline becomes difficult due to behavioral disorders among campers. How counselors deal with these frustrations help determine their job effectiveness, and effective counselors are critical to a camp's success. The box that follows provides a list of strategies that should be useful to any camp counselor who is faced with camper problem behavior.

TEN STRATEGIES FOR CAMP COUNSELORS*
by Ralph Smith

Handling inappropriate camper behavior is one of the most difficult and frustrating tasks faced by camp counselors. The following 10 simple strategies, although far from a cure-all, may help to increase desirable behavior among campers who are difficult to manage.

1. *Reinforce desirable behavior.* It is usually much easier to establish desirable behavior patterns at the beginning of the camp session than to alter problem behavior after it has started. A smile, gesture, or brief word of support is frequently all that is necessary to encourage a camper to maintain or to increase acceptable behavior.
2. *Clearly state privileges as well as rules.* Tell campers what they may do; too many "don'ts" violate strategy #1. If campers clearly understand what is permitted, they will not need to test to determine acceptable limits. Camper participation in establishing rules may help as well.
3. *Tolerate some annoying behavior.* Too much attention to annoying behavior may not only interefere with an activity's effectiveness, but may serve to reinforce undesirable actions. Also, certain annoying behaviors may be typical for the child's developmental stage.
4. *Use nonverbal cues.* Eye contact, accompanied by a frown or gesture, may control undesirable behavior without the possibility of embarrassing the camper in front of his or her peers.

---

*These ten strategies for managing problem behavior of campers were included in Project REACH's *Camp Staff Training Series.* In addition, they were published in an issue of *Camping Magazine* (June, 1980), and appear here in abbreviated form.

5. *Consider redirection to a different task or activity.* The challenges of any activity should be consistent with the camper's skill development, so plan for varying levels of skill and try to individualize tasks to each camper's abilities. Many behavior problems result from activity dissatisfaction or boredom and may be eliminated by "redirecting" the camper to another task or activity.

   NOTE: Despite careful attention to the above strategies, problem behaviors may occur that require immediate intervention. Any disciplinary action should be fair, consistent, and administered in an understanding manner. The next strategies may be helpful when intervention is required.

6. *Clarify consequences of unacceptable behavior.* A camper should clearly understand the personal impact of his or her behavior, such as anticipated disciplinary action. It also may be advisable to encourage the camper to clarify the consequences of his or her own actions by asking, "What things do you think will happen if you continue to act this way?" When clarifying consequences, it is important to avoid using a threatening tone of voice and, above all, the staff member must be prepared to follow through if the undesirable behavior continues.

7. *Clarify benefits of acceptable behavior.* This is the corollary to strategy #6, and may be useful in concert with it. Staff should be reminded, however, that pointing out the benefits of acceptable behavior will be most effective if it occurs immediately after desirable behavior (strategy #1).

8. *Use "time-out" procedures.* It may be necessary to temporarily remove a disruptive camper from the situation in which problem behavior is occurring and place him or her in a location where little or no enjoyable stimulation is received. Once removed, the camper should be allowed to return after a short period of time, but it is important that this return be contingent upon appropriate behavior.

9. *Punishment, if used, should be a last resort.* Punishment (of any kind) does not allow the camper to avoid the consequences by exhibiting acceptable behavior. Thus, attention is directed to the punishment itself, rather than to the problem and alternative forms of behavior. Any form of punishment should be appropriate to the situation and, of course, must conform to camp policies.

10. *If in doubt, seek help.* This strategy should be used whenever the counselor feels incapable of coping with a particular situation or

camper. It should be stressed that seeking help is not a sign of defeat or inadequacy. No one, no matter how experienced, has all of the answers to handling camper behavior problems.

Rodney and Ford (1971) emphasized the unique role of a camp counselor who supervises children:

> The child-adult relationship at camp is a very unusual one, for in this particular setting the adult in the role of camp counselor is considered neither teacher, regulator, disciplinarian, minister, nor parent. Yet, he is a combination of all, and at the same time he is a companion and a pal. (p. 14)

Whether working with children or adults, the qualities, or personality traits, of an ideal camp counselor are almost endless. Some, however, are more important than others. Kimball (1980) emphasized "flexibility, a high degree of perseverence and tolerance for frustration, an ability to empathize, and a sense of humor" (p. 31). Creativity is certainly another vital characteristic, as is good judgment. Of course, knowledge of how to manage the physical needs of dependent campers is essential when a camp includes moderately and/or severely disabled campers. However, the single most important characteristic for any camp counselor is a genuine interest in and love for the campers. When counselors are "into" their campers, the camp's atmosphere is alive and exciting for everyone, and possibilities for personal fulfillment abound.

One experienced director of a special camp confided that he and his administrative staff once sat around a campfire discussing the attributes of previous counselors. "We selected an 'all-star' staff made up of the best counselors we had seen during the preceding 10 years," he said. "Afterwards, we tried to identify what qualities made them so special. Their ages and personalities varied, but one characteristic was common to all—they *loved* being with the campers." These counselors showed their love in a variety of ways; they put the campers' needs above their own desires, they asked for the campers' ideas and tried to implement them, they were alert to risks but never overprotected the campers, and, above all, they established an atmosphere of sharing between themselves and the campers. "They all stayed a few summers and then moved on," the director said, "but their campers will never forget them." After a brief pause, he added, "And I know they will never foregt their campers!"

Good counselors enable a camp to fulfill its potential. They serve as role models for the campers and promote personal growth within their

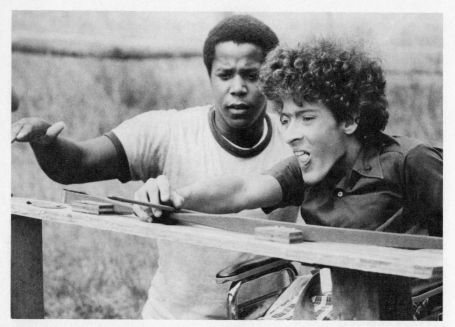

Figure 8–2. Effective camp counselors enable a camp to achieve its objectives. Counselors who are dedicated to the well-being of their campers provide experiences that foster personal growth and self-discovery. (Courtesy of the League for the Handicapped, Baltimore, MD)

group. Successful camps select their counselors wisely, and they provide them with the best possible training. As most camp directors acknowledge, a camp is only as good as its counselors.

Staff Training

In the spring of 1972, a conference was held that underscored the importance of staff training for special camps. The National Conference on Training Needs for Personnel in Camping, Outdoor, and Environmental Recreation for Handicapped Children was held at the Asilomar Conference Grounds in Pacific Grove, California. Sponsored by the Bureau of Education for the Handicapped (BEH—now the Office of Special Education, U.S. Department of Education), this Conference (1) examined current training practices, (2) identified problem areas and needs with respect to training, and (3) developed a series of strategies for staff training methods and materials.

One of the most beneficial outcomes from this conference was the funding by BEH of three special projects to upgrade training techniques in camping and environmental education for individuals with disabilities. Project REACH at the University of Kentucky was one of these projects. Project REACH developed a *Camp Staff Training Series* designed to "assist camp personnel to gain a better understanding of the nature of their jobs and to acquire those skills and competencies needed to perform their duties in an effective and professional manner" (Pearce, Vinton & Farley, 1979, p. 1).

The portion of the *Camp Staff Training Series* devoted to preparing camp counselors was particularly exciting. It included six separate instructional "modules" that were prepared by a variety of experts in the field of special camping. Each module, or unit, was field tested at six different sites. The resulting publication, *Camp Counselor Training Series* (6 Vols.), was packed with useful written materials and learning exercises. The six volumes included (1) An Orientation to Camping and the Camp, (2) Knowing the Campers, (3) Camp Program Planning and Leadership, (4) Camp Health and Safety Practices, (5) Dealing with Camper Behavior, and (6) Evaluating the Camp Experience. There is little doubt that completion of this or a similar comprehensive training program would help any counselor improve his or her skills as a camp couselor in a special camp.

Whether or not a formal training program is used (such as the one developed by Project REACH), staff training is of vital importance. Each training program should do the following: include some "hands-on" experience, provide practical tips and information, specify policies and procedures, stress safety and health, and clarify program philosophy. In short, camp training must prepare staff members for all aspects of their jobs. Of primary importance, however, is preparation for being with the campers.

Knapp (1984) emphasizes the need for staff training to develop interpersonal skills with campers. Reporting the results of a survey of midwestern camp personnel, Knapp listed knowledge of group dynamics, leadership skills, and techniques for building camper self-esteem as the three most important staff training topics. He added:

> Camp leaders recognize that their staff need both people skills and activity skills to perform their roles effectively. Because of time limitations, they are forced to decide what topics are most important to include in pre-camp educational workshops. The results of this study reveal that the respondents viewed the development of people skills as more important than activity skills. (p. 24)

Byrd (1972) outlined three aspects of preparation for being with campers that are unique to camps serving people with disabilities. First, information about disabilities and special needs should be simple and basic. "If a counselor is going to have a camper with muscular dystrophy" wrote Byrd, "he does not need to know the detailed population incidence of MD, its etiology and medical research summaries to date. He does need to know what help the MD camper will need and how best to give it. . . . If he is fed quantities of technical medical and psychological jargon in professional terms in pre-camp, he is apt to think of the impending (carefully chosen word) camper less and less as a person, and more and more as a medical case—thus defeating one of our main purposes in camp" (pp. 140–141).

Byrd's second point was that all areas of difference between campers with disabilities and nondisabled campers need to be specified. The nature of the campers' disabilities or special needs would, no doubt, determine what information should be included in this aspect of camp training. Byrd urged that physical, psychological, social, and emotional differences be specified, but he included a warning that "the danger exists of exaggerating differences and potential individual problems to the point of painting the camper as a potential monster!" (p. 141). The authors of this text strongly support Byrd's caution, and feel that emphasizing differences between disabled and nondisabled campers is generally inadvisable.

The third unique aspect offered by Byrd is the need for "empathy" training. Empathy means that you not only recognize another's situation, but you identify with that person to the point of actually experiencing his or her thoughts or feelings. It means that you *really* understand what someone else is experiencing. Byrd suggested that discussions and role playing (simulations) are two ways to achieve empathy. Some films and videotapes may be effective, too. Whatever techniques are used, however, empathy is one of the most important qualities a counselor can possess. Every camp training program should include activities designed to foster empathy, thus enabling the formation of positive attitudes toward campers who have disabilities. As noted by Stearn (1984), staff attitude is the first aspect to be analyzed when ensuring that a camp is accessible to people with disabilities.

Proper training refines the skills and attitudes of all camp staff members and enables them to offer the best possible experience to campers with disabilities. If campers are to receive the maximum benefit from their stay at camp, a well-trained staff is essential.

Benefits of Organized Camping

Camping offers many potential benefits to individuals with disabilities. Both parents and health professions agree that the camp environment offers a unique setting for personal growth. Many individuals with disabilities have limited life experiences due to the barriers they face.

Camp, however, gives a chance for exploration of oneself and the environment. It allows the flexibility to express creativity, yet provides sufficient structure for feelings of security. Above all, it offers a chance for independence of thought and action to individuals who are, regrettably, too often forced to assume a dependency role. As Feeley (1972) wrote, "We dream of challenges and create actualities by our wit, skill and ability. We live with the quiet of the universe and learn to 'know thy self' " (p. 44).

Advocates attribute numerous benefits to an organized camping experience. Hansen (1972) analyzed 50 references, including research articles, and listed the 5 most frequently mentioned benefits. These included (1) recreational activities, (2) learning opportunities, (3) expanded environment, (4) socialization/informal group participation, and (5) independence/self-confidence. Hansen also divided the statements included in his resources into 2 categories, primary benefits and functional benefits. Table 8–1 shows these categories, as well as the benefits included in each.

Hopefully, camp's many benefits interact to help campers with disabilities increase their own feelings of self-worth. Thus, their self-concepts are strengthened. Lundegren (1976) observed that an individual's self-concept is influenced both by interaction with others (especially significant others) and by interaction with the environment. She added, "Camping has the unique opportunity to contribute in all aspects here" (p. 263). A number of self-concept studies have supported Lundegren's statement (Robb, 1971; Hourcade, 1977; Sessoms, 1979; Shasby, Heuchert & Gansneder, 1984), but the evidence is far from conclusive.

In fact, most of the benefits that are claimed by camping enthusiasts have only limited research support. Weaknesses in research methodology and use of questionable measures have limited the results of many camping studies. Also, some authorities doubt that short camp sessions, with young and often inexperienced counselors, could produce significant changes in campers. Still others caution that returning from camp to an institution may have negative consequences, particularly for those with psychological disorders (Ryan & Johnson, 1972; Polenz & Rubitz, 1977).

There is still much research that needs to be done, but almost everyone who has worked in camps with disabled individuals can cite examples of personal growth among campers. They are convinced, as are the authors of this text, that organized camping programs offer many benefits to campers, irrespective of disabilities or special needs. As Sessoms (1979) concluded, "What is known is that a purely recreationally oriented program does have value and consequences [for disabled campers]. It stands on its own merit; need we say more" (p. 42).

Table 8–1
Benefits of Camping for Handicapped: A Codified Statement*

Primary Benefits	Functional Benefits
Attitudes independence/self-confidence motivation self-awareness heightened morale improved behavior improved discipline improved cooperation respect for others	**Educational** learning opportunities learn new skills and activities opportunity for success improved verbalization higher academic achievement creativity

Social
socialization/informal group
  participation
group identity
relationships with adults of a
  nonprofessional nature
get along with others
opportunity for sharing
	Physical
	activities of daily living
	increased opportunity for participation
	improved coordination and physical
	  fitness
	
	Vocational
	organizing own activities
	camping as possible future
	  employment
	initiating own activities

Environmental expanded environment heightened community interest/ awareness opportunity for normal experiences adapt to community adapt to family	**Recreational** activities fun education for leisure

*From: Hansen, C. C. Content analysis of current literature on camping for handicapped children. In Nesbitt, et al., *Training Needs and Strategies in Camping for the Handicapped*. Eugene, OR: University of Oregon Press, 1972, pp. 34–35.

WILDERNESS-ADVENTURE PROGRAMS

One of the most exciting developments in camping and outdoor-related activities for people with disabilities has been the recent emphasis on wilderness and adventure programs. These programs provide a challenging experience for any action-oriented individual, irrespective of disabling condition. They also offer participants many opportunities for physical expression and personal achievement that is *not* based upon complex language skills or abstract thinking processes. Wilderness-adventure programs include challenges that can be understood in concrete terms, and they take place in an outdoor environment that maximizes feelings of personal freedom. It is precisely these qualities that make wilderness-adventure programs the ideal leisure experience for many people with disabilities.

While wilderness-adventure programs vary in format and techniques, most have been adapted from the model established by the Outward Bound program (Hollenhorst & Ewert, 1985). In the early 1960s, Outward Bound opened their program to special population members by incorporating "delinquent" youth into their program. This program included outdoor skills training, a group expedition, and a three-day solo experience in the wilderness. It was felt that such experiences could help bridge the gap between society and young people who did not behave according to society's norms and values. Golins (1978), for example, wrote that many such young people are "looking for a way to join [society] without losing too much face. Adventure based education becomes a ticket he can buy to integrate himself into society honorably" (p. 27).

By 1978, Outward Bound was offering challenging outdoor experiences to many individuals with disabilities. People with cerebral palsy, paraplegia, multiple sclerosis, amputations, muscular dystrophy, and many other disabilities were being given the chance to participate in Outward Bound groups composed of four nondisabled people and four individuals with disabilities (Goodwin, 1978). Other programs were also emerging, many willing to accept people who were considered too disabled by some Outward Bound programs. Wilderness Inquiry II in Minnesota, C. W. Hog in Idaho, and Paraplegics on Independent Nature Trips (POINT) are a few examples of such programs. Through activities such as rock climbing, white water rafting, canoeing, spelunking (caving), backpacking, and so on, these programs and others like them provide personal challenge while at the same time foster interpersonal interaction and small group cooperation.

Wilderness Experience Components

Philosophy, format, and techniques vary from program to program, but there are some components common to most, if not all, wilderness-adventure programs open to people with disabilities. The following components, although listed separately, are interrelated and combine to form an experience that, hopefully, has life-long meaning to participants.

1. *The experience takes place in the out-of-doors.* Most people in technological societies experience a variety of manmade constraints in their daily lives. Windowless rooms in modern buildings shut out "distractions"; city lights and signs tell people when to cross the street, where to park their cars, what products to buy, and so on; schools restrict movement by insisting that each student sits at a desk until a bell rings its approval to

move (usually to another desk). Examples of these constraints are limitless. People with disabilities experience all of these constraints, of course, plus many barriers that do not limit nondisabled people. Wilderness settings, however, offer a chance to overcome barriers that have not been imposed by other human beings. Adaptive behavior is required by mother nature, not by architects or school officials. For people who have disabilities that do not limit mobility, such as learning disabilities, the wilderness also offers an important chance for freedom of movement and expression while, at the same time, providing a natural, yet orderly, environment.

2. *Small-group cooperation and trust in others is emphasized.* Some disabled individuals by necessity devote much of their daily lives to individual challenges. Not only must they overcome obstacles that do not confront their nondisabled peers, but they also may find their contributions to a group or family effort ignored or devalued. It is little wonder, therefore, that some people with disabilities have limited experience in cooperative efforts. Wilderness-adventure programs, however, provide for group experiences that require cooperation and trust. Each participant has the opportunity to contribute to a clearly defined group goal, and because the group is small, that contribution is evident to everyone. The freshly caught fish frying over an open fire will be shared among those who caught the fish *and* those who gathered the firewood. Everyone learns that his or her efforts were of value—there could not have been a meal without *each* person's contribution. In time, a series of such activities results in a cohesive group characterized by members who not only cooperate with each other, but also trust that everyone will do his or her part. As noted by Hollenhorst & Ewert (1985), "Activities that emphasize the importance of the individual's contribution and responsibility to the group and that involve camaraderie, friendship, group decision making and problem solving should be an integral part of the [wilderness-adventure] program" (p. 33).

3. *Stressful objectives are systematically presented and successfully achieved.* In Robert Frost's poem, *The Death of the Hired Man*, an elderly farm worker is referred to as having "nothing to look backward to with pride, And nothing to look forward to with hope, So now and never any different." Unfortunately, some people feel like they are in the same situation. Their lack of success in the past, whether in school or in other aspects of their lives, has resulted in a feeling of futility toward the future.

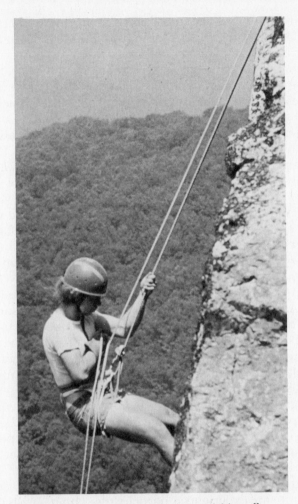

Figure 8–3. Wilderness-adventure activities offer participants personal challenges that demand discipline, concentration, and trust in others. Rock climbing, for example, requires both individual skill and dependence upon fellow participants. (Courtesy of Robert Myers)

As one youth expressed emphatically, "Why should I try, man? I'd just [mess] up again!" Wilderness-adventure programs offer the participant much more than a hodge-podge of outdoor experiences. They are composed of activities that are carefully selected and systematically introduced. Whether these challenges are contrived, as with some Outward Bound activities, or occur naturally in the process of an expedition, each requires the accomplishment of a specific objective. Each objective is challenging enough to induce feelings of stress, but not so difficult that it should result in failure. In order to cross a stream by use of a fallen tree, the young woman with a disability must overcome her fear of falling. As important, however, is the fact that she may also be making progress toward overcoming her fear of *failing*.

4. *The group's leader is critical to program effectiveness.* Leading wilderness-adventure activities requires a great deal of experience and skill, especially when the activities involve stressful situations in unfamiliar surroundings. The leader of a wilderness-adventure group must guide the group so that objectives are achieved *by the group members themselves.* At the same time, the leader needs to remain alert to the optimum (ideal) level of stress for the group. Too little stress prevents a feeling of accomplishment, but too much stress can result in feelings of failure. As noted by Kimball (1980), "There is only a small difference between tension that is creative and growth oriented and tension that is defeating" (p. 12). The leader must be able to anticipate events and likely reactions of group members. He or she must not only know the techniques for accomplishing group goals, but *when* to use them. Leading a wilderness-adventure program is an awesome task! Yet, it provides immense personal reward because behavior changes and personal growth among participants become clearly visible as the experience progresses. The wilderness-adventure program leader is the catalyst who enables these positive results to occur. Fortunately, many wilderness-adventure programs provide an opportunity for experienced participants who have disabilities to assume leadership of groups. Wilderness Inquiry II, which arranges canoe and dogsled trips, presently has several previous participants with disabilities leading their challenging expeditions. C. W. Hog and POINT, on the other hand, were formed by experienced outdoorsmen who have disabilities.

Wilderness-Adventure Activities and Outcomes

Hollenhorst & Ewert (1985) found that the most important activities to nondisabled Outward Bound participants included expeditions and group-oriented challenges. Since people with disabilities generally participate in wilderness-adventure programs for the same reasons as nondisabled individuals (Lais & Schurke, 1982; Richardson, in press), these same activities predominate among programs with participants who have disabilities. Examples include a 19-day trip to the Yukon (Lais, 1985), dogsled rides into the Idaho wilderness (Wittaker, 1984), and the dramatic climb of rugged Guadalupe Peak (8751 ft. in elevation) by a group of POINT members with spinal cord injuries.

Both the Yukon and Idaho trips were integrated experiences in which nondisabled individuals participated along with people who had disabilities. Such expeditions are generally organized with careful attention to group structure. Describing Wilderness Inquiry II canoe trips into the Boundary Waters along the U.S.-Canada border, Lais & Schurke (1982) noted that:

> A usual group would include two people who use wheelchairs, two who are sensory impaired, three 'able-bodied' persons, one who uses crutches and two group leaders. Consideration is given so that groups are intergenerational, balanced in the number of men and women, and

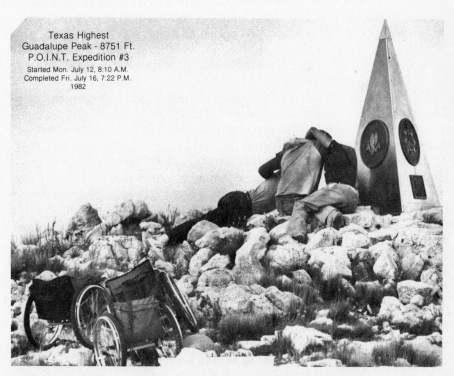

Texas Highest
Guadalupe Peak - 8751 Ft.
P.O.I.N.T. Expedition #3
Started Mon. July 12, 8:10 A.M.
Completed Fri. July 16, 7:22 P.M.
1982

Figure 8–4. Overcoming nature's challenges requires cooperation and interdependence among participants. In addition, such experiences provide unparalleled feelings of personal control and accomplishment. (Courtesy of **POINT**)

include persons from a wide variety of occupations and lifestyles. (p. 25–26)

Such integrated wilderness-adventure programs enable each group member to utilize his or her unique skills and abilities. People with disabilities are generally accepted for their abilities (Lais, 1985), and nondisabled participants accept the responsibility for performing tasks that are difficult or impossible for people who have disabilities. It is a learning experience for everyone, and each person is expected to respond to the challenge at hand. As one participant with cerebral palsy explained, "'You are encouraged to do things you never thought possible but, with a little effort and ingenuity, you find out that you can do them'" (Lais & Schurke, 1982, p. 27).

Some expeditions, such as the POINT climb of Guadalupe Peak, are composed exclusively of participants with disabilities. One goal of such trips may be the feeling that participants receive from successfully "going it alone", or not depending upon nondisabled companions to assist with difficult tasks. Successfully overcoming wilderness challenges can increase a person's self-confidence (Wright, 1983) and overcoming them without the aid of nondisabled participants can provide unparalleled feelings of personal control and achievement. Despite the fact that only three of the six POINT members who began the ascent of Guadalupe Peak actually reached the summit, all participants shared in the joy of accomplishment.

The outcomes of any successful wilderness-adventure program are similar, whether or not they include people with disabilities. Participants enjoy the beauty and wonder of nature, share experiences with other human beings, develop skills, and overcome challenges that enable feelings of self-worth and personal control. The presence of people with disabilities in such programs may intensify these outcomes for everyone. As Corty (1978) wrote, upon returning from one expedition, "Looking around the table at those faces I have come to know so intimately, I realize that we have been voyageurs not only through the boundary waters, but through the hearts of ourselves and each other. . . . It has been a voyage that will continue long after the paddles are put away" (pp. 10–12). Hopefully, the outcomes of a wilderness-adventure experience will help all participants, including those with disabilities, enjoy smoother and more satisfying voyages through life.

—————————— SUMMARY ——————————

Organized camping and wilderness experiences offer everyone, including people with disabilities, unique opportunities for enjoyment and personal growth. Experts have attributed many beneficial outcomes to participation in these experiences, including improved interpersonal skills, increased strength and endurance, greater independence, and enhanced feelings of self-worth. Despite these benefits, however, less than one tenth of people with disabilities in the United States have had the opportunity to participate in organized camping and wilderness programs. As these programs expand to accommodate more people with disabilities, it is essential that they (1) have clearly stated objectives, based on a sound philosophy, (2) provide effective staff training that emphasizes empathy for campers, and (3) offer well-organized and safe activities that are consistent with the skills and interests of *all* campers.

Suggested Learning Activities

1. Identify eight topics that you feel should be included in any orientation program for a special camp. Develop a learning activity for one of these topics.

2. Interview the director of a special camp or wilderness-adventure program. What does he or she feel are the *unique* benefits that can be derived from participating in the program?

3. Vinton, et al., list five basic principles for camps to follow in order to create an appropriate atmosphere for achieving its objectives. Discuss how each of these principles facilitates the personal growth of campers with disabilities.

4. List ten qualities that are important for a camp counselor to exhibit. Discuss the importance of each.

5. Name the four wilderness experience components that are common to most wilderness-adventure programs. Discuss the benefits to participants provided by each component.

References

American Camping Association. *Standards for Accrediting Camps.* Martinsville, IN: American Camping Association, 1980.

American Camping Association. What is the role of camping? *Camping Magazine, 57*(4), 22–24, 1985.

Byrd, J. D. Selecting and training staff in a camp for handicapped children. In Nesbitt, J. A., et al., *Training Needs and Strategies in Camping for the Handicapped.* Eugene, OR: University of Oregon Press, 1972, pp. 136–143.

Corty, J. Disabled blaze new trails in the wild. *The New York Times*, October 21, 10–1, 12, 1979.

Feeley, J. E. Should every handicapped person have a camping experience? In Nesbitt, J. A., et al., *Training Needs and Strategies in Camping for the Handicapped.* Eugene, OR: University of Oregon Press, 1972, pp. 44–45.

Golins, G. L. How delinquents succeed through adventure based education. *Journal of Experiential Education, 1*(2), 1978, 26–29.

Goodwin, G. Outward Bound. *Sports 'n Spokes, 4*(1), 1978, 5–7.

Hansen, C. C. Content analysis of current literature on camping for handicapped children. In Nesbitt, et al., *Training Needs and Strategies for the Handicapped.* Eugene, OR: University of Oregon Press, 1972, pp. 32–37.

Hardt, L. J. *Easter Seal Guide to Special Camping Programs.* Chicago: The National Easter Seal Society for Crippled Children and Adults, 1968.

Hillman, W. A. and M. S. Appel. Camping and environmental education for handicapped children and youth. *Therapeutic Recreation Journal, 12*(4), 6–8, 1978.

Hollenhorst, S., and A. Ewert. Dissecting the adventure camp experience: Determining successful program components. *Camping Magazine, 57*(4), 32–33, 1985.

Hourcade, J. Effect of a summer camp program on self-concept of mentally retarded young adults. *Therapeutic Recreation Journal, 11*(4), 178–183, 1977.

Kimball, R. O. *Wilderness/Adventure Programs for Juvenile Offenders.* Chicago: University of Chicago, School of Social Service Administration, 1980.

Knapp, C. E. Staff education: Balancing people and activity skills. *Camping Magazine, 56*(6), 22–24, 1984.

Lais, G. Paddling the Yukon. *Sports 'n Spokes, 10*(6), 9–12, 1985.

Lais, G, and P. Schurke. Wilderness Inquiry II. *Sports 'n Spokes, 8*(2), 25–27, 1982.

Lyle, B. *Camping—What Is It?* Martinsville, IN: American Camping Association, 1947.

Lundegren, H. Self-concepts of special populations. In van der Smissen, B., compiler, *Research Camping and Environmental Education.* State College, PA: The Pennsylvania State University, 1976, pp. 253–273.

Nesbitt, J. A., C. C. Hansen, B. J. Bates, and L. L. Neal. *Training Needs and Strategies in Camping for the Handicapped.* Eugene, OR: University of Oregon Press, 1972.

Pearce, B. O., D. A. Vinton, and E. A. Farley. *Directory of Agencies Concerned with Camping and the Handicapped.* Lexington, KY: University of Kentucky (Project REACH), 1979.

Polenz, D., and F. Rubitz. Staff perceptions of the effects of therapeutic camping upon psychiatric patients' affect. *Therapeutic Recreation Journal, 11*(2), 70–73, 1977.

Richardson, D. Outdoor adventure programs for physically disabled individuals. *Parks and Recreation,* in press.

Robb, G. M. A correlation between socialization and self-concept in a summer camp program. *Therapeutic Recreation Journal, 5*(1), 25–29, 1971.

Rodney, L. S., and P. M. Ford. *Camp Administration*. New York: John Wiley & Sons, 1971.

Ryan, J. L., and D. T. Johnson. Therapeutic camping: A comparative study. *Therapeutic Recreation Journal*, 6(4), 178–180, 1972.

Sessoms, H. D. Organized camping and its effects on the self-concept of physically handicapped children. *Therapeutic Recreation Journal*, 13(1), 39–43, 1979.

Shasby, G., C. Heuchert, and B. Gansneder. The effects of a structured camp experience on locus of control and self-concept of special populations. *Therapeutic Recreation Journal*, 18(2), 32–40, 1984.

Shea, T. M. *Camping for Special Children*. St. Louis: C. V. Mosby, 1977.

Stearn, S. Accessible programs. *Camping Magazine*, 56(7), 12–15, 1984.

Vinton, D. A., D. E. Hawkins, B. D. Pantzer, and E. M. Farley. *Camping and Environmental Education for Handicapped Children and Youth*. Washington, D.C.: Hawkins & Associates, 1978.

Wilkinson, R. E. *Camps: Their Planning and Management*. St. Louis: C. V. Mosby, 1981.

Wittaker, T. C. W. Hog: A journey into the unknown. *Sports 'n Spokes*, 9(5), 8–11, 1984.

Wright, A. N. Therapeutic potential of the Outward Bound process: An evaluation of a treatment program for juvenile delinquents. *Therapeutic Recreation Journal*, 17(2), 33–42, 1983.

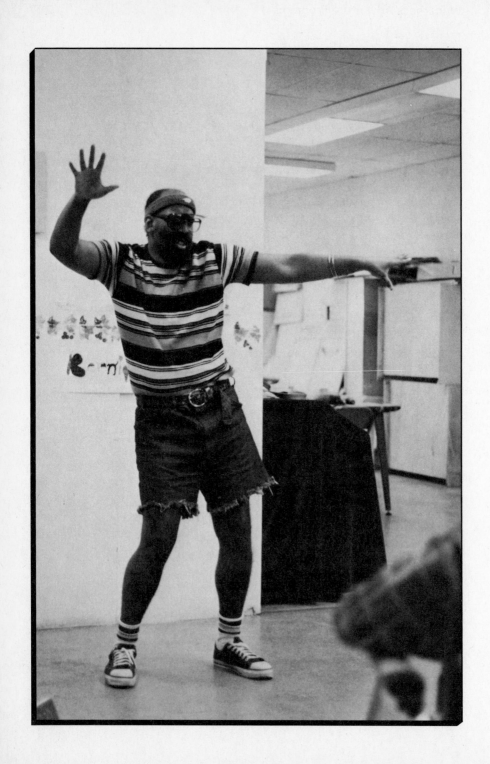

9

The Arts—For Everyone

The more a person travels around the world, the more he or she becomes aware of the cultural differences among human beings. Behaviors that are acceptable, or even rewarded, in one country are taboo in another. Ideas that are received with acclaim by members of one culture are rejected as absurd by people with different heritages. Yet, despite many differences, people throughout the world demonstrate similar desires for aesthetic experiences. Appreciation of beauty, in its many forms, appears to be universal. Enjoyment of manmade beauty is so fundamental to human existence that the right "to enjoy the arts" is included in the United Nations' Universal Declaration of Human Rights. Through the arts, people are offered an opportunity for interaction on an aesthetic level. Such interaction, which is based upon positive feelings for beauty, is a very important part of human society. In fact, much of our knowledge about the customs, values, and beliefs of ancient societies is based upon archeological analysis of their artwork. The arts, it seems, help to form and also to reflect the national character (ethos) of a society.

Because the arts are so essential to a society, they make an important contribution to individual development. Hayman (1969) underscored this importance in the following statement:

> Art can and should be an experience shared by all men every day of their lives; this does not mean that all men must be painters, architects,

209

authors, composers, nor does it mean that they must spend all of their days in museums, their evenings in theatres and concert halls. Rather, it means that man's innate sensitivities to the arts must be allowed to develop and, by early encouragement and education, must be given opportunity for growth so that the whole man can emerge. (p. 11)

In the United States, our "work ethic" background has resulted in less emphasis on the arts than is found in many other nations. Nevertheless, the arts are essential to each citizen's life. From the small child drawing with crayons to the senior citizen reflecting upon a lifetime of experiences through poetry, the arts provide a basis for discovery, self-expression, and human growth. In short, access to and participation in the arts is important for *all* persons in our society.

WHAT CONSTITUTES "THE ARTS"?

The term "the arts" is used frequently in everyday conversation, yet defining this term is exceedingly difficult. As Roehner (1981) pointed out, "On the one hand, the arts are those human endeavors that are known as art, dance, drama, filmmaking and photography, music and writing. On the other hand, the arts is also a whole battery of working methods of styles and constantly developing skills. . . . The arts embody a way of working and learning" (p. 6). "The arts," therefore, has more than one definition. The term refers to a set of creative activities, but it also implies a concept that encompasses many methods and processes.

Regardless of art form, the arts is founded upon one essential element—creativity. Participation in the arts, on any level, provides the individual with an opportunity to organize, interpret, and express his or her *own* perceptions of the world. In other words, the arts offers a uniquely personal experience to everyone, disabled and nondisabled alike. Creativity, as noted by Diamondstein (1974), "involves the capacity to be open to experience, to welcome novelty, to be intrigued by discovery, and to exercise new dimensions of imaginative thought" (p. 15).

Creativity in the arts is not necessarily limited to the act of developing an artistic creation. Someone else's effort, such as a musical score, offers the chance for creativity, too. For example, a pianist may play his or her own interpretation of another's creation. Carrying this idea a little further, some authorities even insist that merely perceiving a work of art is, in itself, a creative act. Paraphrasing one of his friends, Shaw (1980) stated that "once you have really experienced Shakespeare's *King Lear*, you cannot even fry the breakfast bacon in quite the same way again" (p. 73). Perhaps Shaw was exaggerating, but his point is an important one. As shown in Figure 9–1, participation in the arts

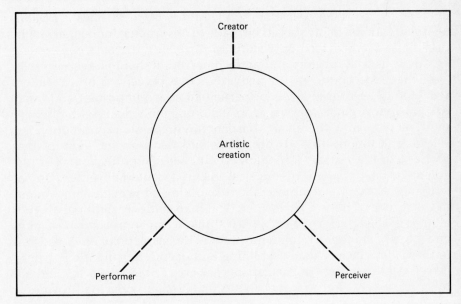

Figure 9–1. Three levels of arts participation.

offers an individual the chance to have an aesthetic experience on one (or more) of three levels—as the *creator*, the *performer*, or the *perceiver* of a work of art.

The *creator* of an art work, no matter what medium is used, is providing an expression of his or her own being. The creator gives form to symbols or objects in such a way that beauty results, and this beauty is shared with (and affects) others. The *performer* takes a creator's efforts and, through his or her own artistic feelings and skill, transmits the work of art to others. As noted above, the *perceiver* views the performance or work of art and experiences it in a creative way. The perceiver "feels" the artistic effort, but unlike the creator and performer does not share with others what is felt. Of course, it is not necessary (nor possible in some cases) for all three levels of participation to be offered by a given work of art. The painter does not need a performer to transmit his or her work of art to an audience. Also, the same person may be involved on different levels, as when a poet recites his or her own poems. Nonetheless, the arts cannot be fully understood without recognizing the presence of these three levels of participation.

It is especially important for people associated with special recreation services to recognize that three levels of participation are offered through the arts. Rehabilitation professionals, advocacy groups, and people with disabilities themselves complain that people who have disabilities are too often spectators while others perform. This is a valid complaint. Every effort should be made to ensure that individuals with disabilities are provided opportunities through the arts to experience creativity as both creators and performers. But it should be recognized, also, that "spectators" of the arts are *active* perceivers of a creative work of art. All three levels of participation are important and offer unique opportunities for everyone, including individuals with disabilities. The woman with mental retardation who paints a sunset provides a lasting testimony to both her talent and her personal view of the world. She is a creator. The blind youth who faithfully practices his guitar lessons may use his musical talents to entertain others. In so doing, he brings the composer's work to life and provides enjoyment to the listeners. He is a performer. The man with cerebral palsy who attends a ballet performance by Baryshnikov can appreciate the agility and grace of another's human movement. He has an emotional reaction to the ballet's beauty that is uplifting and deeply moving. He is a perceiver. All three of these participants are engaged in "the arts," and all three are receiving the many benefits that arts participation provides.

BENEFITS OF ARTS PARTICIPATION

The benefits received from participation in the arts are not necessarily different for disabled and nondisabled individuals. However, barriers may limit opportunities for persons with disabilities to participate in community arts activities. Thus, people who have disabilities may not receive as many personal growth experiences as their nondisabled peers. If arts programs are made available to *everyone*, however, the three levels of arts participation offer limitless opportunities for enjoyment and satisfaction, as well as personal growth. An examination of some of the following five benefits of participation reveals why the arts are so important to everyone in the community.

(1) Self-Discovery. Creativity, which is the cornerstone of arts participation, requires that an individual get in touch with his or her own feelings and perceptions. Participation in the arts, therefore, may enable a person to become more aware of his or her own individuality. Diamondstein (1974) emphasized the importance of self-discovery through involvement in the arts by noting that it can "open new windows on the world and enable [the participant] to perceive his world more richly" (p. 3). Dance, for example, may provide the opportunity for a young man with a psychological disorder to focus on the sensations of muscle relaxation and tension. Once focused on these sensations, the connection between his own emotional feelings and muscular responses may become clearer to him. Such discoveries may not only aid in self-awareness, but may also make future happiness a more realistic goal (Williams, 1977). This view of the arts, as an essential means of self-discovery for people with disabilities is summarized in the following statement by Perks (1979):

> As an arts advocate I believe that music, dance, drama, and art are man's natural and essential means for self-expression. They assist in leading man to an understanding of himself and the world in which he lives. Man expresses his dreams, fears, desires, awe, and wonder of life through the arts. Since the arts are integral to man, they must be central in the educational and life experiences of all people. Creative arts experiences can be a powerful vehicle for providing beauty and joy to people (with) physical, emotional, or mental handicapping conditions. Arts programs for handicapped people assist in developing a heightened awareness of self in relationship to others and life. (p. 27)

(2) Communication with Others. Both the creator and performer levels of arts participation provide unique opportunities for an individual, particularly one with a disability, to communicate with others. For example, people who cannot speak distinctly may use novels, poems, and so on, to share ideas, thoughts, and feelings with others. The late Christy Brown (1932–1981), an Irish author and poet with severe cerebral palsy, was an excellent example of such communication. Able to type only by using the little toe on his left foot, Christy Brown published a renowned novel entitled *Down All the Days*. This book, a fictionalized version of his autobiography, *My Left Foot*, was a powerful personal statement by a talented and perceptive man. In it he was able to express the challenges and frustrations he faced while living with a severe physical disability. As Melville Appell (1978) of the U.S. Office of Special Education stated, "For [people with disabilities] the arts do not only represent learning strategies or economic wherewithal. The arts afford . . . the opportunity to communicate directly on a personal basis with the society in which they live" (p. 16).

Kennedy (1985) provided an example that brings Appell's statement to life. Describing the reaction of a blind Canadian woman in her late twenties when she was asked to draw a picture, Kennedy wrote:

> . . . she protested: 'How can I make a picture? I've never seen anything, let alone a picture, in my life!' But she soon discovered for the first time that she had an ability and a talent she had never used and never suspected she had. She found she could communicate with and learn from pictures—and she did not have to be taught to do so. (p. 165)

(3) Improved Self-concept. The way an individual feels about himself or herself is a critical factor in adjustment to life's many stresses. There-

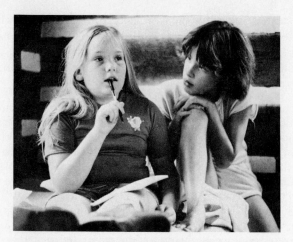

Figure 9–2. Creativity forms the foundation for arts participation. The girl with a disability who writes a poem is offering an expression of her own being; the beauty that results from her creativity may be shared with others. (Courtesy of the League for the Handicapped, Baltimore, MD)

fore, activities that provide for successful participation and offer a chance to exert personal control of a given situation are especially important. Arts activities are ideally suited for both success and personal control. Most, for example, do not have a right or wrong way of doing things. Whether painting on canvas or dancing to music, the participant should be developing his or her own personal sytle. Arts activities encourage individuality and are noncompetitive in nature. There is no winner or loser. Participation itself can be the measure of "success." Perhaps more important than success, however, is a perception of being in control of the situation. The arts offers a unique opportunity for an individual with a disability to be in control. A participant in an arts activity is constantly presented with decision-making opportunities, and the individual himself or herself controls the outcome of each decision. Personal control is reflected in the photographer's adjustment of a camera's lens, the musician's decision to hold a particular note, and the painter's selection of colors. Laureen Summers, a talented weaver who has cerebral palsy, emphasized her perceptions of control before the House Subcommittee on Select Education (May 2, 1977). Summers stated, "When I weave, I feel completely in charge of myself. I think of my accomplishments as statements of myself—my longing to create something real and beautiful." The end product of Summers' artistic effort is not only a work of art, but probably a better self-concept as well.

(4) Skill Development. The many different activities included within the arts offer opportunities to develop and improve upon daily living skills. To cite a few examples, painting and sculpture emphasize fine motor tasks; dance promotes increased coordination, endurance, and flexibility; and literature and drama teach one to communicate through written words and verbal expression. Cognitive, psychomotor, and affective skills may all be enhanced through arts participation. Although the following statement by Smith (1981) refers to children with learning disabilities, it is obvious that it is valid for any child who has a disability.

> Through all the arts forms, a child can be helped to sort out one color, one shape, one form, one sound from another; discriminating through the hands, the body, the eyes, the ears, and all the senses is part of artistic experience. Learning to look, learning to listen, remembering what is seen, remembering what is heard—problem areas for the learning disabled—are emphasized in the arts. These skills help organize experience. They help make sense of the world, make sense of the messages coming in through the senses. That's what perception is all about—making sense of the environment, organizing it to have meaning. (p. 84)

The process of organizing nonverbal experiences is essential, and provides the foundation for subsequent skill development through the arts. Appell (1978) examined research that focused upon the arts and concluded that the effects of arts programs include "improved social response, gains in school achievement, self confidence gained by personal achievement, and a better and more integrated existence" (p. 14). The Arts in Education Project, conceived by the National Committee, Arts with the Handicapped (NCAH), developed a conceptual model that illustrates the use of an arts program for skill development (NCAH, 1981). This model, which has been modified to include literary activities, appears in Figure 9-3. The primary purpose of the model is to show that basic learning abilities and aesthetic development are interrelated, and both are enhanced through participation in the arts.

(5) Societal Recognition and Awareness. The arts have proven especially well suited for people with disabilities to share their exceptional talent with others. Christy Brown (literature—cerebral palsy), Stevie Wonder (music—blindness), Joni Eareckson (art—quadriplegia), Sylvia Plath (literature—psychological disorder), Itzhak Perlman (music—polio), and Phyllis Frelich (drama—deafness) are just a few of the disabled people who have received national and international acclaim

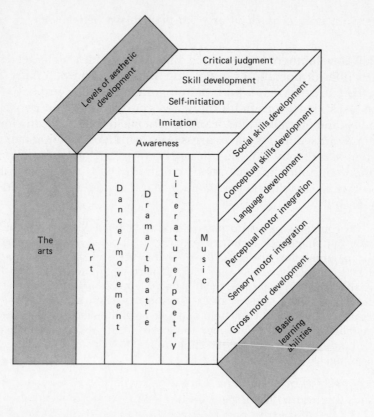

Figure 9–3. Arts for learning conceptual model. Modified from: National Committee, Arts with the Handicapped. *Arts Resource and Training Guide.* Washington, D.C.: NCAH, p. 59.

through the arts. Their successes also have helped make the general public aware that disabled individuals have a great deal to offer society. Such public awareness is of benefit to all special population members, regardless of their artistic talents.

It should be noted also that the arts has proven to be an excellent vehicle for public awareness when the subject (irrespective of the creator and performer) refers to disability. The Kids on the Block, for example, is a puppet troupe that provides outstanding entertainment while at the same time focuses on issues of disability. It is a joy to observe the audience react to these puppets, most of which portray youngsters with disabilities. Teenagers smile with understanding when a girl puppet, wearing leg braces, sings that she is the only kid on the block who can wear braces and chew gum at the same time; adults laugh when the puppet with Downs Syndrome states, "I have my ups and my Downs"; and all of the youngsters in the audience wave their hands in anticipation, hoping to ask questions about the puppets' disabilities during a question and answer session. Janus (1981) emphasized the value of the Kids on the Block program. Advocating the use of a specially prepared kit to aid teachers, she wrote:

> When one considers the implications of Bill 82 in Ontario [Canada] schools, which provides for education for every child in his/her least restricted environment, the problem of immediate integration of disabled people into society becomes apparent. The Kids on the Block Teachers' Kit, used as a medium for the creation of positive attitudes toward disabled peers and their integration into the visible majority, is a move toward the solution. The message is clear. It hits *home.* (p. 35)

The end result of the Kids on the Block is more than mere entertainment for those in attendance. As Malloy (1978) pointed out, "... The arts reflect and inspire the hopes and struggles of society. Struggling for their place in society, handicapped people can infuse the arts with a completely new range of human experiences, and through the arts inspire the public to accept them for their gifts rather than their needs" (p. 39).

The five benefits of arts participation are not all encompassing, of course. Nor, as noted by Ross (1980), should they be interpreted to mean that everyone benefits equally from artistic pursuits. Just as some people will display more artistic talent than others, some will benefit more than others from arts involvement. It was stated previously that the benefits of arts participation are similar for both disabled and nondisabled people. The *degree* of benefit may differ, however. Spencer (1978) described the importance of art lessons in a German concentration camp during World War II, and proposed that the need for art increases during times of crisis. For many people with disabilities the challenges of daily life approach crisis proportions, so their need for arts involvement may be much greater than their nondisabled peers. Regardless of whether their need is greater or the same as everyone else's, however, two important principles should be recognized: (1) Everyone, including people with disabilities, can enjoy and benefit from participation in the arts; and (2) each art form can benefit from the unique perspective offered by disabled participants. After experiencing the following poem by Christy Brown, few could dispute either of these statements:

> *To Helen Keller*
>
> *I heard it on a plain undreaming day*
> *hunched by the squat old toadstool of a radio*
> *that never did give out the news clearly anyway.*
> *You had just died.*

The house lay in Sunday morning silence
Out in the dull pavement-gray day
people sulked or strutted to church
full of their little unholy terrors and persecutions.

I nursed my headful of dreary dissipation
half hearing the erratic static of the gut-twisted radio
that remote disembodied faraway stilted voice
jerking over the crammed and jammed airlanes of
*   man-made mayhem:*
"We regret to announce the death of . . . "

I heard the news alone.
Alone when I most needed someone to share this sorrow
and yet would most certainly have resented that intrusion.
Such a sorrow is never shared
as that kind of triumph is seldom won.
I felt a momentary surprise.
Surprise that so beautiful a life should have a closing
so like any other.
As if beauty can ever know a close.

Yet I knew
and felt envious.
Envious of your life and your dying.

A symphony only you could listen to
throbbing at your fingertips like light.
A vision beyond the crazy charade of sight.
A dream torn from pain
that had in it all the music of all the birds
that ever sang in this deaf-mute world.

You who saw such splendor of light
heard such a marvel of music
conversed and had your being with such beauty.
You shrank my shrill little world to an atom
made me lift my eyes to pain
and not decline the chalice.

(Reprinted with permission of Stein and Day Publishers.)

NATIONAL COMMITTEE, ARTS WITH THE HANDICAPPED*

Because of the many benefits offered by the arts, the Joseph P. Kennedy, Jr., Foundation provided funding in 1974 to support a National Confer-

*This committee changed its name in 1986. It is now known as Very Special Arts.

ence on Arts with the Mentally Retarded. The interest created by this conference eventually resulted in the formation of the National Committee, Arts with the Handicapped (NCAH). An educational affiliate of the John F. Kennedy Center for the Performing Arts, the NCAH receives support from the U.S. Office of Education and the Alliance for Arts Education, as well as from the Joseph P. Kennedy, Jr., Foundation. Its main function is the coordination of nationwide efforts to provide arts programs for individuals with disabilities. This function is reflected in the following mission statement:

> The mission of the National Committee, Arts with the Handicapped is to assure that disabled individuals have equal opportunity to participate in programs which demonstrate the value of the arts in the lives of all individuals and provide opportunities for the integration of disabled people into society.

The NCAH has five goals that demonstrate the Committee's dedication not only to program development and implementation in the arts, but also to research, training, technical assistance, public awareness, and interagency coordination. Each of these goals has stated general objectives that the NCAH feels are both realistic and obtainable. The NCAH goals are:

Goal 1. To support the initiation and expansion of arts-related programs that enhance learning and enrich the lives of disabled persons.

Goal 2. To initiate and support research, development, and evaluation activities relating to programming in the arts for disabled persons.

Goal 3. To provide arts-related training and technical assistance to those agencies and individuals who provide services to disabled persons.

Goal 4. To develop and implement systems that demonstrate effective interagency cooperation and community involvement in providing services in the arts for disabled individuals.

Goal 5. To expand international awareness and to provide a system for sharing information about existing programs in the arts for disabled persons.

Among the many exciting programs supported by the NCAH is the Very Special Arts Festival (VSAF) Program. This program offers opportunities for disabled and nondisabled youngsters to develop their talents in the visual and performing arts. Thus, in preparing to demonstrate their artistic skill before an audience, the children are placed in an ideal situation for promoting integration. All participants are encouraged to express their own individuality in a noncompetitive way. In addition, working toward the annual festival requires a year-round cooperative effort from everyone involved. This unique blending of individual expression with collective cooperation toward a group goal provides the perfect environment for lasting integration of disabled and nondisabled people.

The VSAF Program's impact extends well beyond the young participants, too. Parents, artists, teachers, and spectators all benefit from a variety of arts experiences. Demonstrations, workshops, exhibits, and a multitude of performances are all part of the annual festival that concludes a year of preparation. In-service training is a special emphasis of the VSAF Program, so everyone connected with the festival's educational efforts is well prepared for his or her role. Spectators leave the festival with a new appreciation for the abilities that disabled artists possess, and through such experiences the general public becomes more aware of the valuable contribution made by the arts to the lives of all persons. The VSAF is, indeed, a very special program.

LEADERSHIP IN THE ARTS

The quality of any arts program or activity is dependent upon its leadership. This is especially true if the program or activity is accessible to individuals with disabilities. It has been estimated that only 12 percent of the more than 8 million disabled children and youth in the United States participate in arts programs (Sherrill & Routon, 1980). This fact is staggering when one considers the many joys and benefits that result from participation in the arts, particularly at an early age. As previously mentioned, this situation also deprives the arts of the unique perspective that only participants who have disabilities can provide. The lack of arts programs for individuals with disabilities, whether integrated or segregated in structure, can be overcome only through knowledgeable, energetic, and effective leadership.

In June, 1977, a symposium coordinated by the National Committee, Arts with the Handicapped, and The National Aesthetic Learning Center provided a better understanding of the prerequisities for effective leadership, as well as some competencies that are desirable for arts personnel. The participants at the symposium identified the following key concerns:

■ A comprehensive approach for educating arts education personnel must be developed at all levels: national, state, university.

- Most arts educators are unfamiliar with the special emotional, physical and mental needs of the handicapped child and the resulting programmatic adaptations that must be made in order to provide accessible and high quality creative arts experiences.
- Changes in curriculum materials, teaching techniques, arrangements of classroom space, and so forth, must be considered to integrate the handicapped child into the regular arts education classroom or to develop more individualized and specialized arts education programs.
- Qualified personnel are needed to ensure that handicapped children are no longer denied opportunities to learn about the arts, through the arts, in the arts.
- The current national status of arts education reflects an emphasis on music and the visual arts; equal experiences must be provided by qualified personnel in drama and dance.
- Arts educators are generally unfamiliar with the scope, nature, and impact of the Education for All Handicapped Children Act (Public Law 94–142) and Section 504 of the 1973 Rehabilitation Act.
- Pre-service and in-service training programs for arts educators should systematically identify training resource personnel, including special educators, handicapped and non-handicapped artists, parents of handicapped children, art therapists, state and local arts agencies, and institutional personnel. (NCAH, 1981, 42–43)

The primary implication of the preceding list is clear. Personnel working with persons who have disabilities need adequate training, both in the arts and in how to lead arts activities effectively. It is not possible, within the scope of this chapter, to provide a comprehensive guide for leaders of arts activities that would encompass all art forms and all types of disabling conditions. We may, however, offer a few essential principles for successful leadership of an arts program that includes participants with disabilities. These principles include:

1. Determine program goals. What you are trying to accomplish through your arts program should be expressed as written goals. These program goals, to a large extent, will guide decision making in such matters as the amount of integration desired, leadership style employed, whether cooperative group projects are more desirable than individual efforts, and so on. One area of special concern in the arts is the relative importance of the final product in comparison with the *process* used to achieve the final product. Although there will be some situations that require a strong emphasis upon the finished product, the authors of this textbook agree with the following statement by Roehner (1981):

> . . . a blind child working with finger paint may express a feeling of being loved by making magnificent circles in finger paint. The product may not be aesthetically pleasing but the kinesthetic treatment of the soft paint with circular motions indicates that the student perceives something of emotion, love, and is responding to it and to the medium. It is the art of expressing that is important, not the product. (p. 6)

Putting the final sentence of Roehner's commentary into a written goal statement would help ensure that program leaders approach all arts activities in a consistent way.

2. Encourage Creativity. Moran (1979) contended that the creative talents of individuals are "often thwarted, ignored, or tossed aside by [others] on the grounds that they work against long established human

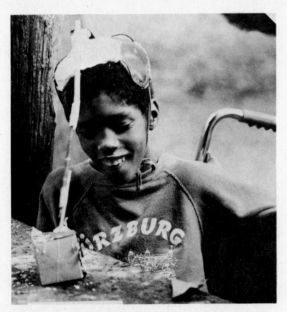

Figure 9–4. Modifications may be required to allow successful arts participation. For example, attaching a brush to a helmet can enable a participant who has upper extremity limitations to experience the joy of painting his *own* crafts project. (Courtesy of the League for the Handicapped, Baltimore, MD)

traditions" (p. 48). The arts, however, should provide activities that encourage, rather than discourage, creative expression. Prefabricated or highly structured arts activities should be minimized or eliminated, and program leaders should emphasize flexibility in each activity. The leader's importance in fostering creativity cannot be overemphasized. The leader can serve as a role model by expressing his or her own individuality while, at the same time, communicating to each participant that there is no such thing as failure in the arts (Kunkle-Miller, 1981). Successful integration is much easier to attain when creativity is emphasized. Children with mental retardation, for example, may be able to achieve high status in an integrated arts group because they do not differ significantly from their nonretarded peers on nonverbal measures of creativity (Sherill & Cox, 1979). Ross (1980) also stressed the importance of creativity and stated that arts leaders should create conditions of creativity by:

1. establishing the sanctity of mutual truthfulness.
2. developing trust (trustworthiness and mutual trustfulness).
3. being free enough to free students to act playfully, to explore and invent an atmosphere that is nonjudgmental, where error is essential to trial.
4. providing conditions of psychic safety—being compassionate.
5. being devoted to the child's learning and growth. (p. 110)

Unless creativity is allowed to flourish, many of the benefits of arts participation will be lost.

3. Individualize Activities. Each arts activity should be geared, as much as possible, to the skill level and personal needs of each participant. The demands of a given activity should be compared with the participant's capabilities, and modifications made when appropriate. The following are a few considerations for offering arts activities to participants with disabilities:

1. Time, space, and materials may need to be limited in order to meet specific needs.
2. Emphasis should be placed on the senses by using appropriate materials—i.e., sand, finger paints, soft cloth or yarn, aromatic fragrances, audible devices, etc.
3. Small group size is often preferable to larger groups, and forming a circle increases feelings of unity in some activities, such as dance.
4. A logical progression of skill development should occur, starting with tasks that have been mastered and proceeding to more difficult ones.

5. Reinforce accomplishments with appropriate praise. This rewards participation and gives the individual a feeling of success.

Ananda Coomaraswamy, an Indian writer, is credited with stating that "the artist is not a special kind of man, but every man is a special kind of artist" (Shaw, 1980, p. 73). Individualizing arts activities brings out the "specialness" in each participant, irrespective of disability.

4. Plan for Access. In their 1975 publication *Arts and the Handicapped: An Issue of Access*, the Educational Facilities Laboratories (EFL) and the National Endowment for the Arts (NEA) stated, " . . . the vast majority of handicapped people still perceive the arts as an inconvenient obstacle course strewn with rules, regulations, revolving doors, and inaccessible opportunities" (p. 6). Public laws have helped improve this situation (see Chapter 12), but it often is necessary to make special preparations to ensure that arts programs are accessible to and usable by people with disabilities. Architectural barriers often limit participation by those who have disabilities, but public attitudes are important, also, when planning for access. The EFL and NEA (1975) noted that the use of "tactile" art galleries, which allow artifacts to be handled by blind individuals, is criticized by some museum officials because "they fear that artifacts will be at worst destroyed and at best soiled by repeated handling" (p. 20). Sadly, such attitudes serve to prevent people with disabilities from becoming patrons of the arts. Access depends upon both removal of physical obstacles *and* change of attitudinal barriers.

5. Attend In-service Training Programs. As the arts participant increases in skill, his or her changing needs may require a change in teaching methods and materials. Similarly, the leader of an arts program should continue to grow by seeking relevant and informative in-service training opportunities. Unfortunately, many such programs focus solely on awareness or sensitivity training in one specific arts area. Selecting *quality* in-service programs, however, can result in benefits. The NCAH (1981) cautions potential in-service participants, " . . . the frequency and length of individual training sessions has much less to do with effectiveness, than the quality of the instructor, format and resources" (p. 169). Careful selection is required, but in-service training for arts leaders can result in better arts programs for participants who have disabilities.

ARTS PARTICIPATION—TWO EXAMPLES

This chapter has provided information about the arts and people with disabilities, but to really understand the *personal* nature of arts involvement we need to examine actual examples of arts participation. Rather than give superficial information on many of the excellent programs around the country, we have selected two in-depth examples. One of these focuses on an individual participant, Claudia Fowler, and the deep personal fulfillment she received from writing poetry. The other, Theatre Unlimited, presents group participation in the arts (theatre), and highlights creative expression, attitude change, and integration through the arts.

Claudia Fowler

Claudia Fowler died on December 11, 1981. In most ways Claudia's life was not exceptional, but she had cerebral palsy and scoliosis which, for all of her 32 years, resulted in almost complete dependency upon others. She could not walk; neither could she dress, bathe, eat, nor use the toilet unassisted. Claudia could speak, but only people who spent a great deal of time with her could understand. Many whose lives touched Claudia's thought she had severe mental retardation—they did not take the time to find out if she could comprehend what they were saying. "Claudia couldn't understand why people who knew her, even some relatives, would speak to her as if she were a child," commented her mother, Catherine L. Fowler. "That's something I will never understand, either," she added, slowly shaking her head.

> *Feelings*
>
> *People are not just specimens of the physical anatomy,*
> *   they consist of mysterious and unpredictable things which*
> *   are known as feelings.*
> *Feelings aren't something that we can control*
> *   although sometimes we'd give anything if we could;*
> *   they're a part of life which is involuntary.*
> *Occasionally, we become timid about expressing our feelings,*
> *   and they grow into a whirlpool of frustrations within us.*
> *To share our feelings with someone,*
> *   is like releasing a herd of wild mustangs;*
> *   it places our innermost soul in a state of tranquility*
> *   and freedom.*
>
> *(Claudia, 1978)*

Claudia attended "special" elementary and junior high schools in the Baltimore, Maryland, area. It was many years before P. L. 94–142 (Education for All Handicapped Children Act), however, so the regular high schools were not accessible to individuals using wheelchairs.

Denied the right to attend high school, Claudia was taught by home tutors until she received her high school diploma in 1968. Home instruction did enable Claudia to develop her cognitive abilities, but it deprived her of one very important aspect of the teen years—social interaction with peers.

Remedy for Loneliness

Today, pearl-gray clouds fill the sky,
  making the solitude seem more intense,
Loneliness is the most agonizing sickness,
  with no chemical pain reliever known;
    it is the slowest form of suicide
Being lonely and withdrawn from people,
  is just as poisonous as any
    type of malignancy.
This senseless illness has the simplest remedy in the world,
  a friend.
One other thing is also needed,
  a willingness to trust your fellow man.

                                              (Claudia, 1977)

Community programs developed exclusively for individuals with physical disabilities became Claudia's primary source for social interaction. Many of these programs, however, required that she conform to the leader's plans, rather than allowing her the freedom to pursue her own interests. "Claudia became very frustrated with some of the programs she attended," her mother recalled. "A woman at one program *insisted* that she participate in a cooking class. After the class Claudia said to me, 'Mother, I'll never be able to cook! Why can't I be allowed to do what I want?'" Few of these programs could offer her the freedom she desired—the freedom to express her individuality in her own way. This need for self-expression was met when Claudia began to write poetry.

"My first attempts at writing poetry began in 1974," wrote Claudia. "It is a bit difficult to describe just how I come up with a poem. It builds up inside of me, but not in my mind, until I start to type. The words just keep coming 'til I type the last word in a poem. It is sort of like giving birth." Most of the thoughts included in Claudia's poems evolved while she lay in bed at night reflecting on her favorite themes of animals, nature, and human emotions. In the morning, her poems were "born" at an electric typewriter. Claudia could not use her arms and hands to type, of course, but she did have some control of her head movements. She painstakingly pecked at the typewriter keys using a metal pointer attached to a head band. As with most severely disabled people with cerebral palsy, the amount of muscular control Claudia possessed varied from moment to moment. The more relaxed she was, the better she was able to type. She wrote, "To type a poem takes me anywhere from half an hour to a week depending on the length of the poem and how nervous I feel. Of course, some days are better than others." Claudia could relax best when she was able to spend time out of doors. Whether she was sitting behind her rural home overlooking acres of fields and woods, or on a hike at the resident camp she loved, Camp Greentop, Claudia was fascinated by the wonders of nature.

> *Perfect Day*
>
> *If a mystical person suddenly materialized to grant me one*
>   *perfect day,*
>   *I know exactly the things I would order.*
> *It would be a bright, warm, late Spring day,*
>   *with the birds singing their songs in the meadow-green shade*
>   *of the rich, new foliage of the trees;*
>   *as the honeybees and butterflies dart and dash from flower*
>   *to flower as though they were on a city-wide shopping*
>   *spree.*
> *The first thing I'd wish to do would be to soar through the clouds,*
>   *and let the golden eagle act as my guide.*
> *To have the creatures of the forest as my teachers,*
>   *so I may learn their many secrets;*
>   *and I promise not to tell a single soul.*
> *Let me follow the wild mustangs*
>   *as they race with the wind of the plains.*
> *May I be given the privilege of accompanying the white-tail deer,*
>   *while they quench their thirst at a clear, spring-fed stream.*
> *I would observe as many activities of nature as time would allow,*
>   *and request that you share it all with me.*
>
>   *(Claudia, 1979)*

It was at Camp Greentop, a resident camp located in western Maryland, that Claudia met Peter Setlow and his wife, Barbara. Pete, the camp's Program Director, appreciated Claudia's intellect and took a sincere interest in her. The friendship between Claudia and the Setlow family, particularly Pete, continued year-round until Claudia's death. The importance of friendship in anyone's life cannot be overestimated, but to someone with a severe disability the joy of having a genuine friend may transcend all other emotions. Pete, Barbara, and later their children, Barry and Jenny, added much happiness to Claudia's life. But, as the Setlows are quick to point out, knowing Claudia also enriched their lives immensely.

Never a Stranger, Again

When I first saw you,
*   you were just a stranger to me.*
But you, along with time have,
*   in some mysterious way;*
*   claimed a segment of my life.*
Unlike most of life's gifts which fade with time
*   the treasure of you in my life will last forever.*

(Claudia, 1976)

What You Mean To Me

To peer into your autumn leaf-brown eyes and perceive how much
*   you care without a single word being spoken,*
*   is something mystical which only you possess.*
When you arms tenderly encompass me,
*   it is as though an invisible fortress materializes to obstruct*
*   life's annoyances and disappointments.*
You have taught me many important things,
*   but among the most invaluable is that someone does care about*
*   me as a person.*
Uncertain of whether you are aware of what you mean to me,
*   I yearn for the day when everything is as tranquil as a*
*   mid-winter's morning;*
*   and there will be time for you to listen to my memorized*
*   inventory of all the wonderful ways that you*
*   supplement my life.*

(Claudia, 1978)

Two Important Arrivals
(dedicated to Barry and Jenny Setlow)

The sky is the color of the robin's broken egg shell,
*   given to me by someone very special.*
This fragile gift rests in a small, gray-blue box on
*   my reference book shelf,*
*   where it becomes a welcome sight from*
*   typewriter*
*   keys, papers and books.*

> Looking into my dresser mirror,
>   two, important, little people gaze down at me
>   from
>   a photograph held tightly by the mirror's
>   frame.
> It is possible to see you both grow up again and
> again.
>   simply by glancing at the row of photographs
>   spread
>   along the middle shelf of my bookcase.
> From a Halloween dog and a little hobo,
>   to two, bright elementary school students.
> While looking through some old photographs the
> other
>   night,
>   I came across a couple of baby pictures.
> It is difficult to realize that so many years have
>   come and gone since the two of you first entered
>   this world,
>   but I didn't know what I was missing until
>   your arrival.
>
> *(Claudia, 1980)*

The last few months of Claudia's life were spent in the hospital. She was not physically strong, but her faith and friendships sustained her. Finally, however, in late 1981, respiratory failure claimed Claudia's life.

> Life
>
> Life is a strange thing,
>   which can't be explained in just a few words.
> It is the happiness found in a new healthy baby,
>   or the sadness of a senseless death.
> The gleam in the eyes of a child as he tried to
>   blow out the candle on his first birthday cake
>   or the empty look in the eyes of a lonely old
>   man as he gazes out the window on his ninety-first
>   birthday.
> That hard struggle of a young intelligent girl lifting
>   herself from the apathy of the slums,
>   or the wealthy sophisticated debutante;
>   who has her desires and goals handed to her
>   without having to strive for them.
> It is seeing and appreciating the beautiful wonders of nature,
>   and not taking them for granted.

> *Life is made of these things and so much more,*
> *but above all else, it is the most precious thing*
> *that we will ever have and*
> *it should be cherished.*
>
> *(Claudia, 1976)*

Final Comment

Claudia Fowler was not included in this chapter because she possessed exceptional literary talent. Until now, none of her poems has been published, although a friend did have some of them bound into a volume entitled *A Bridge to My Thoughts*. Claudia was unique because every individual, whether disabled or nondisabled, is unique. The arts simply provided Claudia with a meaningful way of expressing her individuality. A British woman, who had a disability that distorted her facial features and prevented speech, once wrote, "It's my body you see, not my mind." Through her poems, we get a glimpse of Claudia Fowler's bright and sensitive mind.

Theatre Unlimited*

Theatre Unlimited is a dramatic ensemble that shatters popular myths about mental retardation. Composed of half developmentally disabled and half nondisabled actors, the company is dedicated to a creative process that provides a vision; the vision is that of a community of spirit, where love sparks the transformation process allowing the performer to risk and the viewer to perceive in new ways. Through visual and corporeal images, a spectrum of pain and exhilaration is revealed. The company sustains the life of those who live and work with the denials of severe limitation. Theatre Unlimited is changing the context and aesthetics of theatre. Performances throughout the nation provide a model for artists, educators, recreators, and therapists, and present new attitudes and approaches to the general public.

Process. Theatre Unlimited's work is based on transformation and revelation. The ensemble addresses many of its members' needs—physical, emotional, and intellectual—while offering society a model for the

*Theatre Unlimited is a program of the San Francisco Recreation Center for the Handicapped, Inc. The Company's publication, *Theatre Unlimited*, was funded by a grant from the Evelyn J. and Walter Hass, Jr., Foundation, and the Sandy Foundation. The booklet was written by David Morgan, Herb Felsenfeld, and Richard Heus, and appears in modified form with permission of the authors and the San Francisco Recreation Center for the Handicapped, Inc.

future. In addressing these needs, the actors approach a nurturing quality of spirit, which when viewed by an audience has applications in many realms.

The persona of the actor is central to this process. The actor transforms images of sound/movement and quantities of time/space for the single purpose of exposing a soul in public. As one audience member discovered, "There is someone up there, who is beyond labels, beyond pity and fear—someone who is more like myself than I ever realized."

The roots of Theatre Unlimited lie in developmental theatre. A relatively new approach, this form seeks to prepare the actor physically and vocally, with an extra emphasis on emotional development and group process or ensemble work. Theatre Unlimited defines an ensemble as "a group of supporting players who work together to create a single effect." The struggle towards this goal is unifying in ways that go beyond performance and artistic product. This ensemble process is reflected in all aspects of the company's work and play. The ensemble is able to sustain a flow of energy throughout warm-ups, rehearsals, discussions, and performances. Concentration and focused interactions are nurtured and find expression through sound, movement, and physical contact. Like improvisational theatre (another approach utilized by Theatre Unlimited), ensemble process demands the development of trust, support and cooperation. Through this approach emerges a level of honesty and caring that has allowed the company to clearly mature from year to year.

Developmental theatre builds on the critical ability of the actors much more than on the ability of the director. Actors' contributions lead the director and the playwright. This method draws its content from personal experiences and self-discoveries.

While it is true that a nondisabled actor can express a movement or a dramatic gesture with more fluidity than a performer with cerebral palsy, it is equally true that sincerity of ensemble effort achieves artistic excellence. Theatre Unlimited has forged its own identity, and there is much that can be done only by the artists in Theatre Unlimited. The work is built on discipline and imagination, the principal ingredients of theatre art. As one participant expressed:

> Well, my disability is also in the head.
> Most of the time I do
> have seizures. When I have seizures I completely
> black out. I don't even know where I am, or
> if I'm in room, in the room, in the
> Most of the time when I have a real big seizure
> my speech I can't even see what I'm doing
> or when I'm standing I fall down

on the floor. And sometimes I could hit my head
and knocked out.
But, this work, well Yes
People are nice pleasant funny
sometimes they're bossy
sometimes not
and learning to act
Being an actress is not easy
but I am still learning
Also interesting How drama
I have a very good imagination and
· I can imagine a lot of things.
I didn't use to have a good imagination. Before.
Now I do. I've learned what time to come and
when to go. I'm going to a few classes for jobs.
I'm also a volunteer for serving foods on tables.
Yes Theater helped for responsibility.

Rehearsal. Theatre Unlimited first met on September 19, 1977, and decided that initially each three-hour rehearsal would consist of a full hour of physical warm-ups, followed by a half hour of partnered exchanges such as mirror exercises and give-and-take games, an hour for the introduction of ensemble activities, and a half hour at the end for group discussion and sharing. It turned out, however, that too-much-structure-too-soon inhibited both growth and the possibility of new discoveries.

While building and maintaining a ritual of starting with group warm-ups, and closing with a circle for discussion and sharing, the company loosened the time in between to allow for spontaneous occurrences and to accommodate specific rehearsal needs.

The warm-up routine incorporates traditional theatre exercises along with the company's collective knowledge of techniques from yoga, T'ai Chi, mime, and dance. The first year was challenging work for everyone. Nothing came easily. Through the basic techniques of task analysis and physical sensitivity training, Theatre Unlimited determined what steps contributed to the learning of each skill. As individual movement began to come more easily, self-confidence grew. A common vocabulary of movement and sound was developed from activities that encouraged risk taking, trust, and initiative.

Particularly important was the time taken to study and learn the essential skill of relaxation. From a calm basis, sessions continually maintained a flow of energy that rarely demanded a break. From the beginning, energy was high and the intensive level of training produced slow yet steady progress. The abled to disabled ratio of the company allowed the participants to become close working partners. At first, some members were confused by the abstract nature of the work. To them drama meant putting on a play. Common questions were: "What's this mirror for?" or "Why am I relaxing?" Then and today, it is necessary to continually struggle for a common vocabulary, one accessible to all company members. The group concentrated on the basic building blocks of actor training, sound and movement, and began to put more and more imagery to its physical work. By connecting concrete images to movement, understanding began to increase and entire movement combinations were assimilated.

Much early work focused on building the trust necessary to function well as an ensemble. Games and exercises were introduced that demanded this response. Actors leaned on each other with full body weight. They formed a tight circle and took turns falling into waiting arms. One partner led the other, blind-folded, through strange environments. Because these games placed few cognitive demands, success was easily noted.

Learning is frequently divided into three categories: cognitive, affective, and physical. While research shows that those with normal intelligence score significantly higher in verbal measures of creativity—or the cognitive domain—there are no significant differences between retarded and nonretarded on nonverbal measures of creativity. Developmentally disabled often show strengths in imaginative behavior and willingness to trust, take risks, and be spontaneous. From its inception, Theatre Unlimited's process has been built on this research and on the belief that a creative theatre form that relies on nonverbal activity can evolve.

The mirror game is the best example of this kind of nonverbal activity. With its many variations, it has been an essential part of ensemble training. A partnered exercise of follow-the-leader, the mirror exercise demands great concentration. Often performed to slow, flowing music, it involves both precise imitation, as well as creative initiation. As roles are reversed and partners changed, actors begin to know each other as individual expressive people.

At the end of each three-hour session the ensemble sits in a circle and talks. When pressed for reactions to the evening's rehearsal, disabled members often find it difficult to articulate specific feelings. It has been particularly gratifying for the company to become close enough for all to share reactions and feelings.

While progress seemed slow in the areas of physical conditioning and cognitive understanding, the company never remained frustrated. Something very exciting was happening on an effective awareness level. As David Morgan remembers, "We were having a great time playing together. The company was growing in its feelings for one another. We cared." Sharing, especially in nonverbal ways, began to balance in importance with the pace of Theatre Unlimited's skill building. One participant stated:

> Here I've learned about timing—after ten years of working with disabled people. I've finally allowed myself the time to wait. It's different timing than I would use. But when someone else uses it, it's unique. Here, I find that disabled people 'can do'. For years we've been told that they can't. The progression is amazing—people are expressing themselves, they are saying things to each other, to the audience. I can take that knowledge of slow steady growth back to my job and use that with my hope that people will change. It may take 2 or 3 weeks, maybe 2 or 3 years.

Performance.   Theatre Unlimited views its approach to performance as a direct and logical outgrowth of rehearsals and workshops. Performance is looked at as a way station along a developmental continuum and the audience is invited to participate in the viewing of this process.

Nondisabled actors are often anxious at the thought of public viewing, especially when the piece is in embryo form. Fear stalks the rehearsal floor. During that beginning time the members who have disabilities take a different approach. They are primarily concerned with what will happen next—just the daily schedule, not a grand design. It is okay that the score has not been completed. A lesson slowly takes hold; anxiety grows into trust, if faith is there to slow the process, so a form may develop that can enclose the whole scope of the work.

The company's first performed score (an outline of events that occur in sequence around a theme) was called "The Initiation." Its theme involved two groups of strangers learning each other's rituals, and eventually coming together. The score was also an accurate reflection of the company's stage of development. Tensions, anxieties, and mistrust existed. Instead of being looked at as problems, these fears were incorporated into the creative process, and solutions, developed through rehearsal, were shared in public.

"The Initiation" was given its first performance in May 1978, at the Fort Mason Center in San Francisco. Technical aspects of the piece remained simple—as much out of choice as out of financial necessity. Performing barefoot in leotard tops and drawstring pants against a dark backdrop, the group utilized masks and live percussion accompaniment.

The outcome of the first year's exploration involved work that was primarily in sound and movement. Work was at a level of physical interaction akin to dance-theatre. Because of its grounding in improvisation, the company was able to transform mistakes, missed cues, and delayed entrances into appropriate happenings. A style was beginning to evolve. The audience saw that support could be a demanding and exciting physical discipline.

In January 1979, the group began working on a new piece. Another level of development happened during that second year. The score grew in complexity. New elements included performing parts of the sequence in American Sign Language; creating a particular place, a playground, through the actors' imaginative skills; refining the company's sound/movement skills to extend into the area of physical and spatial transformation; and integrating song and poetry into the sequence.

As in the first year, anxiety grew in direct proportion to the complexity of the work. A group of actors not knowing what is going to happen next can lead to the artistic equivalent of a haunted house. In getting through this year, reserves of faith were tested. The proof of the work's value was in the public reaction. Audience response—especially during moments when the planned "next move" did not occur—gave the company reassurance. People were once again genuinely intrigued by what they saw. The awkward, the amateurish, were transformed into the deeply human, the deeply affecting. The audience participated in the event. The act of faith *played*.

For Theatre Unlimited, performance is a laboratory where the group can explore and reveal greater understanding of the developmental process. The performance laboratory is a place where ideas, not personalities, dominate.

Workshops. Workshops are the way Theatre Unlimited reaches out and opens its process to the audience. Here the momentum of performance winds down, the fourth wall between viewer and actor opens and the empty space fills with the activities of revelation.

It is during these activities, at least from the perspective of the viewer, that the way the company works is more exposed. When the public can see the company members' interrelationships, which are the core of performance training, then the model becomes accessible for replication.

People—from school-age children on up—are involved in an intensely physical experience. What begins as two groups, actors and viewers, soon coalesces into one group that functions on different levels. The line starts to blur. What of the disability? Does it make any difference?

Here the viewer is put into a unique situation: for example, working with a man who has Down's Syndrome, is almost nonverbal, and is engaged in bending over to touch the top of his head to his toe. Not knee. Toe. Perception shifts, and the mind moves on to the next level of wonder. A woman with mental retardation shows a university professor how to master an isolation exercise. Ground is broken, and the meaning of the word "disabled" changes.

The essential role of workshops in the company's comprehensive program is skills-building in such areas as: physical and vocal flexibility, assertiveness and leadership, and social awareness and personal responsibility. The co-leaders demonstrate activities in a way that is free of self-consciousness and embarrassment. As each participant finds a level of success, the group becomes increasingly more spontaneous. A developmental model has been designed for these activities to ensure progression at an individually determined rate. Moving from relaxation to awareness of personal resources, each person connects with the environment and with a partner. The process continues through to the beginning of ensemble work.

As the activities are co-led, attitudes among lay people are challenged, and professionals in the field find themselves among the learners. Institutional staffs, especially, are often victims of their own form of disability—that of losing sight of the humanity of the people they serve. With the infusion of Theatre Unlimited, their energy is expanded and their perspectives are altered. The effect is tonic-like, and the company is a refresher to workers deserving strength and encouragement.

The most uninhibited reactions, and in many ways the most challenging and gratifying, are those involving school children. Students in the second and third grades have not learned to label and stereotype. They can hardly wait to share energy and games. As they look to all company members as equals, their learning is accelerated and they are soon involved in a joyful experience. The workshop atmosphere is exciting, with a sense of wonder that is barrier-free, as the following quote attests:

> What I want from the general public is honesty. I see how our process has changed people in our company, because now people are together with those they can trust, we can confide in each other, talk and really feel like we're getting honest feedback. There was not communication, before, between some of these people. You could sit down and listen to people talk, and one person would be talking and the other person would respond on a totally different subject. There was no real communication, there was no feeling. Now I sit and listen to our company talk and it's amazing. It's almost too much. It's 'you know, I really like you.' All this out front stuff.

Theatre Unlimited functions as a reflection of our particular time and culture, in addition to acting as a model of events about to happen.

As long as the model remains healthy, it will point toward a time of unobstructed access to creative tools for all people.

―――――――――――――――――― **SUMMARY** ――――――――――――――――――

The arts help to form and also to reflect the national character of society. As a result, it is essential that *all* members of society be provided the opportunity to participate in the arts. Such participation may be through the creation of an original work of art, but it also may be through performing the work of another artist, or even perceiving the artistic efforts of another in a creative way. These three levels of art participation offer limitless opportunities for enjoyment and satisfaction, as well as personal growth. This is especially true for people who have disabilities because their opportunities for personal growth experiences may be more limited than those of nondisabled individuals.

Suggested Learning Activities

1. Name the three levels of participation in the arts, and give (from your own experiences) specific examples of each.

2. Interview a community recreation arts specialist and determine the ways in which individuals are encouraged to participate in all three levels of arts participation.

3. Write a poem that expresses your feelings concerning the arts for everyone.

4. Examine the activities offered by a local recreation center. Specify five arts activities that could be incorporated into the program, and discuss the benefits of each activity.

5. Discuss why it is important for nondisabled individuals to experience the artistic efforts of people with disabilities.

6. Discuss ways that community recreators can use the arts as a tool to allow individuals with disabilities to express their own feelings or needs.

References

Appell, M. J. An overview: Arts in education for the handicapped. In National Committee, Arts for the Handicapped, *The Arts and Handicapped People: Defining the National Direction*. Washington, D.C.: NCAH, 1978, pp. 13–17.

Diamondstein, G. *Exploring the Arts with Children*. New York: MacMillan, 1974.

Educational Facilities Laboratory and the National Endowment for the Arts. *Arts and the Handicapped: An Issue of Access*. New York: Educational Facilities Laboratory, 1975.

Hayman, d'A. Introduction. In UNESCO, *The Arts and Man: A World View of the Role and Functions of the Arts in Society*. Englewood Cliffs, NJ: Prentice-Hall, 1969, pp. 11–26.

Janus, C. The Kids on the Block: An effective medium for positive attitude change. *Journal of Leisurability*, 8(4), 32–35, 1981.

Kennedy, J. Insight into blindness. In Bernstein, E., ed. *1985 Medical and Health Annual*. Chicago: Encyclopaedia Britannica, 1985, pp. 154–165.

Kunkle-Miller, C. Handicapping conditions and their effect on the child's ability to create. In Kearns, L. H., M. T. Ditson, and B. G. Roehner, eds. *Readings: Developing Art Programs for Handicapped Students*. Harrisburg, PA: Arts in Special Education Project of Pennsylvania, 1981, pp. 8–20.

Molloy, L. Public facilities and handicapped patrons. In National Committee, Arts for the Handicapped, *The Arts and Handicapped People: Defining the National Direction*. Washington, D.C.: NCAH, 1978, pp. 37–39.

Moran, J. Mainstreaming severely and profoundly handicapped children. In *Creative Arts for the Severely Handicapped*. Springfield, IL: Charles C. Thomas, 1979, pp. 47–56.

National Committee, Arts for the Handicapped. *Art Resource and Training Guide*. Washington, D.C.: NCAH, 1981.

Perks, W. Self expression through the arts: A human right. In Sherrill, C., ed. *Creative Arts for the Severely Handicapped*. Springfield, IL: Charles C. Thomas, 1979, pp. 25–28.

Roehner, B. G. What is an arts program? In Kearns, L. H., M. T. Ditson, and B. G. Roehner, eds. *Readings: Developing Arts Programs for Handicapped Students*. Harrisburg, PA: Arts in Special Education Project of Pennsylvania, 1981, pp. 5–7.

Ross, M., ed. *The Arts and Personal Growth*. New York: Pergamon Press, 1980.

Shaw, R. Education and the arts. In Ross, M., ed. *The Arts and Personal Growth*, New York: Pergamon Press, 1980, pp. 69–78.

Sherrill, C., and R. Cox. Personnel preparation in creative arts for the handicapped: Implications for improving the quality of life. In Sherrill, C., ed. *Creative Arts for the Severely Handicapped*, Springfield, IL: Charles C. Thomas, 1979, pp. 3–11.

Sherrill, C. and J. R. Routon. Arts for the handicapped: Legislation, funding and programs. *Therapeutic Recreation Journal*, 14 (3), 34–41, 1980.

Smith, S. The arts in the education of learning disabled children. In National Committee, Arts for the Handicapped, *A Collection of Interest*, Washington, D.C.: NCAH, 1981, pp. 80–90.

Spencer, M. J. A case for the arts. In The Rockefeller Foundation, *The Healing Role of the Arts*, New York: The Rockefeller Foundation, 1978, pp. 1–9.

Williams, R. M. Why children should draw. *Saturday Review*, September 3, 1977, 101–106.

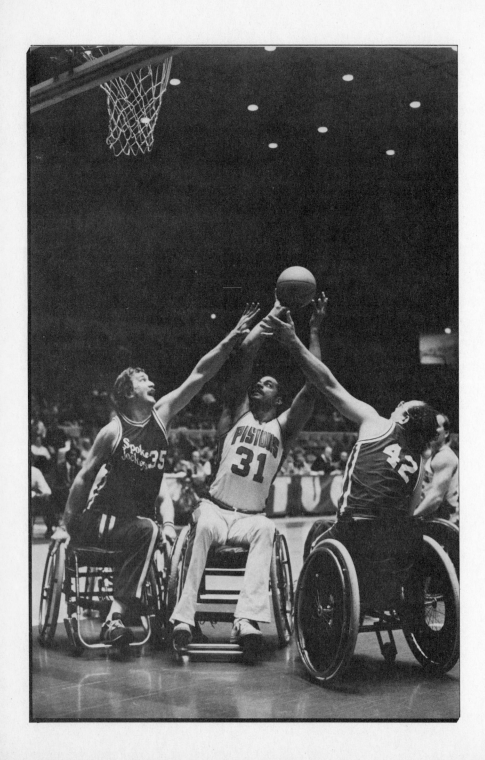

10

Competitive Sports for Individuals With Disabilities

You only have to pick up a newspaper or turn on a television to be reminded of the importance of competitive athletics in the United States. Game results for local sports teams are often noted on the front page of major metropolitan newspapers, and it is not unusual for local television news programs to devote twenty percent or more of their air time to sports topics. But the influence of organized sports upon our culture goes much deeper than merely the reporting of athletic events by the mass media. Indeed, sports and sports-related matters permeate our society, and in order to fully understand the importance of competitive sports for individuals with disabilities it is necessary to note the extent to which sports affects all of our lives.

George Sage, a noted sports sociologist, emphasized the massive influence sport has upon our way of life. In his book, *Sport and American Society: Selected Readings*, Sage (1974) states:

> Sport is such a pervasive human activity that to ignore it is to overlook one of the most significant aspects of contemporary American society. It is a social phenomenon which extends into education, politics, economics, art, the mass media, and even international diplomatic relationships. Involvement in sport, either directly as a participant, or indirectly as a spectator, is almost considered a public duty by many Americans. It has been observed that if there is a religion in America today, it is sport. (p. 5)

Although Sage's statement may be a slight exaggeration, there is little doubt that even the most disinterested citizen finds himself or her-

241

self influenced by the world of competitive athletics. Everyday expressions, which have their roots in organized sport, are commonplace. For example, you may feel that the decision between studying for an upcoming exam and going to see the latest hit movie (which, incidentally, may have a sports theme) is a "toss up," or you might approach the nice looking redhead in your English class with a good "game plan," but later discover that you have "struck out." The list of such expressions seems endless, including such well-known phrases as "jumping the gun," "hitting below the belt," "laying the ground rules," and "playing dirty pool." In fact, it is rare to complete a day without having heard or used at least one verbal expression that has its origin in organized sport.

Probably the most dramatic examples of sport's influence upon society have occurred in the political arena. The combined characteristics of (1) a team concept; (2) an objective system of performance evaluation (or, at least, the *appearance* of objectivity); and (3) a clearly defined winner and loser, make sporting events a natural outlet for national, regional, or community pride. No American who witnessed the stunning upset of the powerful and heavily favored Russian ice hockey team by a young but enthusiastic United States team in the 1980 Winter Olympics could question the power of a sporting event for inspiring intense feelings of nationalism. When this remarkable U.S. team went on to capture the gold medal by defeating Finland, a highly emotional nation imagined itself standing with the players on the victory platform.

In addition, sport has found its way into the arts by providing themes for countless books, plays and movies. Sport also has considerable impact on the economy. Not only do sport related products crowd the shelves of department stores, but sports "consumers" spend considerable sums of money each year through both direct (attendance) and indirect (radio, TV, magazines, etc.) consumption of sporting events. Additionally, education and sport are closely related in the United States, where the provision of sports teams by public schools is considered to provide students with a valuable preparation for adult life. Indeed, there are few areas of modern society which are not influenced in some way by the presence of sport.

SPORTS FOR DISABLED PERSONS

Despite the widespread influence of sport in our society and the recognition of its contribution to an individual's growth and development, the role of sport in the lives of persons with disabilities has received relatively little attention. In his interesting and widely read book, *Sports In America*, James Michener (1976) covered many fascinating aspects of sport. In-depth chapters are included on the role of sport in the lives of children, minorities, and women. Yet, though Michener's book is more than 500 pages long, the subject of sports for people who have disabilities is virtually ignored. Occasional articles on sports for athletes who are disabled may appear in newspapers or other publications, but they rarely appear in the sports sections and are usually treated as "human interest" stories rather than genuine examples of competitive sporting events. Even the major network television sports shows, which seem anxious to televise almost anything *remotely* resembling sport, have generally failed to provide coverage of organized and highly competitive sports competition among athletes who are disabled.

Why, with sport's influence so important in our culture, has society's acceptance of competitive sports programs for disabled athletes been so slow developing? Perhaps one reason is the comparative newness of organized sports for people with disabilities. Although sports historian Earle Zeigler (1979) dated the first recorded sports competitions as occurring during the Early Dynastic period of the Sumerian civilization (3000–1500 B.C.), organized sports for people with disabilities is largely a twentieth-century phenomenon. In fact, most sports programs for individuals who are disabled are less than twenty-five years old.

Newness alone does not account for the lack of public attention, however. Probably a more fundamental reason for the absence of public awareness and interest in sports for people with disabilities is the widespread belief that such programs are solely "therapeutic." The needs and motivations of disabled athletes are often viewed as different from their nondisabled counterparts, and the primary emphasis of such competition is seen as rehabilitation. While the rehabilitative potential of sports involvement is undeniable, emphasizing this aspect to the exclusion of the other benefits to the individual participant is unfortunate. Such emphasis merely strengthens the public's view of individuals with disabilities as "different" or "abnormal." Rather than stressing differences, the desire for sports participation among many people who have disabilities is, in fact, a classic example of the *similarity* of all people—whether disabled or nondisabled.

Professor Timothy Nugent (1969), long-time Director of the University of Illinois Rehabilitation-Education Center until his retirement in 1985, emphasized this point in the following statement:

> Let us recognize that, individually and collectively, [disabled people] have the same aspirations, interests, talents and, in most instances, the

same skills as all people. They have the same basic social-psychological needs and would like to travel the same avenues that you and I have been privileged to travel in fulfillment of these needs. It is the fault of our society as a whole, and more particularly, of the apathy, lack of awareness and sensitivity of our professional leaders that these individuals have not been privileged to travel these avenues. It is not the fault of the disability or the individual with the disability. (pp. 20–21)

As discussed earlier, sports is an important part of our society and, as such, it is one of the major "avenues" for needs fulfillment mentioned by Professor Nugent. Providing sports opportunities for athletes who are disabled is not necessarily rehabilitation, but it is a contribution that enables the participant to receive the same physical, social, and psychological benefits that organized, competitive sports programs offer to *all* participants.

Fortunately, there is evidence that athletes with disabilities are beginning to receive the recognition they deserve. In the 1980s two wheelchair athletes, George Murray and Doug Heir, have appeared prominently on boxes of Wheaties, "The Breakfast of Champions"; a U.S. postage stamp was issued paying tribute to athletes who compete in the Winter Special Olympics; the 1984 International Games for the Disabled received prominent, and generally appropriate, media coverage as a sporting event; and Sharon Rahn Hedrick became the first athlete with a disability to receive the prestigious Southland Olympia Award.

Common Goals of Sports Participation

As noted by Rarick (1984), there are many sports opportunities throughout the United States and Canada available to people with disabilities. Football, racquetball, softball, track and field, basketball, and tennis are just a few of the many wheelchair sports providing outlets for athletes with mobility limitations. People with visual impairments, sometimes using sighted guides, can participate in such sports as beep baseball, golf, archery, bowling, and many winter sports (Montelione & Mastro, 1985; Rarick, 1984; Spraggs, 1984). The Special Olympics offers opportunities for winter and summer competition among people with mental retardation. In addition, both disabled and nondisabled senior citizens compete in the Senior Olympics. Each of these programs, as well as others providing sports competition for special populations, makes unique contributions to participants. Each differs from the others in many ways, including administrative procedures, type of athletic contests offered, basic rules of competition, fund-raising techniques, and so on. Yet, there are a number of things that competitive programs for people with disabilities have in common. Most, if not all, of these programs:

- Provide a method of informing the public about the unique *abilities* that participants possess.
- Promote independence, sports skill development, and increased physical fitness among their participants.
- Promote maximum participation by offering local or regional events, but also provide for recognition of outstanding performances through national and international competition.
- Have some system of classification, such as degree of disability, etc., in order to make the competition in events as "fair" as possible.
- Use the classification system as a method of increasing participation opportunities among individuals with severe disabilities.
- Offer some unique competitive events, or modified activities, that provide the participant with a chance to display special skills not usually associated with nondisabled competition.

Criticism of Segregated Programs

In addition to sharing some common goals and procedures, sports programs for athletes who are disabled also receive similar criticism. One of the most frequent complaints about these programs is that they "segregate" participants who have disabilities from nondisabled athletes. Most of the programs mentioned previously have regulations that prohibit nondisabled participants from competing against athletes who have disabilities. It is argued, therefore, that the participants with disabilities do not get the chance to meet, talk to, and become friends with nondisabled individuals who share similar interests in sport. Logically, this lack of opportunities for social interaction with nondisabled peers fails to provide the competitor who is disabled with social skills that are necessary in everyday life. Although many of these programs do use nondisabled volunteers, the role of a volunteer often places the nondisabled person "above" the competitor. To be effective, social interaction between disabled and nondisabled peers should be on an equal level.

Advocates of programs for athletes with disabilities, however, counter the above criticism with several logical points. First, they note that sports programs are but one aspect of a person's life. Fundamental changes are needed in other societal institutions, such as education, transportation, and so on, to promote integration of individuals with disabilities into society. In effect, sports programs for individuals with disabilities are a reaction to a segregated society, not a cause of it. Secondly, supporters of these programs urge that providing the disabled athlete with a fair chance for success in sporting events may require excluding nondisabled individuals from competition. Having nondisabled peers serve as volunteers may also offer the chance for social interaction in a cooperative, rather than competitive situation. Thirdly, it is maintained that segregated sports participation enhances the development of social and physical skills in an environment of acceptance and understanding. This social and physical development, which is enhanced by successful competitive experiences, promotes confidence and self-esteem among participants.

Brian Nettleton (1974), from Australia, observed that social acceptance of people with disabilities is often low, thus limiting the possibility for integration. He stated, however, that "it is possible, via carefully structured experiences in various sporting activities (provided sport is defined widely), to increase social acceptance and all that goes with it" (p. 9). The Canadian sports system gives credence to Nettleton's statement. In provinces such as Ontario and Alberta, athletes with disabilities routinely compete against each other at the same time and in the same physical location as nondisabled athletes. This "parallel" concept enables mutual sharing of the competitive spirit among *all* athletes, but avoids the inequities that might result from direct competition between disabled and nondisabled athletes. McClements (1984) described Saskatchewan's effort to offer parallel competition among athletes with mental retardation and their nondisabled peers. He stated that parallel competition allows athletes with disabilities "a greater choice in athletic activities and programs and the opportunity to meet, interact with and most importantly, participate with their [nondisabled] fellow athletes" (p. 23).

Stan Labanowich, the Commissioner of the National Wheelchair Basketball Association, is a strong advocate for parallel competition in sporting events. In 1981, Dr. Labanowich optimistically predicted that by 1988 wheelchair basketball, and perhaps other events for athletes with disabilities, would be incorporated as a part of the Olympic Games (AAHPERD, 1981, p. 5). Four years ahead of Labanowich's prediction, the 1984 Olympic Games in Los Angeles included two "exhibition" wheelchair track events: the 800-meter dash for women and the 1500-meter dash for men. These events were telecast nationally and provided the viewing audience with an example of sports competition at its finest.

Disabled Sports Humor

In recent years, the development of organized sports opportunities for disabled athletes in the United States has been accompanied by a very

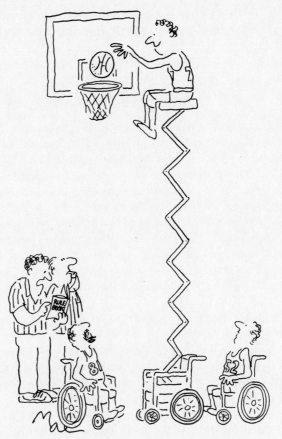

Figure 10–1. "Here it is, Nugent . . . rule 27, section 7: No player shall . . . " (Courtesy *Accent on Living,* Spring, 1982)

healthy phenomenon—the growth of disabled sports humor. *Sports 'n Spokes, Accent on Living,* and other publications dedicated to the interests of individuals with disabilities have provided their readers with sports-oriented cartoons designed to bring out humorous aspects of both disability and sports for people with disabilities. The purpose of these cartoons is consistent with Thomas Fuller's statement, "He is not laughed at that laughs at himself first." By laughing at themselves first, athletes with disabilities help to reveal the normalcy of sport for disabled people. Figure 10-1 provides an example of a cartoon that depicts athletes who are disabled.

Interestingly, *National Lampoon,* a humor magazine not usually concerned with issues of disability, was one of the first publications to include cartoons about athletes with disabilities. In their May, 1974, issue, they provided a section entitled "Handicapped Sports." Although several of the cartoons in *National Lampoon* were of questionable taste, many athletes with disabilities appreciated the attention they provided.

Competitive Programs

As mentioned above, there are many sports programs offering a variety of competitive opportunities to people with disabilities. For example, the Committee on Sports for the Disabled, within the U.S. Olympic Committee (U.S.O.C.), is composed of seven different organizations that govern competitive sports for various disabling conditions (Rarick, 1984). These organizations include the American Athletic Association for the Deaf (AAAD), National Association of Sport for Cerebral Palsy (NASCP), National Handicapped Sports and Recreation Association (NHSRA), National Wheelchair Athletic Association (NWAA), Special Olympics, Inc., United States Amputee Athletic Association (USAAA), and United States Association for Blind Athletes (USABA). Among the criteria for membership on this U.S.O.C. Committee is the stipulation that each organization must govern competition in more than one sport. Ironically, this rule has excluded many sports organizations, including the National Wheelchair Basketball Association (NWBA), from U.S.O.C. representation. The NWBA is the oldest, and arguably the most democratic, among all of the organizations governing sports for people with disabilities.

Obviously, it would be impossible to describe in this chapter all of the sports programs for athletes with disabilities throughout the United States and Canada; however, two widely known programs have been selected to serve as examples: (1) *wheelchair sports* for people with mobility limitations; and (2) the *Special Olympics* for children and adults with mental retardation.

WHEELCHAIR SPORTS

Historical Development

The wheelchair sports movement in the United States owes its beginning and continued growth to three primary factors: (1) advances in medical technology, which have resulted in an increasing life expectancy for individuals with physical disabilities; (2) the competitive spirit and determination of disabled athletes who always manage to find ways to overcome personal and organizational difficulties in order to participate in competitive sports; and (3) farsightedness among several determined professionals who have provided the leadership "spark" needed for establishment and continued expansion of wheelchair athletics.

Prior to World War II, wheelchair sports was virtually nonexistent. Although the needs of people with physical disabilities were becoming increasingly recognized by concerned United States citizens and organizations, few people thought that athletic competition was appropriate for so-called "cripples." By the Second World War, however, medical technology and battlefield evacuation methods had improved to the point where severely wounded soldiers were kept alive in increasing numbers. These soldiers, including amputees and spinal cord-injured young men, would have died in prior wars, but now they returned home to veterans' hospitals throughout the United States. Despite their injuries, these men desired the same competitive sports opportunities that they enjoyed prior to going overseas.

The desire for competition in organized sports grew as these veterans, many of them athletes prior to injury, progressed from playing catch, table tennis, and bowling to the more active physical demands of waterpolo, softball, and touch football. But, it was basketball that really caught the imagination and competitive spirit of these veterans. It was rough, strenuous, and highly competitive. Don Swift, one of the early wheelchair basketball players, was quoted as describing the game as "a combination of football and basketball in that there was considerably more contact than exists now . . . a much rougher game" (Labanowich, 1975, p. 34).

Soon just playing basketball against other patients within the hospital was not satisfying enough. By 1948 there were at least six organized veterans teams in the United States and the famous "Flying Wheels" from California began their cross-country tour playing wheelchair basketball against other teams. The wheelchair sports movement in North America was underway.

Formation of Associations

Among the many people who were aware of wheelchair basketball's start, as well as the potential for other wheelchair sports, were Timothy Nugent and Ben Lipton. These two men were to become the driving force for wheelchair sports as we know it today. Tim Nugent, from the University of Illinois, not only formed the first college wheelchair basketball team in 1948, but he organized the first National Wheelchair Basketball Tournament in April, 1949. This tournament provided the basis for development of the National Wheelchair Basketball Association, which Nugent headed as Commissioner for 25 years. When he retired as NWBA Commissioner in 1973, Tim Nugent could proudly boast that the modest beginning of six NWBA teams had grown to almost 100 teams throughout the United States.

While wheelchair basketball was blossoming in the 1950s, Ben Lipton, from Bulova School of Watchmaking, recognized the need for other types of competitive opportunities for individuals with disabilities. At the time, basketball was dominated by men, and ball-handling skills required fairly good use of most upper body muscles. Track and

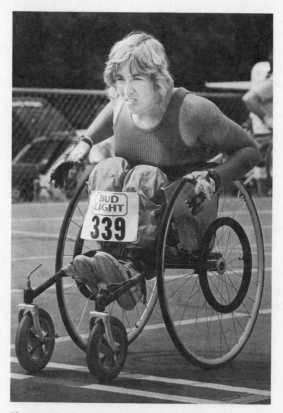

Figure 10–2. In the 1950s, wheelchair sports events like track and field, table tennis, and swimming offered competitive opportunities for women with spinal cord injuries. Today, women with disabilities compete at a high level in all aspects of wheelchair sports programs. (Courtesy of PVA *Sports n' Spokes* Magazine)

field events, table tennis, swimming, and other competitive activities, however, offered new avenues for women and individuals with high spinal cord injuries. In 1957, Lipton followed the lead of his European counterpart, Sir Ludwig Guttmann of Stoke Mandeville, England, by initiating the first U.S. Wheelchair Games. These games, which included many of the forenamed events, were a resounding success and Lipton became the Chairman of the newly formed National Wheelchair Athletic Association in 1958. Like Nugent, Ben Lipton presided over the growth of his organization, the NWAA, for well over 20 years.

Thus, the development of organized wheelchair sports in the United States has been stimulated by two simultaneous, but separate, organizational movements: The National Wheelchair Basketball Association and the National Wheelchair Athletic Association. A brief examination of each organization's sports program will help explain the state of wheelchair sports in the U.S. today.

National Wheelchair Basketball Association

Following Nugent's retirement in 1973, Dr. Stan Labanowich became the second and, to date, only other National Wheelchair Basketball Association (NWBA) Commissioner. Labanowich has overseen a continued growth in wheelchair basketball. There are well over 160 teams currently in the NWBA.

History and growth do not give a complete picture of wheelchair basketball; that can only come from watching one of the fast and exciting games played between two highly skilled teams. Wheelchair basketball is played according to National Collegiate Athletic Association rules, although a few modifications to these rules are made to accommodate the use of wheelchairs. Each game is played on a full-sized high school or college court and the baskets remain at the 10-foot level. The amount of strength and skill required by wheelchair basketball players can be easily demonstrated by trying to shoot accurately at a 10-foot basket from 15 feet away *while sitting on a chair!* And shooting is just *one* of the many skills required to excel in wheelchair basketball. As any of the nondisabled people who have tried to compete against wheelchair basketball players can tell you, being able to shoot means very little if you cannot move the wheelchair with speed and agility. As one TV sports commentator noted, "I thought I was a pretty good basketball player but those guys (wheelchair team members) put me to shame. I was zero for twelve from the foul line, and they ran, er, wheeled circles around me on the floor."

Some of the important aspects of wheelchair basketball and the National Wheelchair Basketball Association that should be mentioned are as follows.

Rules. As noted earlier, NCAA rules serve as the standard for wheelchair basketball, but modifications are made when special situations dictate. For example, contact between chairs was not originally considered to be a personal foul. Bob Miller, the first president of the NWBA, described the result:

> Wheelchair Bulldozers we called ourselves, the reason being that in those days before the rules were refined, you could ram a guy all you wanted—when you caught him sitting dead with the ball. You could ram into him and take the ball away from him. And so we picked the name Bulldozers—Wheelchair Bulldozers (Labanowich, 1975, p. 34).

As a result of such tactics, the wheelchair is now considered to be a "part" of the player. Throughout the years, the sophistication of wheelchair basketball rules has increased to the point where today's Official NWBA Rules and Case Book is over 25 pages long. The Case Book portion of this document gives rule interpretations for more than 45 actual game situations.

Classification System and Team Balance. Wheelchair basketball requires a great deal of balance, upper body strength, and overall coordination. Players with lower spinal cord injuries (in general, the lower the injury, the more muscle function a player has) or disabilities only affecting the lower extremities (legs) usually have a competitive advantage over players with more severe disabilities. Some wheelchair basketball players are actually able to walk, but on their feet could not keep pace with nondisabled players. In order to provide opportunities for the higher spinal cord–injured individual to compete in basketball, a classification system was devised based upon, but separate from, the one used by National Wheelchair Athletic Association competitors (see Figure 10-3 in the next section of this chapter). Wheelchair basketball players are currently placed into one of three "classes" according to the following system:

Class I. Complete motor loss at T-7 or above or comparable disability where there is total loss of muscle function originating at or above T-7.

Class II. Complete motor loss originating at T-8 and descending through and including L-2 where there may be motor power of hips and thighs. Also included in this class are amputees with bilateral hip disarticulation.

Class III. All other physical disabilities as related to lower extremity paralysis or paresis originating at or below L-3. All lower extremity amputees are included in this class except those with bilateral hip disarticulation (see Class II).

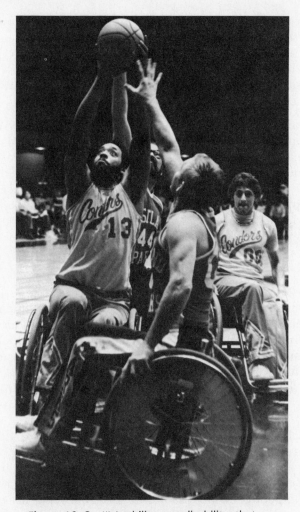

Figure 10–3. "It's ability, not disability, that counts." Wheelchair basketball offers an athlete with a lower extremity disability the chance to demonstrate great skill and physical ability to the nondisabled public. (Courtesy of PVA *Sports n' Spokes* Magazine)

Basketball is a team sport, so merely classifying individuals according to the above system is not enough. Each classification (I, II, and III) is given a numerical or point value as follows:

  Class I. 1 point
 Class II. 2 points
Class III. 3 points

Current NWBA rules prevent a team from placing five players on the floor at the same time whose "point" totals exceed 12 points. Since no more than three Class III's are allowed at one time, many NWBA teams use three Class III's, one Class II, and one Class I. Thus, the more severely disabled Class I player is provided an opportunity to play thanks to the NWBA's "team balance" concept.

Scope. Although originally limited exclusively to males, NWBA teams have been open to participation by both sexes since 1974. Women may join any one of the teams in the Association, which includes a number of all-women teams. In addition to the annual National Wheelchair Basketball Tournament for the "final four" top teams, the Association also helps to support the National Women's Wheelchair Basketball Tournament and the Intercollegiate Wheelchair Basketball Tournament. Although most of the teams in the NWBA are located in the continental United States, there are also several Canadian teams that have chosen to affiliate with the Association.

Democratic Representation. One of the more favorable aspects of the NWBA is its policy that the players establish all rules, including rules of play and the Association's Constitution and By-Laws. This is accomplished at an annual meeting of team delegates where all of the Association's business is conducted. The idea of recreation consumer input from persons with disabilities is relatively new in the U.S., but the NWBA has been practicing this policy since its formation in 1949.

National Wheelchair Athletic Association

The National Wheelchair Athletic Association (NWAA) was formed almost 10 years after the NWBA, but it quickly took on a very important role in wheelchair sports development. Since it was not limited to a single sport, the NWAA became the representative body for a varied group of competitors with disabilities. The following list of sporting events, currently governed by the NWAA, gives some idea of this variety: track events (100-yard dash, to distance events), field events (shotput, javelin, discus), swimming, weightlifting, archery, and slalom (an obstacle course event in which competitors compete for the best time).

Under the leadership of Ben Lipton, the NWAA became the wheelchair sports organization that organized and supervised U.S. participation in most major international competitions. These international events, including the well-known "Paralympics," became a prized goal for every NWAA competitor. Jon Brown, holder of the world heavyweight weightlifting record, underscored the personal importance of international competition by stating, "I don't remember walking. I've never climbed a stair. I've never run. So for me these games are a dream come true" (Weisman and Godfrey, 1976, p. 121).

As with wheelchair basketball, the National Wheelchair Athletic Association, the events it governs, has several aspects that should be highlighted:

Classification System. Since NWAA events generally feature *individual*, rather than team, competition, some form of classifying the severity of a person's disability is essential. As noted previously, individuals with lower extremity injuries may have a competitive edge over those with injuries that also affect stomach, chest, back and/or arm muscles. By placing an athlete into one of five classification categories (six for swimming events), it is possible to provide a better "match" for equal competition. Some competitors have questioned the NWAA spinal cord levels selected for classifying athletes, but a study by Dr. Robert Steadward (1978) seems to support the present system. Steadward used films to analyze each of the NWAA classes and, with the exception of some confusion between Class IA and Class IB, he found the present method to be justified. As noted by Lindstrom (1985), however, "No classification system in competitive sports, for able-bodied or for disabled, will ever be totally fair to each individual: those being near the upper limit of the class definition will have an advantage over those being near the lower limits" (p. 48). Table 10–1 provides an explanation and diagram of the present system used by the NWAA to classify participants with spinal paralysis, along with the classification categories of several other prominent programs for athletes with disabilities.

Scope. The NWAA's regional, national, and international competitive activities provide a wide range of events for many males and females with mobility limitations. Unlike wheelchair basketball, the NWAA's format of individual competition within medical classifications offers almost unlimited competitive opportunities for persons with very high spinal cord injuries (quadriplegics). Individual competition also provides athletes with disabilities who live in rural areas an opportunity to compete since team membership is not necessary.

Slalom Event. All of the events governed by the NWAA parallel closely the rules and format of sports for able-bodied participants, except for the slalom event. The slalom course requires a competitor to demonstrate exceptional wheelchair handling skill by going over, under, and around numerous obstacles. Speed and wheelchair agility are the qualities needed to excel in this event, and the finalist in each class with the best time is declared the winner. Since this event is unique to wheelchair sports, it generates a great deal of spectator interest. It also provides many wheelchair athletes with the motivation to master difficult, but important, wheelchair handling skills, for example, "wheelies" and curb jumping. The uniqueness of the slalom event has also resulted in

Table 10–1
Competitive Classification by Disability*

The classification system currently utilized for competition in sports for the disabled is the result of years of careful study and adaptation. The classifications are based upon the type of disability, the degree of disability, and the functionality of the disability.

Amputee Classifications

The system is based on acquired and congenital amputations.

Abbreviations

AK = Above or through knee joint
BK = Below knee, but through or above talocrural joint.
AE = Above or through elbow joint.
BE = Below elbow, but through or above wrist joint.

Classification Code

Class A1 = Double AK
Class A2 = Single AK
Class A3 = Double BK
Class A4 = Single BK
Class A5 = Double AE
Class A6 = Single AE
Class A7 = Double BE
Class A8 = Single BE
Class A9 = Combined lower plus upper limb amputations.

Blind Classifications

B1

No light perception at all in either eye up to light perception, but inability to recognize objects or contours in any direction and at any distance.

B2

Ability to recognize objects or contours up to a visual acuity of 2/60 and/or a limitation of field of vision of 5 degrees.

B3

2/60 to 6/60 vision and/or field of vision between 5 and 20 degrees.

Cerebral Palsy Classifications

Class I

Severe involvement in all four limbs. Limited trunk control, unable to grasp a softball. Poor functional strength in upper extremities, necessitating the use of an electric wheelchair.

Class II

Severe to moderate quadriplegic, normally able to propel wheel chair with legs or if able, propels wheelchair very slowly with arms. Poor functional strength and severe control problems in the upper extremities.

Class III

Moderate quadriplegic, fair functional strength and moderate control problems in upper extremities and torso. Uses wheelchair.

Class IV

Lower limbs have moderate to severe involvement. Good functional strength and minimal control problems in the upper extremities and torso. Uses wheelchair.

Class V

Good functional strength and minimal control problems in upper extremities. May walk with or without aids, but for ambulatory support.

Class VI

Moderate to severe quadriplegic. Ambulates without walking aids, fewer coordination balance problems when running or throwing.

Class VII

Moderate to minimal hemiplegic. Good functional ability in nonaffected side. Walks/runs with a limp.

Class VIII

Minimally affected hemiplegic. May have minimal coordination problems. Able to run and jump freely. Has good balance.

Les Autres (Other) Classifications

L1

Wheelchair user. Reduced functions of muscle strength, and/or spasticity in throwing arm. Poor sitting balance.

L2

Wheelchair user with normal function in throwing arm and poor to moderate sitting balance. Or reduced function in throwing arm, but good sitting balance.

Table 10–1 (*Continued*)

Les Autres (Other) Classifications

L3
Wheelchair user with normal arm function and good sitting balance.

L4
Ambulant with or without crutches and braces; or problems with the balance together with reduced function in throwing arm.

Note
An athlete is allowed to use orthosis or crutches if he so wishes. The throw can be done from a standstill or moving position in L4 and L5.

L5
Ambulant with normal arm function in throwing arm. Reduced function in lower extremities or balance problem.

L6
Ambulant with normal upper extremity function in throwing arm and minimal trunk or lower extremity disability. A participant in this class must be able to demonstrate a locomotor disability that clearly gives him or her a disadvantage in throwing events compared to able-bodied sports men or women.

Spinally Paralyzed Classifications

To compete in the wheelchair sports, athletes must have significant permanent neuromuscular-skeletal disability (spinal cord disorder, polio, amputation, etc.).

Class IA
All cervical lesions with complete or incomplete quadriplegia who have involvement of both hands, weakness of triceps (up to and including grade 3 on testing scale) and with severe weakness of the trunk and lower extremities interfering significantly with trunk balance and the ability to walk.

Class IB
All cervical lesions with complete or incomplete quadriplegia who have involvement of upper extremities but less than 1A with preservation of normal or good triceps (4 or 5 on testing scale) and with a generalized weakness of the trunk and lower extremities interfering significantly with trunk balance and the ability to walk.

Class IC
All cervical lesions with complete or incomplete quadriplegia who have involvement of upper extremities but less than 1A with preservation of normal or good triceps (4 or 5 on testing scale) and normal or good finger flexion and extension (grasp and release) but without intrinsic hand function and with a generalized weakness of the trunk and lower extremities interfering significantly with trunk balance and ability to walk.

Class II
Complete or incomplete paraplegia below T1 down to and including T5 or comparable disability with total abdominal paralysis or poor abdominal muscle strength (0–2 on testing scale) and no useful trunk sitting balance.

Class III
Complete or incomplete paraplegia or comparable disability below T5 down to and including T10 with upper abdominal and spinal extensor musculature sufficient to provide some element of trunk sitting balance but not normal.

Class IV
Complete or incomplete parplegia or comparable disability below T10 down to and including L2 without quadriceps or very weak quadriceps with a value up to and including 2 on the testing scale and gluteal paralysis.

Class V
Complete or incomplete paraplegia or comparable disability below L2 with quadriceps in grades 3–5.

SWIMMING EVENTS ONLY

Class V
Complete or incomplete paraplegia or comparable disability below L2 with quadriceps in grades 3–5 and with up to and including 39 points on the point scale.

Table 10–1 (*Continued*)

SWIMMING EVENTS ONLY (cont.)

Class VI
Complete or incomplete paraplegia or comparable disability below L2 and with 40 points and above on the point scale.

Swimming Point Scale
Each of the muscle groups in the lower extremities (legs) is rated according to power on a scale of 1 through 5. There are 10 muscle groups in each leg or 20 in all. Therefore, a 1 rating on all 20 muscle groups would score 20 points. A 5 rating on all 20 muscle groups would score 100 points. Athletes can score anywhere along the point scale from 20 to 100.

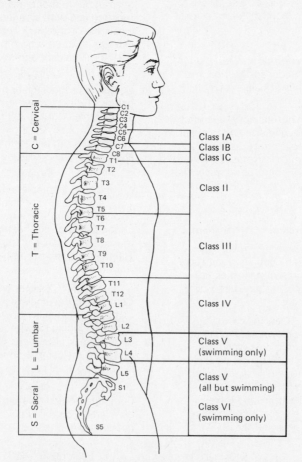

Figure 10–A. Medical Classification. (Modified and reproduced with permission of Challenge Publications, Inc.)

*Modified and reproduced with permission of Challenge Publications, Inc.

criticism from some authorities because it is believed to violate the concept of normalization. Efforts to eliminate this event from wheelchair sports competition have not been successful, however, and the slalom continues to be a popular addition to most wheelchair games.

Benefits of Wheelchair Sports

There is no doubt that participation in organized wheelchair sports, whether through the NWBA or NWAA, requires a large personal commitment—one involving time, effort, and *money*. The present cost of most sports-adaptable wheelchairs, which are lighter and more durable than conventional chairs, is well over $1,000.

The investment needed to establish a wheelchair basketball team may exceed $20,000, including wheelchairs, uniforms, equipment, and one season's travel and game expenses. Why, since it is so expensive, do individuals and some organizations provide their financial support to wheelchair sports? The answer to that question can be found in an explanation of three of the benefits that wheelchair sports offer. They are:

1. Participant Growth and Development. Sports for nondisabled individuals are claimed to offer great physical and mental benefits. This claim is also made about wheelchair sports because, as Stein (1982) observed, disabled and nondisabled athletes share the same goals, objectives and motivations. Many studies and journal articles have stressed the importance of wheelchair sports for individuals with physical disabilities. Jochheim and Strohkendl (1973), for example, noted the physical problems caused by poor conditioning in paraplegia, and urged participation in several wheelchair sports events to overcome these problems. Likewise, Loiselle (1979) stressed the benefits of wheelchair sports participation, with particular emphasis on the psychosocial effects. Research studies by Guttmann and Mehra (1973), Spira (1967), Zwiren and Bar-or (1975), and many others have provided evidence in support of participant benefits. Increased physical fitness and strength, a better self-concept and social adjustment, and greater awareness of the world through travel are all positive aspects of wheelchair sports participation.

2. Public Awareness. Wheelchair athletes often quote the expression, "It's ability, not disability, that counts," and wheelchair sports offer the individual who has a disability an excellent chance to display great skill and physical ability to the nondisabled public. Watching the exciting action of a wheelchair basketball game, or observing a disabled athlete wheel more than 26 miles in a marathon event, cannot help but increase a nondisabled person's appreciation of people with disabilities. The myth of "dependency" is quickly dispelled by watching displays of athletic skill, and the wheelchair sports spectator may walk away with a newly formed attitude of appreciation and respect toward people with disabilities.

3. Motivation for Others. The skill displayed by wheelchair athletes often provides much needed motivation for youth or individuals who have been recently disabled. During the 28th National Wheelchair Basketball Tournament (NWBT) in Baltimore, for example, a large number of young people with physical disabilities attended the games. Later, the director of the tournament was informed by local school personnel that the 28th NWBT resulted in renewed enthusiasm for physical activity and adapted physical education programs. The publicity and excitement of the tournament was "just what the doctor ordered" for the youth of Baltimore. Today, several of the young spectators at the 28th NWBT in 1976 are regulars on Baltimore's wheelchair basketball teams.

Expanding Opportunities

The wheelchair sports movement has not only experienced phenomenal growth; it has provided the model for others to promote sports for individuals with disabilities who are ineligible for competition against or not on a competitive level with the "traditional" wheelchair athlete. Multiple disabilities or those affecting the upper extremities often limit or prevent participation in NWBA or NWAA events. The National Cerebral Palsy Games, and their preliminary competition on local, state, and regional levels, have helped to fill the void in competitive sports opportunities for people with such disabilities. These games, held by the National Association of Sport for Cerebral Palsy, have classification categories for competitors who use wheelchairs, but also have classes for ambulatory and semi-ambulatory (users of crutches and other walking aids) competitors (see Figure 10–3). Events held at these games include but are not limited to archery, horseback riding, weightlifting, table tennis, soccer, bowling, rifle shooting, and track and field.

The acceptance of competitive sports for all athletes, including those with severe and/or multiple disabilities, was evidenced by the success of the International Games for the Disabled held in New York in 1984. Nearly 2,000 athletes competed in these widely publicized games, which drew 900 media representatives from around the world (McCann, 1985). Sherrill and Canabal (1985) reported that 620 events were held in 18 different sports across 26 separate classification categories. In addition, 11 research projects, coordinated by Dr. Julian Stein, gathered scientific data at the Games. Stein, from George Mason University, stated, "Most of the research at the Games centered on observation of functional abilities and interviews concerning sociological and psychological aspects of sport. Hopefully the findings will reach scholars and practitioners around the world" (Sherrill & Canabal, 1985, p. 29).

A Decade of Change

The following chronology, modified from *Sports 'n Spokes'* 10th anniversary issue, illustrates some of the many dramatic events that occurred in wheelchair sports from 1975 to 1985.

1975 ■ *Sports 'n Spokes* publishes its first issue.
■ Bob Hall becomes the first wheelchair competitor in the Boston Marathon.
■ First Women's National Wheelchair Basketball Tournament is held.
1976 ■ Six countries decline to participate in the Toronto Olympiad due to South Africa's inclusion in the Games.
1977 ■ First National Wheelchair Marathon is held in conjunction with the 81st Boston Marathon.
■ The Cerebral Palsy sports movement emerges, separate from the NWAA, and develops its own classification system.
■ First National Wheelchair Softball Tournament is held.
1978 ■ First U.S. National Cerebral Palsy Games are held.
■ Canada's University of Alberta in Edmonton establishes a research and training center for athletes with physical disabilities.
1979 ■ Gold Cup, the world championship of wheelchair basketball, is held in the U.S.
■ U.S. Olympic Committee forms Committee on Sports for the Disabled.
■ Peter Axelson develops first controllable sled for snow skiers with spinal cord injuries.
1980 ■ First National Wheelchair Tennis Championships are held.
1981 ■ First National Amputee Games are held.
■ Ben Lipton steps down as Chairman of the NWAA.
1982 ■ Amateur Racquetball Association's National Championships feature exhibition wheelchair racquetball division.
1983 ■ U.S. Handicapped Ski Team is formed.
■ Canada hosts Gold Cup in Halifax, Nova Scotia.
■ National Wheelchair Racquetball Association is founded.

1984 ■ VII World Wheelchair Games, to be held at the University of
Illinois, are cancelled due to financial problems.
   ■ International Games for the Disabled are held in New York.
   ■ Wheelchair track exhibition events are held as part of the
Olympic Games.
   ■ First National Junior Wheelchair Games are attended by
youngsters from the U.S. and Canada.
1985 ■ First NWBA "old-timers" game is held in conjunction with the
National Wheelchair Basketball Tournament.
   ■ Mono-ski competition is included in the 14th National
Handicapped Ski Championships.
   ■ First issue of *Palaestra: The Forum of Sport and Physical
Education for the Disabled* is published.

The above chronology shows the diversity of wheelchair sports, as
well as many of the changes that have occurred in recent years. One
dramatic change not included above, however, is the evolution of the
sports-model wheelchair. Prior to 1978, wheelchair athletes competed
in "standard" wheelchairs with, at most, minor modifications such as
smaller handrims and lowered seats. At the 22nd National Wheelchair
Games in 1978, however, George Murray introduced two innovations
that would forever alter the design and use of sports-model wheelchairs. LaMere and Labanowich (1984) noted that Murray modified the
wheelchair to elevate "his knees excessively high to compensate for his
lack of sitting balance owing to the [high] level of his [spinal cord]
lesion. . . . Through compensating for his lack of sitting balance, Murray
was able to generate a complete stroke and follow through" (p. 12). This
alteration, plus Murray's use of steering handles on the front casters of
his wheelchair, directly resulted in a liberalization of the NWAA's rules
regulating competitive wheelchairs.

Today, there are at least 10 manufacturers who produce quality
sports wheelchairs that incorporate Murray's modifications, plus many
additional innovative features. Probably the most striking difference
between present wheelchairs and those of 10 years ago, however, is
their weight. The wheelchair George Murray used in 1978 weighed
about 50 lbs; today, his sports wheelchair weighs less than 14 lbs!

Technological advances in the sports-model wheelchair, both in
weight and design, have also helped to make life easier for nonathletes
who use wheelchairs. Today's lighter and more maneuverable "standard" wheelchairs were made possible by advancements in wheelchair sports technology. Hopefully, wheelchair sports will continue to
be at the forefront of wheelchair technology, as well as competitive
sports for people with disabilities.

SPECIAL OLYMPICS
Historical Development

Unlike wheelchair sports, the Special Olympics was not formed because the participants themselves created a demand for the programs. The characteristics of mental retardation often prevent effective consumerism without the aid and assistance of nondisabled "advocates." These advocates work to ensure that the needs, desires, and rights of mentally retarded people are met within society. The formation of the Special Olympics is an example of such advocacy.

Early in the 1960s, President John F. Kennedy's administration stressed the importance of physical fitness activities for all United States citizens, and many studies were conducted that clearly established the need for such activities. By 1967, research on physical fitness revealed a lack of physical proficiency among people with mental retardation. The primary cause of this shortcoming was felt to be a lack of programs that stressed physical activities. Haskins (1976) noted that these studies revealed 45 percent of school children in the U.S. who had mental retardation received *no* physical education instruction, and only 25 percent received as much as one hour per week. The Chicago Park District, responding to the obvious need for athletic programs for youth who were mentally retarded, developed the idea of a nationwide competition stressing track and field events.

In 1967, the Chicago Park District sought the assistance of the Joseph P. Kennedy, Jr. Foundation in order to finance their idea for a national track meet for youngsters who were mentally retarded. The idea was well received, no doubt in part because the Kennedy family had personal experience with mental retardation. A daughter of Joseph and Rose Kennedy has mental retardation. Rather than expending a lot of money and effort on a program that might not succeed, the Kennedy Foundation and the Chicago Park District agreed to test their new idea by holding and then evaluating the success of a single national meet. That meet, held in 1968, included participants from only 24 states, but the enthusiasm and enjoyment displayed by the 1000 competitors overshadowed the failure of many states to organize teams. Mrs. Eunice Kennedy Shriver represented the Kennedy Foundation at that premier meet, and the joy she saw among competitors convinced her that the concept of a national sports program for people with mental retardation was a solid one. Following that first event, Special Olympics, Inc., was formed with Mrs. Shriver serving as President. During the years that followed, the Special Olympics grew in participation, competitive events, and public recognition. Today, it is estimated that more than one million children and adults with mental retardation participate in Special Olympics programs throughout the world, and the number of local, chapter, regional, national, and international events exceeds 10,000 each year.

Organization and Events

Special Olympics competition is organized to assure that as many people with mental retardation as possible get an opportunity to participate. Spring track and field competition, for example, is offered in a large number of "local" meets that do not require a lot of travel by participants. Holding local events close to the communities where the participants live means that event organizers are usually familiar with local agency or school personnel. Such agency or school professionals can be very helpful in recruiting and training Special Olympics competitors. Thus, local rivalries may be promoted, local customs observed, and local resources utilized at this initial level of track and field competition. All of this helps to produce maximum participation among eligible citizens within the community.

In addition to local events, Special Olympics offers a chance to participate in games that draw competitors from larger areas. These may lead to international competition, which is held every four years. The 6th International Special Olympics Summer games held in the United States, for example, drew 4300 competitors from 52 countries. The Canadian delegation, with over 100 competitors, was the largest international representative, and each of the 50 U.S. states sent a delegation. The host state, Louisiana, entered 350 Special Olympians in the competition (Mills & Barnes, 1984). International Special Olympics competition is also offered in winter sports, and the 1985 Winter Games drew a record number of competitors from around the world (Shriver, 1985).

The 1980s have been very exciting times for Special Olympics participants because the number of competitive events has grown dramatically. The traditional events are track and field activities, but Special Olympics now offer much more to athletes. Fall events and winter sports are becoming commonplace in many states, and the number of official Special Olympics sports and events continues to grow. In addition, official sports and events are complemented by "demonstration" sports and events, which may become official activities in the future. A list of Special Olympics official and demonstration sports and events is included in Table 10-2.

Classification and Eligibility

Most sports programs for individuals with disabilities develop a competitive classification system that requires that participants compete in

Table 10–2
Special Olympics Sports and Events*

Official Special Olympics Sports and Events.

(a) The following are official Special Olympics sports or events:
   (1) Basketball
      (aa) Team Competition
      (bb) Individual Run, Dribble and Shoot Competition
   (2) Bowling
   (3) Floor Hockey
   (4) Frisbee Disc
   (5) Gymnastics
      (aa) Free Exercise
      (bb) Tumbling
      (cc) Balance Beam (female competition)
   (6) One-Meter Diving
   (7) Poly Hockey
   (8) Soccer
      (aa) Team Competition
      (bb) Individual Skills Competition
   (9) Slow-Pitch Softball
  (10) Swimming
      (aa) 25-Meter Freestyle
      (bb) 50-Meter Freestyle
      (cc) 25-Meter Backstroke
      (dd) 25-Meter Breaststroke
      (ee) 25-Meter Butterfly
      (ff) 100-Meter Freestyle Relay
  (11) Track and Field
      (aa) 50-Meter Dash
      (bb) 200-Meter Dash
      (cc) 400-Meter Run
      (dd) Mile Run
      (ee) 400-Meter Relay
      (ff) High Jump
      (gg) Standing Long Jump
      (hh) Softball Throw
      (ii) Pentathlon
  (12) Volleyball
  (13) Wheelchair Events
      (aa) 25-Meter Race
      (bb) 30-Meter Slalom
      (cc) 100-Meter Relay
  (14) Winter Sports
      (aa) Alpine Skiing
  (11) Giant Slalom
  (22) Slalom
  (33) Downhill Race
      (bb) Nordic Skiing
  (11) 100-Meter Sprint
  (22) One-Kilometer Race

Table 10–2 (*Continued*)

Official Special Olympics Sports and Events. (*Cont.*)

---

    (33) Three-Kilometer Race

      (cc) Ice Skating

    (11) 50-Meter Race

    (22) 100-Meter Race

    (33) 400-Meter Race

    (44) Figure Skating

(b)   Rules for official sports and events are found in the "Official Special Olympics Sports Rules."

Demonstration Sports and Events.

(a)   Up to three of the following sports are eligible for inclusion in Chapter Games.

(1) Badminton	(7) Rhythmic Exercise and Dance
(2) Cross Country	(8) Synchronized Swimming
(3) Equestrian Events	(9) Tennis
(4) Field Hockey	(10) Touch Football
(5) Golf	(11) Water Polo
(6) Physical Fitness Events	(12) Wrestling

(b)   The following events are also classified as demonstration sports or events.

    (1) Gymnastics—low horizontal bar, side horse vault, low parallel bars, vaulting horse, still rings and pommel horse.

    (2) Swimming—100-meter freestyle, 50-meter backstroke, 50-meter breast-stroke, 100-meter individual medley, and 100-meter medley relay.

    (3) Track and Field—100-meter dash, 800-meter run (16 and older), 200-meter race walk, running triple jump (16 and older), shot put, hurdles (16 and older) and running long jump.

---

*From: Official Special Olympics General Rules

categories based upon the degree of their disability (e.g., wheelchair sports programs). Although the Special Olympics does use the I.Q. score of an individual to establish eligibility for participation, no attempt is made to further classify competitors according to their level of mental functioning. Rather, events are structured so that participants generally compete against others who are (1) the same sex, (2) similar in chronological age, and (3) at approximately the same level of performance. The last classification category is determined by examining actual scores, times, or distances recorded during prior meets or practice sessions. Thus, a 12-year-old girl with an I.Q. of 40 might compete in the same 50-meter dash as another girl of similar age, but with an I.Q. that is 25 points higher. Despite this rather large gap in I.Q. level, the race should still be a close one because previous 50-meter dash times, not I.Q. test scores, were used to place these girls in the same race. Exceptions to the above three categories for equalizing competition may be made occasionally, but only to ensure that there are enough athletes to enable a sport or event to be held.

Special Olympics originally offered athletic opportunities exclusively for children with mental retardation, but today there is no upper age limit for participation. Events are open to any individual with mental retardation who is 8 years of age or older. Since Special Olympics events are restricted to persons classified as having mental retardation, there is a maximum I.Q. score that serves as a guide for participant eligibility. Competitors generally have I.Q. scores of 75 or less. Interestingly, athletes who are members of established interscholastic or intramural teams are not eligible for Special Olympics events. This policy does limit some youth with mental retardation who wish to take part in as many athletic opportunities as possible, but it is consistent with the idea of mainstreaming. Persons with mental retardation who are able to compete in "regular" programs and activities do not require segregated experiences, such as Special Olympics events.

Important Aspects

There are many aspects of Special Olympics that deserve special recognition. A few of these are as follows.

The 10 Percent Rule. Equality of competition is a very important part of Special Olympics sports and events. A closely matched contest provides a more exciting and enjoyable time for both spectators and athletes. But the reason for ensuring basic competitive equality goes much further than just enjoyment: the self-esteem of a participant may be harmed if he or she is entered against athletes at vastly greater skill levels. Even physical injury could result from such situations, particularly if the less skilled competitor tries to duplicate a difficult maneuver without prior experience and training. In order to avoid physically and psychologically harmful situations caused by competitive imbalance, Special Olympics has the 10 percent rule. Basically, this rule requires that participants should be matched for competition with other athletes who perform within approximately 10 percent of each other. A 15-year-old boy who usually throws the softball about 30 meters should be grouped for competition with boys of similar ability who generally throw approximately 29 to 32 meters. Although this rule is obviously a flexible guideline and cannot always be enforced, it serves as an excellent standard to alert event organizers to the importance of equality of competition.

Wheelchair Competition. Special Olympics does offer a chance for individuals with multiple disabilities to experience sports competition, and many of these individuals use wheelchairs for mobility. The wheelchair competition within Special Olympics should not be confused with "wheelchair sports," however. The athletes participating in Special Olympics must conform to appropriate eligibility rules, including a diagnosis of mental retardation. Since the only restriction for participation in wheelchair sports is a lower extremity disability, Special Olympics wheelchair events offer a chance for *equal* competition for wheelchair users who have mental retardation that might not be available in conventional wheelchair sports programs.

Year-round Training and Participation. In 1979, the current mission statement for Special Olympics was adopted. One emphasis of this mission statement is "to provide year-round sports training and athletic competition in a variety of well-coached Olympic-type sports (Special Olympics, 1980). In its early development, Special Olympics received criticism because many participants were poorly trained and were often ill-prepared for competitive events. Although this situation still may exist in many cases, chapters such as New York, California, Pennsylvania, and the District of Columbia have led the way toward providing professional training for Special Olympics athletes. These and other Special Olympics Chapters recruit qualified volunteer leaders to train competitors and offer events in the fall, winter, and spring to ensure year-round fitness through Special Olympics participation.

Normalization Principles. One of the controversial aspects of Special Olympics is its traditional lack of conformity to the principles of mainstreaming and normalization. The program itself is a segregated experience and many Special Olympics events have featured child-oriented activities along with the competitive events. Face painters, clowns, and other well-meaning volunteers often provide an atmosphere not normally associated with athletic competition, particularly adult competition. Awards are frequently given to all competitors, not just those who succeed in their events. Volunteers are traditionally referred to as "huggers," a demeaning term that fosters an attitude of dependency. With the increasing professionalism of Special Olympics employees and volunteers, however, these situations appear to be changing. The District of Columbia Special Olympics (D.C.S.O.), for example, has established normalization as one of its most important goals. The staff of D.C.S.O. works closely with area group home residents. According to Steven L. Mason, D.C.S.O. Director of Training, "We feel that sports participation is a very important avenue for achieving the goal of normalization." He further notes that Special Olympics adheres as closely as possible to the spirit of regular Olympic Games, and points with pride to Loretta Claiborne, a young woman from Pennsylvania who got her start in Special Olympics. Ms. Claiborne has successfully completed over 10 marathon races.

Outcomes of Special Olympics

Special Olympics provides a unique training ground for children and adults with mental retardation. Through physical training and competition, particularly if these are conducted according to normalization principles, the participant learns behaviors that aid his or her adjustment in society. Physical fitness has been shown to improve, particularly when year-round opportunities are available (Texas Tech University, n.d.), and the increasing number of physical education programs inspired by Special Olympics should result in future gains in this important area. But Special Olympics offers more than physical fitness. The chance to experience success is essential to everyone, and Special Olympics offers successful experiences to many athletes with mental retardation, particularly those who work hard to get the most from their efforts. The following observation of one volunteer stresses the importance of effort and success:

> I remember one Special Olympian in particular. Her name was Christian. For an hour, from the time the games had begun at 9:15 A.M., she had been trying to complete a single [high] jump. After beginning her approach, she would stop two feet in front of the bar. There she stood, tense and rigid, either frightened or unsure, but always backing away, not attempting the jump. Other participants continued to take their turns. Some were successful, some weren't. And all the while Christian studied her jump. After an hour, she ran once more toward the bar with strong, even strides. She didn't balk this time. She jumped and cleared the bar, and the crowd roared its praise. Christian had cleared the high jump, a mere 1.1 meters (3'7"), but the blue ribbon I pinned on her made her feel at least 1.9 meters (6') tall. (Cassell, 1981, p. 519)

Increased levels of fitness, plus recognition that effort and self-discipline lead to success, are valuable outcomes of Special Olympics participation. In addition, research has demonstrated that many Special Olympics participants show (1) more recreation participation after involvement in the Special Olympics (Rarick, 1978), (2) improvement in a variety of recreational skills, including throwing, running, and jumping (Texas Tech University, n.d.), and (3) a more favorable attitude toward school and physical education (Texas Tech University, n.d.).

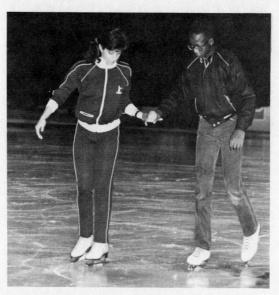

Figure 10–4. Skill development, under the guidance of qualified volunteers, in an important aspect of Special Olympics programs. Ice skating, for example, can be enjoyed after the competitive events are over. (Courtesy of District of Columbia Special Olympics)

Of course, not all aspects of Special Olympics are viewed as yielding positive outcomes for participants. Unless properly conducted, such programs may be more harmful than beneficial. Rarick (1978), for example, lists several undesirable features of Special Olympics, including: "(1) overemphasis by some on winning, with traumatic effects on the loser, (b) inappropriate grouping for competition, (c) program and meets being too long (inefficient administration), (d) inadequate safety precautions, and (e) parental apathy" (p. 245). As previously noted, however, Special Olympics leaders, under the direction of Mrs. Eunice Kennedy Shriver and Dr. Thomas Songster (Special Olympics' Director of Sports and Recreation), have made much progress toward overcoming prior weaknesses in programs throughout the nation. The key to overcoming the problems noted by Rarick is effective volunteer training, and this is the thrust of current Special Olympics efforts. As Steven Mason from D.C.S.O. commented, "Our *emphasis* has turned toward training for both athletes and volunteers." Despite some shortcomings, Special Olympics, Inc., is a rapidly growing organization that offers many valuable experiences to more than one million people with mental retardation.

—————————— SUMMARY ——————————

Despite widespread emphasis upon sports in North America, relatively little attention has been given to sports for people who have disabilities. One reason for this may be overemphasis upon the rehabilitative benefits of sports participation, rather than recognition that the needs and motivations of *all* athletes are basically the same. Providing opportunities for "parallel" competition is one way to emphasize these similarities without creating inequities that might result from direct competition between disabled and nondisabled athletes. Disabled sports humor in the form of cartoons also helps to reveal the normalcy of sports participation among athletes with disabilities. The phenomenal growth of programs such as wheelchair sports and the Special Olympics emphasizes the need for and benefits of sports competition among people who have disabilities.

Suggested Learning Activities

1. Observe (or participate in) a competitive wheelchair sports event and write a two-page report on the experience. Try to include both positive and negative reactions.

2. Interview an athlete who has a disability and determine what personal benefits he or she attributes to sports participation.

3. Make a list of 10 topics that you would consider when preparing and training volunteers for a Special Olympics event.

4. Discuss the benefits of participation in competitive sports for disabled individuals.

5. Choose one undesirable feature of Special Olympics cited by Rarick and determine at least three ways the problem could be resolved.

6. Using the cartoon pictured in Figure 10–1 as an example, create a cartoon illustrating sports for people with disabilities.

References

American Alliance for Health, Physical Education, Recreation and Dance. Labanowich sees olympic future for wheelchair basketball. *Journal of Physical Education and Recreation, 52*(6), 5, 1981.

Cassell, K. D. A special time for special children. *Phi Delta Kappan*, 62(7), 519, 1981.

Guttmann, L. and N. C. Mehra. Experimental studies on the value of archery in paraplegia. *Paraplegia, 11*, 159–165, 1973.

Haskins, J. *A New Kind of Joy*. Washington, D.C.: Joseph P. Kennedy Jr. Foundation, 1976.

Jochheim, K. and H. Strohkendl. The value of particular sports of the wheelchair-disabled in maintaining health of the paraplegic. *Paraplegia, 11*, 173–178, 1973.

Labanowich, S. *Wheelchair Basketball: A History of the National Association and an Analysis of the Structure and Organization of Teams*. Unpublished doctoral dissertation, University of Illinois, 1975.

LaMere, T. J. and S. Labanowich. The history of sports wheelchairs—Part III. *Sports 'n Spokes, 10*(2), 12–16, 1984.

Lindstrom, H. An integrated classification system. *Palaestra, 1*(2), 47–49, 1985.

Loiselle, D. Sport and the physically disabled. *Journal of Leisurability, 6*(1), 3–6, 1979.

McCann, H. The 1984 International Games for the Disabled. *Palaestra, 1*(2), 21–27, 1985.

McClements, J. Integration '84: Access to generic sports competition. *Journal of Leisurability, 11*(2), 20–23, 1984.

Michener, J. A. *Sports in America*. Greenwich, CT: Random House, 1976.

Mills, A. and L. K. Barnes. A world of winners: International Special Olympics. *Palaestra, 1*(1), 6–10, 1984.

Montelione, T. and J. V. Mastro. Beep baseball. *Journal of Physical Education, Recreation and Dance*, 56(6), 60–61, 1985.

Nettleton, B. Self confidence and sport for the handicapped. *Rehabilitation in Australia, 11*(4), 7–11, October, 1974.

Nugent, T. J. Precepts and concepts on research and demonstration needs in physical education and recreation for the physically handicapped. In *Study Conference on Research and Recreation for Handicapped Children* (proceedings), University of Maryland, 1969, pp. 20–23.

Rarick, G. L. Adult reactions to the Special Olympics. In Smoll, F. L. and R. E. Smith, eds., *Psychological Perspectives in Youth Sports*. New York: John Wiley & Sons, 1978.

Rarick, G. L. Recent advances related to special physical education and sport. *Adapted Physical Activity Quarterly, 1*(3), 197–206, 1984.

Sage, G. H. *Sport and American Society: Selected Readings*, 2nd ed. Reading, MA: Addison-Wesley, 1974.

Sherrill, C. and J. Canabal. A kaleidoscope of faces and feelings from the 1984 International Games. *Palaestra, 1*(2), 28–32, 1985.

Shriver, E. K. Tracing the growth of the Special Olympics winter sports program. *Palaestra, 1*(2), 15–18, 1985.

Special Olympics. *Official Special Olympics General Rules*. Washington: Special Olympics, Inc., 1980.

Spira, R., ed. *Influence of Sport Activities on Rehabilitation of Paralytic Subjects*. (Final Report, Project V.R.A.—Isr. No. 22–64), Tel Aviv, Israel, 1967.

Spraggs, S. Archery with the sightless sight system. *Palaestra*, *1*(1), 38–39, 1984.

Steadward, R. D. *Wheelchair Sports Classification System*. Unpublished doctoral dissertation, University of Oregon, 1978.

Stein, J. New vistas in competitive sports for athletes with handicapping conditions. *Exceptional Education Quarterly*, *3*(1), 28–34, 1982.

Texas Tech University. *The Impact of Special Olympics on Participants, Parents and the Community*. Unpublished Study, n.d.

Weisman, M. and J. Godfrey. *So Get On With It*. Garden City, NY: Doubleday, 1976.

Zeigler, E. F. *History of Physical Education and Sport*. Englewood Cliffs, NJ: Prentice-Hall, 1979.

Zwiren, L. D. and O. Bar-or. Responses to exercise of paraplegics who differ in conditioning level. *Medicine and Science in Sport*, *7*(2), 94–98, 1975.

RESOURCES, LEGISLATION, AND TRENDS

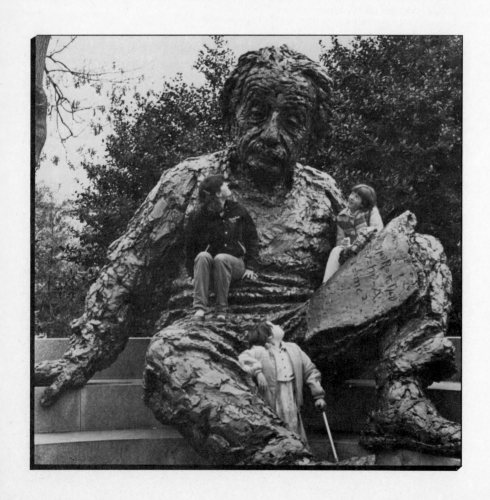

The thought that communities are made up of individuals who function together in applying their resources toward the common good is basic to Chapter 11, *Community Resources.* A process by which citizens collaborate to bring about change in the well-being of the community, referred to as community development, is discussed in the chapter. Particular emphasis is placed on (1) community resources as they relate to recreation for special populations and (2) understanding the community from a sociocultural perspective.

In Chapter 12, *Legislation Affecting Community Programs and Services,* legislation related to community recreation and special populations is presented and interpreted. Special attention is given to the Architectural Barriers Act of 1968, the Rehabilitation Act and its amendments and extensions over the years, the Education of All Handicapped Children Act of 1975, and the Developmental Disabilities and Facilities Construction Act. Implications for recreation for special populations are given for the various pieces of legislation.

In Chapter 13, *Trends in Community Recreation for Special Populations,* an attempt is made to look into the future in order to come to an understanding of things to evolve in the area of leisure services for special populations. Drawing on the views of experts, the literature of the field, and personal intuition, trends for the future are discussed in terms of programming, new approaches, community relations, financial matters, and professional concerns. The chapter concludes on a positive note regarding an increased acceptance of special recreation services by those directing leisure service delivery systems.

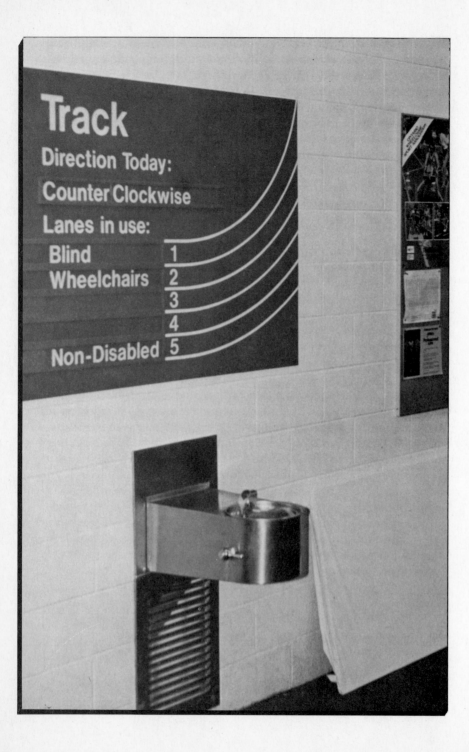

11

Community Resources

What are community resources? How do community resources help provide for special recreation services? What basic knowledge of and skills in community development are helpful in establishing community services for special populations? It is intended that this chapter will address these questions. To do so, perhaps the best way to begin is by defining the term *community resources.*

Webster's New Collegiate Dictionary defines community as "a unified body of individuals." It goes on to clarify by stating that people in a community may have common interests, interact with one another, and live in a particular geographic area. Although the dictionary stipulates the term may also be utilized to describe persons linked by a common interest (e.g., academic community, religious community), it is not in this sense that it is employed in this chapter. Sessoms' (1980) sociologically based definition provides as complete a definition of community as is found in the recreation literature. He has written:

> Sociologists define a community as a collection of individuals who live within a specific geographical area, share a common bond of interdependency and commitment, and function as a group in achieving and fulfilling human needs and wishes. More simply stated, a community is people, geographically living and working together, sharing the benefits of their labor and other endeavors. (pp. 120, 121)

Resources, according to *Webster's New Collegiate Dictionary* are "a source of supply or support: an available means." Resources are persons or things that can be drawn upon as they are needed in order to meet an end. They may include:

- Human Resources
- Informational Resources
- Financial Resources
- Facility and Equipment Resources
- Transportation Resources.

All five types of resources will be discussed in this chapter as they relate to a community providing special recreation services. Community resources, as used here, then are those available means by which communities meet the recreational needs of special populations.

THE IMPORTANCE OF COMMUNITY RESOURCES

Why is an understanding of community resources necessary for leisure service professionals? The answer to this question is relatively straight-forward. Resources are required to accomplish any goal the leisure service professional may have. Without a knowledge of potential resources and how to use them, it is unlikely that goals will be realized. Recreation and park professionals need to develop a working knowledge of existing resources and to know how to draw upon these to achieve goals. The goal of fulfilling the recreational needs of community members from special population groups requires developing particular types of community resources.

HUMAN RESOURCES

Human resources that may be employed in conducting programs for persons with special needs include volunteers, existing agency staff, students completing professional field experiences, personnel from related agencies, and consultants who have skills that may add to the program. Some may assist with the special recreation program on a sustained basis, others may become involved only as they are needed. For example, some individuals may volunteer regularly to work with a particular activity or participate as a member of an advisory council. Others may become involved only with special events or at times calling for their particular skills.

Developing and cultivating human resources is a primary task of the professional coordinating community special recreation services. There are, or course, many ways to go about locating people who may serve as resources. Once an advisory council is formed, its members can be a ready source of information in identifying individuals to fulfill needed roles. Similarly, members of interagency councils can supply names of individuals who may be resources. In some communities, directories of social services will be available. Contacts at colleges and universities are another source of human resources. Many colleges and universities have student volunteer bureaus through which students may give of their talents. Faculty members may have students wishing to complete field experiences and may also serve as consultants, identifying human service personnel in the community. Labor unions and civic clubs offer additional sources of human resources.

No matter what approaches are used to identify human resources, the information collected should be organized in a way that is systematic and easily retrievable. The individual's name, address, telephone number, and how he or she could be a potential resource should be recorded on a card for future reference each time a person is identified.

Volunteers

Budget-conscious administrators may utilize volunteers to enable them to effectively meet the needs of persons with disabilities, while providing services under limited budgets. Volunteers offer a way to stretch an agency's resources. But volunteers supply far more than inexpensive labor in the absence of paid staff. They offer a wealth of diversity in backgrounds and skills that would rarely be available within regular staff. Volunteers also share a dedication to service. Because of their diversity and dedication, they can accomplish tasks that would be difficult or impossible without their efforts.

Janet Pomeroy, Founder and Director of the Recreation Center for the Handicapped in San Francisco, has spoken of the wide base of community support found on the Center's Board of Directors (Pomeroy, 1974). Among those on the Board were:

- several medical doctors
- a social worker
- several attorneys
- a real estate and insurance broker
- a superior court justice
- a recreation educator
- a physical educator
- a member of the Social Services Commission
- a food broker
- a product executive
- an architect

- other business men and women
- parents representing the Auxiliary.

Because of their diverse talents, the Center's board members were able to take on a number of assignments including fund raising, transportation, insurance, recruitment of staff and volunteers, reviewing legislation for funding sources, obtaining supplies and equipment, assisting with preparation of grant applications, and contacting city officials regarding contractual services for the Center (Pomeroy, 1974).

Every community has a number of persons who desire to volunteer their services to meaningful projects. These persons may wish to serve on a board or advisory council for the special recreation program, to do face-to-face leadership, or to work in a supportive capacity in administration, promotion, transportation, or some other aspect of the program.

Recruiting Volunteers. Pomeroy (1974) has employed a number of means to recruit volunteers at the Recreation Center for the Handicapped. She feels that a primary means is to get potential volunteers to visit the Center. Pomeroy states, "We can show the need for the program; we can demonstrate the benefits of recreation; and we can stimulate interest—all of which makes them want to help" (p. 11). Promotion is a second means used by Pomeroy to secure volunteers. The Center provides presentations to service clubs, fraternal organizations, and other groups, and conducts planned campaigns in newspapers and on radio and television. Finally, program volunteers are recruited through contacts with junior high schools, hospitals, youth service agencies, volunteer bureaus, and participants in the Center's program.

The concept of using volunteers from among the Center's participants merits further discussion. Volunteer service can be an especially meaningful leisure pursuit for persons with disabilities. *The Source Book for the Disabled* (Hale, 1979) states:

> This (volunteer work) is a particularly satisfying involvement for people with disabilities because it puts them on the giving, rather than the receiving, end of the "care package." Sighted people with physical disabilities can do much to help the blind by learning braille (or the braille musical code) so they can transcribe printed material, by reading aloud to the blind or by acting as "guide eyes" for them on excursions. Older people who have physical disabilities are often particularly successful at establishing warm and trusting relationships with mentally and physically handicapped children and are able to help them to learn some skill, craft or sport. (p. 355)

Keys to Successful Volunteer Programs. Three key elements must exist in any successful volunteer program. These are (1) involving volunteers in the program; (2) recognizing the volunteers' contributions; and (3) providing proper training for volunteers. Volunteers must be made to feel a part of the program by being included in on decisions. Volunteers, who give freely of themselves, do not wish to be "told what to do." They want to have a voice in the program. Volunteers also need to receive positive feedback when it is deserved. This praise should be given on a daily basis, with special recognition shown through an established awards program. Finally, volunteers must be provided with orientation and training to enable them to succeed.

An outline for the in-service training of volunteers is contained in the Project LIFE (Life is for Everyone) resource and training manual produced at the University of North Carolina (Bullock et al., 1982. pp. 106, 107). Topics include:

1. Characteristics of various disabilities, noting possible limitations and special considerations (emergency and health care procedures should be outlined here also);
2. General activity and equipment modification techniques;
3. Overview of the least restrictive environment concept and how it is being implemented in the department;
4. Assessing existing attitudes of recreation professionals (and volunteers) toward individuals with handicapping conditions;
5. Creating peer acceptance;
6. Use of instructional aides and volunteers;
7. Where to find additional resource information for a specific disability.

Existing Agency Staff

Existing agency staff can add greatly to programming for special populations. Of course, these staff members need to have an in-service training program similar to that outlined for volunteers in the preceding section. Vaughan and Winslow (1979) have written of the advantages of providing regular recreation and park department personnel with such in-service training. They have stated, "Such a program would train regular recreation program personnel to work effectively with the handicapped program participants and would also help them to work with any handicapped participants that they might have in their regular recreation programs" (p. 10).

Students Completing Professional Field Experiences

University departments providing professional preparation for parks and recreation service have students who are required to complete

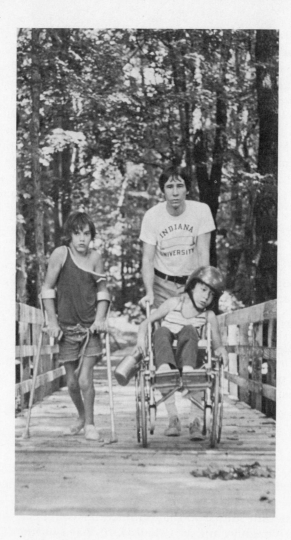

Figure 11–1. A student intern can be a valuable resource.

professional field experiences. These may take the form of practicums or internships. Most practicum experiences are organized to be accomplished during a few hours each week. Full-time internships or field work experiences are often done over a quarter (10 weeks) or semester (15 weeks). Both practicum and internship students can make valuable contributions, provided the agency is willing to offer professional supervision for them. While most students should have some educational preparation regarding special recreation, it is important that agencies complete an early assessment of each student's competencies so that appropriate responsibilities may be assigned and gaps in knowledge or skills may be filled through additional training.

Contracting for Services

Another means of obtaining necessary human resources is to contract for the services of individuals who perform specific tasks. It may be most feasible during the initial stage of program development to enter into contractual arrangements for the services of personnel to consult with regular staff and to actually conduct programs for special populations.

Consultation services can be arranged with administrators of existing recreation programs for special populations, with university faculty who have experience in working with special recreation programs, or with private consultants with expertise in community special recreation programs. Personnel from other community agencies often have the competencies necessary to provide direct service functions. These persons may be employed on a part-time basis to lead special recreation programs. For example, therapeutic recreation specialists for local hospitals or rehabilitation centers may be contracted to offer programs within community park and recreation facilities.

Studies (Edginton et al., 1975; Austin et al., 1978; Vaughan & Winslow, 1979) have identified the lack of trained program personnel as a major hurdle to clear in order to establish community special recreation services. The creative use of human resources may offer a vehicle by which to launch needed community recreation programs for members of special population groups.

INFORMATIONAL RESOURCES

Many resources exist that can offer information valuable to establishing and developing community recreation services for special populations. These range from local resource persons to national computer retrieval systems.

Local Resources

In many communities, or in close proximity, will be colleges and universities that have faculty members with backgrounds in recreation for special populations. Secondly, therapeutic recreation specialists in local hospitals, rehabilitation centers, associations for retarded citizens, mental health centers, and other facilities are often anxious to assist in the development of special recreation programs. Finally, park and recreation staff in neighboring communities, or park districts, may be able to share information concerning leisure services for special populations.

Literature

Although few books have been published on recreation for special populations, a number of journal articles have appeared on the subject. Two journals in which articles have regularly appeared have been *Leisurability* and the *Therapeutic Recreation Journal*. *Sports n' Spokes* provides information on wheelchair athletics. Computer information retrieval systems offer a means to identify a full spectrum of articles, books, and papers that apprise the reader of recent developments. Most major university libraries have access to computerized retrieval systems through which may be obtained an abstracted list of publications in any area of interest.

Organizations

Another source of information on special recreation services is through various organizations. State and local professional park and recreation societies often have committees or individuals who may provide information to practitioners. National professional organizations may also offer assistance. Two of the major organizations in the United States are the American Alliance for Health, Physical Education, Recreation, and Dance (AAHPERD) and the National Recreation and Park Association (NRPA). AAHPERD has offered consultation and literature on programs for persons with disabilities. NRPA offers useful publications such as *Guidelines for Community Based Recreation Programs for Special Populations*, edited by Vaughan and Winslow (1979).

Athletic and recreational organizations for persons with disabilities such as the National Wheelchair Basketball Association, National Wheelchair Athletic Association, Special Olympics, American Blind Bowling Association, and other similar organizations, offer information regarding their particular area of recreational interest. These organizations are listed in Appendix D. Appendix C lists organizations concerned with specific disabilities. Among these, several have been particularly active in promoting special recreation programs, including the American Foundation for the Blind, the Epilepsy Foundation of America, and the National Easter Seal Society for Crippled Children and

Adults. An example of the efforts of such groups has been the publication of *Recreation Programming for Visually Impaired Children and Youth* (Kelley, 1981), an extensive book produced by the American Foundation for the Blind. Finally, youth-serving agencies have attempted to serve the needs of special populations. Two are the Girl Scouts of the USA and the YMCA of the USA. Of particular note has been the Mainstreaming Activities for Youth (MAY) project, conducted by the YMCA Office of Special Populations (Box 1781, Longview, Washington 98632), which brought together 10 youth-serving agencies in a collaborative effort to enhance their mainstreaming efforts.

Conferences, Institutes, and Workshops

Continuing education opportunities abound today. The largest providers of conferences, institutes, and workshops are professional societies and universities. Both the AAHPERD and the NRPA annual conferences regularly offer educational programs on recreation for special populations. In recent years, NRPA has also conducted an annual institute on special recreation programs. Universities provide workshops and institutes for the development of community-based services for special populations. Recreation and leisure studies curricula are the usual sponsors of these programs.

While information on special recreation services has been relatively limited in the past, its growth has been inspired by the desire of many professionals and citizens to establish community-based programs. It is likely that the amount of information available will grow as interest in the area builds.

FINANCIAL RESOURCES

Perhaps no one resource area attracts as much attention as that of financial resources. Without adequate financial support no program can continue to exist. Those concerned with developing programs for special populations must be knowledgeable about financial resources.

Vaughan and Winslow (1979) found that the major funding source for special recreation programs is the general tax fund. Slightly over 87 percent of all park and recreation agencies surveyed used the general tax as a source of funding. Fees and charges were the second greatest source, used by 44.2 percent of the agencies. The types of sources utilized beyond these depended largely on the size of the community. Communities of under 100,000 tended to fund 30 percent to 40 percent of their program from donations. Government grants were a major source of funding for those cities over 250,000 people. Other sources of funds were special taxes, private grants, and contractual agreements.

Vaughan and Winslow state that the major funding source for special recreation programs should be the general tax fund. We concur that special recreation programs should be supported to the largest degree possible through existing tax structures. However, in a time of budget limitations, professionals must be aware of alternative sources as well. This is particularly true when beginning new programs. Once established, special recreation programs usually are supported by the citizenry. Special appropriations may be needed, however, to initiate services.

Special Taxes. Park districts and municipalities in the State of Illinois have been highly successful in establishing special population programs. One reason for the success in Illinois has been legislation that allows park districts and other governmental bodies to cooperate by forming special recreation associations and to levy a special tax up to $.02 for $100 of assessed valuation for special recreation programs. The publication *Guidelines for the Formation and Development of Special Recreation Cooperatives in the State of Illinois* (Robb, 1976) contains specific information regarding the Illinois special tax. Thus, at least one state has used legislation to establish financial means to support special recreation programs.

Fees and Charges. Fees and charges can provide another financial resource for special recreation programming. Just as other public park and recreation programs are supported by fees and charges, similarly those for special populations can apply fees. These should, of course, be in line with other fees charged by the agency.

Contractual Agreements. Park and recreation agencies can enter into contractual agreements with schools, nursing homes, and other agencies to provide recreation services for special populations. While contractual agreements are likely to be a minor financial resource, they offer an additional means of support.

Fund Raising. Fund-raising projects are another means to obtaining revenue for special recreation programs. Many techniques may be used in fund raising. These include governmental and foundation grants, memorial giving, house-to-house and direct mail solicitations, capital fund campaigns, and special events (Mirkin, 1972). Information on governmental and foundation grants is covered in the section that follows. A good source of general information on fund raising is Mirkin's (1972) book, *The Complete Fund Raising Guide.*

Grants. Grants may be made by a governmental agency or through a private foundation. In the past, federal grant monies have been available through a number of sources including Title IV of the Social Security Act for Aid to Families with Dependent Children, Title XIV of the Social Rehabilitation Act, the Developmental Disabilities Services and Facilities Construction Act (PL 88–164) and Amending Law (PL 91–517), The Architectual Barriers Act of 1968 (PL 90–480), and the Rehabilitation Act of 1973 (PL 93–112). Since the governmental grant picture is constantly changing, it is wise to refer to recent information sources when seeking grant funding. The sources that follow provide basic information on where to apply to receive both governmental and foundation grants.

Some possible information sources on grants are:

Annual Register of Grant Support. Academic Media, Marquis Who's Who, Inc., 4300 W. 62nd Street, Indianapolis, Indiana 46268. (Most useful as a guide to private sources of support.)

Catalog of Federal Domestic Assistance. Superintendent of Documents, U.S. Government Printing Office, Washington, D.C. 20402. (Provides a listing and description of federal programs.)

The Corporate Fund Raising Directory. Public Services Materials Center, 415 Lexington Avenue, New York, NY 10017. (Lists 550 corporations and corporate foundations.)

The Foundation Directory. The Foundation Center, 888 Seventh Avenue, New York, NY 10106. (Lists by state 3,363 major foundations in the USA.)

Handicapped Funding Directory. Research Grant Guides, P.O. Box 356, Oceanside, NY 11572. (Lists foundations, associations, and agencies that have funded programs for persons with handicaps.)

Taft Corporate Information System. Taft Corporation, 1000 Vermont Avenue, N.W., Washington, DC 20005. (The system has three components: a newsletter, a regular series of reports on corporations and corporate foundations, and a directory of the major corporate giving entities in the USA.)

It is important to know as much as possible about the governmental agency or foundation. Once potential sources have been identified and information gathered about them, a well-prepared proposal must be developed. What makes a good proposal? There are a number of books to aid in the preparation of sound grant proposals. Some sources of information on how to prepare a grant proposal are:

Dermer, J. *How to Write Successful Foundation Presentations.* New York: Public Services Materials Center (355 Lexington Avenue, New York, NY 10017), 1974.

DesMarais, P. *How to Get Government Grants.* New York: Public Services Materials Center (355 Lexington Avenue, New York, NY 10017), 1975.

Hall, M. *Developing Skills in Proposal Writing*, 2nd ed. Portland: Continuing Education Publications (1633 S.W. Park, P.O. Box 1491, Portland, Oregon 97207), 1977.

Kurzig, C. M. *Foundation Fundamentals: A Guide for Grantseekers*, rev. ed. New York: The Foundation Center (888 Seventh Avenue, New York, NY 10106), 1981.

Lefferts, R. *Getting a Grant in the 1980s*, 2nd ed. Englewood Cliffs, NJ: Prentice-Hall, Inc., 1982.

Margolin, J. B. *About Foundations: How to Find Facts You Need to Get a Grant.* New York: The Foundation Center (888 Seventh Avenue, New York, NY 10106), 1962.

Proposal Writers Handbook: A Step by Step Process. Washington, D.C.: National Association of State Directors of Special Education, 1976.

White, V. P. *Grants: How to Find Out About Them and What To Do Next.* New York: Plenum Press, 1975.

As we have seen, there are many different potential financial resources available for special recreation programs. Funding can come from general taxes, special taxes, fees and charges, contractual agreements, fund-raising projects, governmental grants, or foundation grants. The point should be reiterated, however, that the primary funding for special recreation programs should come from the normal funding source of parks and recreation and not from grants or other special sources.

FACILITY AND EQUIPMENT RESOURCES

Potential facilities for special population programs include parks, forests, pools, community centers, gymnasiums, bowling lanes, athletic fields, and other places where organized recreation commonly takes place. Equipment includes lasting articles or apparatus needed to conduct programs. While adapted equipment is necessary for a few activities, standard recreational equipment is frequently employed in special recreation programs.

Facilities

The major facilities for special recreation programs should be those controlled and programmed by the agency. Of course, existing facilities have to be evaluated to make certain they are accessible and usable by persons with disabilities before they are scheduled for special population programs.

Most communities have a wide array of potential facilities that may be utilized for special recreation programs. In addition to those of the park and recreation department, facilities may be made available through schools, voluntary and youth-serving agencies (e.g., YMCA, YWCA), bowling lanes, churches, hospitals, rehabilitation centers, and other public and private organizations. As a general rule, programs should be conducted in facilities normally used for programming by the park and recreation department or park district.

A facility resource file should be maintained so that a current list of facilities is available. Included should be the name and address of the facility, the agency controlling it, accessibility information, special equipment available at the facility, any cost for use, the contact person, and a phone number. Many communities have published accessibility guides that would be useful in establishing such a resource file. Advisory councils and interagency councils are also potentially rich sources of information in identifying suitable facilities for special recreation programming.

Equipment

It may be necessary to purchase or construct adaptive devices or equipment for some recreation activities to be used by persons with disabilities. Adapted equipment, however, can take on a gimmicky quality if it is not well conceived. It is usually best to consult with an expert before purchasing or building equipment when unsure about the type of equipment or the necessity to have it. Therapeutic recreation specialists often can provide expert advice regarding adaptive equipment. Program participants may also have expertise regarding adaptive equipment.

Examples of adaptive equipment include handle-grip bowling balls (handles automatically retract to be flush into the ball when released), bowling rails to guide visually impaired bowlers, bicycle buddy bars (permit two regular bicycles to ride side-by-side), tricycle body supports (enable children with poor balance to use tricycles), and floor sitters (resemble chairs without legs that allow children to sit up during floor play) (Austin & Powell, 1980). There are, of course, scores of pieces of adapted equipment that may be purchased or constructed. A number of commercial suppliers list adaptive equipment in their catalogues. See Appendix E for a list of potential suppliers.

TRANSPORTATION RESOURCES

Transportation of participants is viewed by many park and recreation departments to be the greatest problem in providing special recreation programs (Vaughan & Winslow, 1979). Major resources suggested by Vaughan and Winslow to solve transportation problems include the following.

■ *Car Pooling.* Participants, families, and friends may serve as resources for developing car pools organized by the park and recreation system.

- *Service Clubs and Social Service Agencies.* Groups such as the Red Cross, Kiwanis, and Lions Clubs may provide transportation for participants. Service clubs may also possibly purchase vans for the park and recreation department.
- *Federal Funding to Purchase Vans.* In the past, federal legislation has provided funding sources for transportation. The Federal-Aid Highway Act of 1973 (PL 93–87) and the Developmental Disabilities Services and Facilities Construction Act of 1971 (PL 91–517) are examples of federal laws for the allocation of funds for transportation.
- *Contractual Agreements.* Contractual agreements may be drawn with schools, health agencies, or other organizations. Such agreements have the added advantage of possibly bringing more participants into the special populations programs from the contracting agency.
- *Public Transportation.* New buses, such as the low floor, heavy duty bus designed by Skillcraft Industries, have features that make them accessible to persons with physical disabilities. The Cleveland Greater Regional Transit and Portland Regional Transit have been using the Skillcraft buses, which have manual wheelchair ramps and low, wide entrances (Ryder, 1982). If public transit systems can be persuaded to obtain such buses, mass transit will offer a viable resource to assist in solving transportation problems for special recreation programs.

The effective use of existing community resources can enable the leisure service professional to meet the recreational needs of persons from special population groups. Creative utilization of community resources, of course, presumes a knowledge of available resources. The first, and largest, segment of this chapter has provided information to permit the location of potential resources. The final portion of the chapter deals with the basic skills in and understanding of community development* that is needed to establish services for persons with disabilities.

KNOWING THE COMMUNITY

Communities are diverse, each being uniquely different from the next. The terms sociocultural, demographic, and ecological have been

---

*The term community development, as used in this chapter, refers to the process by which citizens collaborate to take action to improve the well-being of the community.

employed to categorize the essential features that make communities distinctive. Primary sociocultural variables are social organization and culture. Demographic variables include population size; age, sex, and race composition; birth and death rates; and migration to and from the community and within its boundaries. The ecological perspective is concerned with the interrelationship between the citizens of the community and the geographic setting (Edwards & Jones, 1976).

Sociocultural Variables

The material that follows deals with the sociocultural variables of concern to the leisure service professional wishing to initiate special recreation services. Analysis of the social organization and culture of the community is critical to success in working with structures that bring individuals, agencies, and organizations together to cooperatively achieve common goals.

Features of the social structure in the sociocultural facet of community life are: social groups; social stratification; community subsystems such as the family, the economy, education, religion, government, and social welfare; and normative structures dealing with social norms and values (Edwards & Jones, 1976).

Social Groups. Groups can be formal or informal. Formal groups are those that have structural rules and regulations to govern relationships. Because of their structure, they can utilize formal communications systems that reach relatively large numbers. Examples of formal groups are labor unions, service organizations, and golf and tennis clubs.

Informal groups revolve around interpersonal relationships between group members. Informal groups are relatively small and allow members to meet emotional needs through intimate interactions. Examples are family groups and peer groups (Edwards & Jones, 1976).

Social Stratification. Social stratification deals with social prestige and power. Social prestige is concerned with social class structure. Power deals with the ability to control others and to effect change. Often those in the higher social classes have the most power, although there is not always a direct correspondence since some of the "better" families (high social class) may not hold power due to diminished wealth and political influence. In most communities, however, those with the most influence are those in the upper social classes, or those who hold high status in one of the subsystems such as government or religion (Edwards & Jones, 1976).

Three approaches may be applied to determine holders of power in the community. These are the reputational, positional, and decisional approaches. To determine power by the reputational approach, one must ask the question: Who do you check with before acting? What individual(s), formal groups, or informal groups do you consult on communitywide decisions? The positional approach assumes that those in positions of authority hold the power. Examples would be the mayor and the superintendent of parks and recreation. The final approach, the decisional approach, takes for granted that those involved in making decisions for the community hold the power (Sessoms, 1980).

Sessoms has discussed two situations of power in the community. The first is the *power elite*. The power elite exists in communities where the power is in the hands of a few individuals. In contrast to this monolithic approach is the *multiple pyramid system* in which no one group holds power. Instead, it is a pluralistic system in which the power is held by many.

Jewell (1983), in an article on power structures as they relate to the recreation integration of disabled persons, has discussed four types of communities originally proposed by McCarty and Ramsey (1971). These have been termed the: (1) dominated or restricted power community, (2) functional or conflict-dissipated power community, (3) pluralistic or accordant power community, and (4) inert or power-avoidance community. Jewell has stated that the ability to analyze the community for these power structures is more important than any other aspect of community analysis.

The first of the community power structures presented by Jewell is similar to the power elite community discussed by Sessoms (1980). In the *dominated or restricted power community*, power is maintained by a single individual or a small group of people. Many times the person or persons who are in control run an industry that dominates the community. Citizen boards simply "rubber stamp" the decisions made by the power elite, so the park and recreation department is likewise apt to be under their control. In the case of the community with dominated or restricted power structure, it is necessary to gain the support of the power elite in a way that they will not perceive as threatening.

The second of the community power structures is the *factional or conflict-dissipated power community*. Under this structure long standing factions of the community constantly fight for power. Governing boards are split by factionalism and therefore have great difficulty agreeing on issues. This is a difficult power structure with which to work. The professional must attempt to make progress with both factions, yet not appear to be siding with one group against the other. Hopefully, the creative professional can enable both groups to see how they would beneifit from the new program so their support will be forthcoming.

The *pluralistic or accordant power community* is similar to Sessoms' (1980) multiple pyramid system. Here Jewell states, " . . . sanity and reason do reign and . . . issues and community welfare are important" (p. 27). Petty thinking does not override the decision-making process. Groups debate in a democratic manner to arrive at a consensus on what is best for the community. The leisure service administrator is likely to be viewed as a knowledgeable resource when making decisions. Therefore, the administrator should have thoroughly researched information on the establishment of community services for special populations so he or she can properly brief those in authority of the rationale and procedures for establishing the service.

The least common power structure is the *inert or power-avoidance community*. Both those in positions of authority and the citizenry are apathetic. Here the leisure service administrator ends up making decisions that are, in turn, "rubberstamped" by the board. The problem here is getting the community out of its dormant state and into something new. Even in the most inert of communities, there are a few individuals who are capable of responding given the right motivation.

Knowing the likely community power structure allows the professional to choose the best strategy when approaching those holding power. The professional who is not cognizant of the local power structure will likely have problems in establishing special recreation services, particularly when the integration of disabled persons into ongoing programs is a goal, since integration brings other participants into direct contact with individuals with disabilities.

Community Subsystems. The third aspect of the sociocultural facet involves community subsystems such as the family, the economy, the government, religion, education, and social welfare. Those who hold high status in the various subsystems are likely to have influence within the community. Knowing these persons and their possible interest in community recreation for special populations can be very helpful in establishing new services. This is particularly true with the social welfare subsystem.

The social welfare subsystem, as defined by Edwards and Jones (1976), deals with three major types of community services. These are social work, health care, and recreation. Often social welfare agencies organize themselves for joint action. Community organization structures can take the form of wide-based cooperation such as a council of human service agencies. In other instances agencies with particular thrusts may form councils. For example, a local recreation council may form. Recreation councils are usually made up of nongovernmental agencies such as Boy Scouts, Girl Scouts, Young Men's Christian Association, Young Women's Christian Association, Hebrew Association, and governmental agencies such as park districts, or city or county park and recreation departments. In beginning special recreation services it becomes necessary to know what councils exist in the community so that their support may be gained.

Smaller communities will, of course, be less likely to have coordinating councils. Nevertheless, individual social welfare agencies, churches, service clubs, educational systems, and advocacy groups (e.g., parents groups) are potential allies to initiating special recreation programs. It is therefore just as important to understand these independent agencies as it is to be knowledgeable of coordinating councils in larger communities.

Normative Structures. The final aspect of the sociocultural facet is the normative structure of the community. Social norms are extremely important to the community, as Edwards and Jones (1976) state:

> The social structure of the community—as described above through social groups, social stratification patterns, and subsystems—gets its stability and order from the fact that it exists within a normative structure. The normative structure is made up of norms, i.e., rules and standards that define what people should and should not do in various facets of their community living; sanctions, in the form of penalties applied for violation of, and rewards offered for conformity to, the norms; and values that represent the priorities people attach to material and nonmaterial features of their culture. (p. 89)

Of particular importance to community development are the social norms and values of the community toward change. Some communities will be slower than others to accept any innovation. Resistance to innovation may be lessened if the change fits the existing community value system (Edwards & Jones, 1976). For example, a community that prizes athletic competition may be led to understand how persons with disabilities also need opportunities for sports participation and how the provision of such opportunities can strengthen the athletic image of the community.

Summary: Sociocultural Facet.

The sociocultural facet of community life deals with informal and formal groups, social stratification and power, the varied community subsystems, and norms and values. The normative structure gives the community stability and order. It gives the community its "character." Actions leading to community development transpire through the social groups, social stratification patterns, and subsystems of the community. Familiarity with the sociocultural facet of the community can be of great assistance when initiating any new program, including special recreation services.

SUMMARY

This chapter has discussed community resources as they pertain to the provision of special recreation services. Community resources, including human, informational, financial, and transportation, are necessary to accomplish any goal the leisure service provider may have. Thus, it is important that recreation and park professionals are knowledgeable of such resources and know how to use them in achieving their goals. The use of volunteers and the seeking of additional funding are two aspects which are highlighted in this chapter. Also important to the establishment of special recreation services is understanding the community from a sociocultural perspective. Knowing the community power structures as they relate to the recreation integration of disabled persons enhances the ability of the leisure service professional to provide services for all people, including those individuals who may be disabled.

Suggested Learning Activities

1. Volunteer in a special recreation program. If this is for a single event (e.g., wheelchair basketball game), report your observations in class from your perspective as a volunteer. If you volunteer over a period of time, keep a log of your experiences and reactions. Prepare a brief report based on your log.

2. Interview a disabled person who is volunteering. Ask him or her how he or she became involved as a volunteer and the benefits derived. Bring your notes to class for discussion.

3. Invite several disabled athletes to class to discuss sports organizations with which they are affiliated.

4. Compile a resource file on organizations in your home town that might have interest in community recreation programs for persons with disabilities.

5. In a group, discuss why it is important for recreation professionals to be familiar with organizations related to special populations.

6. Interview a recreation administrator regarding funding for special recreation services. Take notes on your discussion and report to the class.

7. Work on the following problem in a small group. You are in charge of a camp that integrates disabled and nondisabled campers. What alternatives can you identify for funding your

camp, in addition to having parents pay a fee for their child? Use library resources in preparing your response. Report your conclusions to the class.

8. Compile a resource file on national leisure organizations for persons with disabilities. To do this, divide the task among the class members. Organize the brochures and other items you collect so that they may be placed in the library for future reference by other students.

9. Working with a small group of students, analyze the community power structure in your home town, college community, or some other community chosen with your instructor. Write a report of no more than 10 pages on your findings. Then make a presentation in class to highlight your findings.

References

Austin, D. R., J. A. Peterson, and L. M. Peccarelli. The status of services for special populations in the state of Indiana. *Therapeutic Recreation Journal 12* (1), 1978, 50–56.

Austin, D. R. and L. G. Powell, eds. *Resource Guide: College Instruction in Recreation for Individuals with Handicapping Conditions.* Bloomington: Indiana University, 1980.

Bullock, C. C., R. E. Wohl, T. E. Webreck, and A. M. Crawford. *Life is for Everyone Resource and Training Manual.* Curriculum in Recreation Administration, University of North Carolina at Chapel Hill, 1982.

Edginton, C. R., D. M. Compton, A. J. Ritchie, and R. K. Vederman. The status of services for special populations in park and recreation in the state of Iowa. *Therapeutic Recreation Journal 9* 109–116, 1975.

Edwards, A. D., and D. G. Jones, *Community and Community Development.* The Hague, Netherlands: Mouton & Co., 1976.

Hale, G. *The Source Book for the Disabled.* New York: Bantam Books, Inc., 1979.

Jewell, D. L. Comprehending concepts of community power structure. Prerequisite for recreation integration. *Leisurability 10* (1), 24–30, 1983.

Kelley, J. D., ed. *Recreation Programming for Visually Impaired Children and Youth.* New York: American Foundation for the Blind, 1981.

McCarty, D. J., and C. E. Ramsey. *The School Managers.* Westport: Greenwood Publishing Corporation, 1971.

Mirkin, H. R. *The Complete Fund Raising Guide.* New York: Public Services Materials Center, 1972.

Pomeroy, J. One community's effort. *Institute on Community Recreation for Special Populations.* North Texas State University and the Texas Recreation and Park Society, 1974.

Robb, G. M., ed. *Guidelines for the Formation and Development of Special Recreation Cooperatives in the State of Illinois.* Office of Recreation and Park Resources, Department of Leisure Studies and the Cooperative Extension Service, University of Illinois at Urbana-Champaign, 1976.

Ryder, K. Skillcraft bus builder—inventor of the year. *Sun Coast Gondolier,* Venice, Florida, December 25, 1982, p. 24.

Sessoms, H. D. Community development and social planning. In Lutzin, S. G., ed., *Managing Municipal Leisure Services.* Washington, D.C.: International City Management Association, 1980, pp. 120–139.

Vaughan, J. L. and R. Winslow. *Guidelines for Community Based Recreation Programs for Special Populations.* National Therapeutic Recreation Society, a branch of the National Recreation and Park Association, 1979.

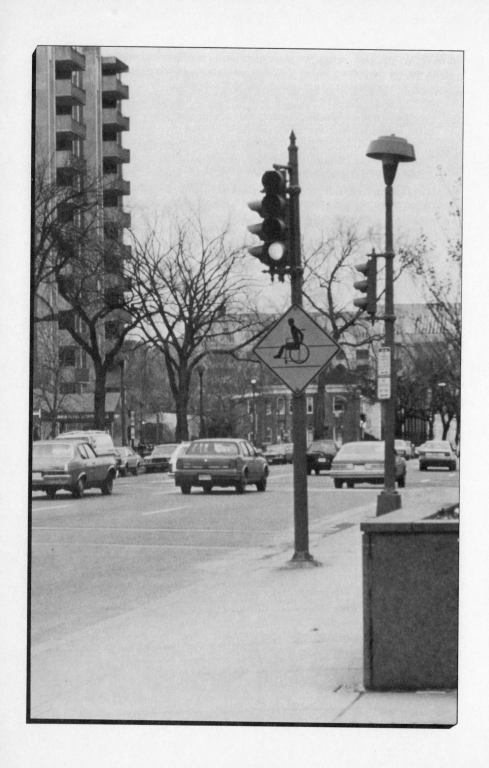

12

Legislation Affecting Special Recreation Services

Over the past three decades, concern for equal rights for individuals who are disabled has been developing and changing. Legislation pertaining to equal access as well as rights to educational and recreational services has evolved. This chapter presents a selection of legislative acts which, to varying degrees, have had impact on the delivery of recreation services to persons with disabilities who reside in the United States.

ACCESSIBILITY

In Webster's *New World Dictionary* (1970), the adjective "accessible" is defined as (1) that can be approached or entered, (2) easy to reach, and (3) obtainable. Federal and state legislation as well as local ordinances have been passed in an attempt to make certain buildings and facilities accessible to and usable by individuals who are physically disabled. This section will discuss legislation dealing with accessibility.

The Architectural Barriers Act of 1968, PL 90–480

Public Law 90–480 is commonly known as the Architectural Barriers Act. It has been amended twice since its initial enactment in 1968: once to cover construction of transportation facilities in the Washington metropolitan area in 1970; and in 1976, to strengthen the language of the

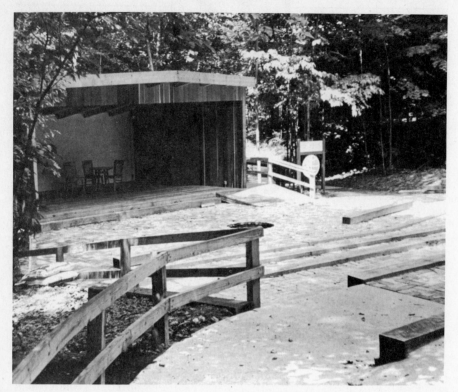

Figure 12–1. Much legislation deals with making facilities accessible.

original bill and to include buildings of the United States Postal Service under PL 90–480 coverage.

While PL 90–480 does not reference recreation, it has had a significant impact on the provision of recreational opportunities for persons who are disabled. In essence, the act ensures that certain buildings financed with federal funds are so designed and constructed as to be accessible to and usable by those with physical disabilities. By 1973, all 50 states had passed similar legislation, and many local governments had passed local ordinances relating to accessibility.

The standards used in PL 90–480 are those developed in 1961 by both the President's Committee on Employment of the Handicapped and the National Easter Seal Society. These guidelines were published in a document entitled *American National Standard Specifications for Making Buildings and Facilities Accessible to and Usable by the Physically Disabled People* and were adopted by the American National Standards Institute (ANSI). The specifications, of course, focus on access to buildings and facilities. Definitions are presented along with wheel-chair specifications, site development (grading, walks, parking lots), and specifications for such items as ramps, entrances, toilet rooms, and public telephones are highlighted. (See Chapter 5 for detailed information on accessibility standards.)

There are several guidelines and legislative acts prepared by governmental bodies that relate to PL 90–480. For example, *The Rehabilitation Act* of 1973 (PL 93–112) established the Architectural and Transportation Barriers Compliance Board to ensure adherence to PL 90–480. The Veterans Administration (VA) in its VA Construction Standard CD–28 (1973), entitled Accommodations for the Physically Handicapped, designates some of the ways that VA facilities need to be altered or designed to accommodate disabled persons. The Building Officials and Code Administrators (BOCA) Building Code was modified in June, 1974, to add provisions for physically disabled and elderly persons (Park, 1980).

State Legislation

It should be noted that nearly half (24) of the states had passed legislation pertaining to accessibility of public buildings prior to the passage of PL 90–480. Application of state legislation usually covers publicly funded buildings. Acts ensure that buildings financed with state monies are constructed accessible to and usable by physically disabled and elderly persons. As stated earlier, *all* states have legislation comparable to PL 90–480. Table 12–1 outlines some aspects of the legislation for three states: Indiana, Maryland, and Pennsylvania.

Summary

As is reflected in this section, the laws pertaining to Architectural Barriers are aimed at making buildings and facilities accessible to and usable by persons with physical disabilities. Acts apply to those buildings that have been constructed with state and/or federal monies.

REHABILITATION ACTS AND AMENDMENTS

The original Vocational Rehabilitation Act was passed in 1954. The primary purpose of this Act was to rehabilitate disabled veterans. Programs included direct medical assistance and vocational training. Nine years later, in 1963, the Rehabilitation Act Amendments included the phrase "recreation for ill and handicapped." Soon after this addition,

Table 12–1
Examples of State Legislation Relating to Architectural Barriers*

State	Legislation Date Effective	Application of Act	Compliance Adopts ANSI Standards	Covers Remodeling	Covers Leased Buildings	Enforcement			Inspection of New Buildings
						State	School	Local	
Indiana	Leg. Act Chap. #49 (10/24/69)	Pub. owned buildings	Yes	Yes	Yes	Admin. Bldg. Council			Yes
Maryland	Leg. Act Senate Bill #404 added new Section #51 to Article #78, A (7/1/68)	Pub. funded bldgs.	Yes	Yes	Yes	Gen Ser Adm	State Dept Ed	Pol Subdiv	Yes
Pennsylvania	Leg. Act #348 Act of Gen. Assem. #235 (9/1/65)	Pub. funded bldgs.	Yes	Yes	Yes	Dept. of Labor and Industry			Yes

*(Taken from U.S. Dept. of HUD, Barrier Free Site Design. Appendix C, pp. 71–75, 1975.)

several colleges and universities received federal monies from the Rehabilitation Services Administration (RSA) to initiate and/or develop master's degree programs to prepare recreators to work with persons with disabilities. Sessoms (1970) has stated that during the first five years of RSA support, 217 traineeships were awarded to 11 universities and colleges. Park (1980) suggested that over 140 colleges and universities had received financial support by the end of the 1970s. Thus, hundreds of students received financial assistance through the RSA program. It is difficult to judge accurately the impact that the RSA traineeship program in recreation has had on either the profession of recreation or the number and quality of leisure services rendered to individuals with disabling conditions. However, it may be surmised that the impact has been significant. In addition, these academic programs laid the framework for the eventual development of therapeutic recreation options and emphases within recreation and park curricula.

Rehabilitation Act of 1973, PL 93–112

The 1973 amendments (PL 93–112) added new directions to recreation services. The "Vocational Rehabilitation Act" was changed to the "Rehabilitation Act." Thus, the concept of rehabilitation was broadened. This act continued the authorization of recreation services in both training and research but added new sections that have had impact on recreation services for persons with disabilities. Selected segments of the Rehabilitation Act follow.

1. Title II—*Research and Training.* This title continued to authorize funds for training recreation personnel to work with handicapped persons and for research monies for projects in recreation.
2. Title III—Section 304—*Special Projects and Demonstrations.* This section made monies available for grants for "operating programs to demonstrate methods of making recreational activities fully accessible to handicapped individuals." Several projects in recreation, such as the Parks and Recreation Commission in Wood County, West Virginia, which developed a recreation complex that is accessible to disabled individuals, have had impact on the delivery of recreation services.
3. Title V—Section 502—*Architectural and Transportation Barriers Compliance Board.* Section 502 created the Architectural and Transportation Barriers Compliance Board (A&TBCB) whose main function is to seek compliance with Public Law 90–480. Any citizen may file a complaint with this agency if a barrier is confronted in a public building or facility, particu-

larly with respect to monuments, parks, and parklands covered by Public Law 90–480. Regulations entitled "Compliance with Standards for Access to and Use of Buildings by Handicapped Persons," were published by this agency in the Federal Register, Tuesday, November 25, 1980. Another function of the A&TBCB required by the Rehabilitation Act Amendments of 1978 (PL 95–602) was to establish minimum guidelines and requirements, which were published in the Federal Register on Friday, January 16, 1981, for the four federal standard-setting agencies. These four agencies designated by the Architectural Barriers Act are: the General Services Administration, Department of Housing and Urban Development, Department of Defense, and the United States Postal Service. These agencies had one year from the effective date of the regulations (January 6, 1981) to issue final revised standards that have as a minimum the guidelines that were published. Many of the A&TBCB provisions were adopted from ANSI (A 117.1–1980). The 1980 ANSI code was not adopted by the A&TBCB; therefore, each federal agency will be issuing new accessibility codes; different design standards are issued by the many diverse federal agencies.

4. Title V—Section 504—*Nondiscrimination Under Federal Grants.* Section 504 is acknowledged to be landmark legislation for disabled Americans. It is commonly referred to as the Civil Rights for the Handicapped. The Department of Health and Human Services (formerly Department of Health, Education and Welfare) is the lead agency for Section 504 compliance. The Department of HHS published the first set of Section 504 regulations for recipients of HHS funds in the Federal Register, Wednesday, May 4, 1977, entitled "Nondiscrimination on Basis of Handicap: Programs and Activities Receiving or Benefiting from Federal Financial Assistance."This section states that "No otherwise qualified handicapped individual shall, solely by reason of his handicap, be excluded from the participation in, be denied the benefits of, or be subjected to discrimination under, any program or activity conducted by an executive agency or by the United States Postal Service."Failure to comply with the law can result in the withholding and/or withdrawal of federal financial assistance.

The impact of the Rehabilitation Act on public recreation services has not been determined. The issue of discrimination has been made unclear by attempts to soften legislation. For instance, the Architectural and Transportation Barriers Compliance Board (A&TBCB) adopted a softened plan on December 1, 1981, when members realized their original proposal faced certain rejection by the Administration and Congress. Dropped were rules requiring renovation of older transit stations and federally leased buildings, including thousands of postal offices. In the final analysis, such actions mean that fewer elevators, rails, ramps and other special requirements will be built in either old or new buildings constructed with federal monies.

Rehabilitation Act Amendment of 1974, PL 93–516

The Rehabilitation Act Amendment of 1974 authorized the planning and implementation of the White House Conference on Handicapped Individuals, which was convened in May of 1977. Recreation was one of 16 major areas of concern at the White House Conference. The final report* noted the importance of recreation for individuals with disabilities and called for the expansion of recreation services, as well as an increase in the number of professionally trained individuals employed in the field of recreation.

Recreation and leisure services, outdoor recreation for disabled persons, and recreational programs and facilities are mentioned in the report. Generally, the main points of the report included funding incentives, accessibility, community-based recreation programs, and employment and training of recreation professionals. In addition, under the heading of "Social Concerns," recreation was listed. The following is an abbreviated list of concerns dealing with the design of recreational services:

- Accessibility
- Program Variety
- Leisure Skill Development
- Handicapped Lobby

- Transportation
- Program Integration
- Funding for Recreation
- Public Awareness

Rehabilitation Act of 1978, PL 95–602

As with many federal programs, the 1973 Rehabilitation Act and the programs it authorized expired at the end of five years. In 1978 legislation was introduced to extend and amend the 1973 act. The 1978 act contained six separate sections that called for recreation and leisure services as part of the rehabilitation process. PL 95–602 authorized the continuation of training programs, although training funds for recrea-

---

*The White House Conference on Handicapped Individuals, Volume Two: Final Report, Part C. Washington, D.C.: Superintendent of Documents, U.S. Government Printing Office, 1977.

tion were curtailed in several regions of the country. The act included recreation as a service to be provided in rehabilitation facilities as well as in special public projects and demonstration programs such as the Regional Activities and Recreation Center for the Handicapped in Wood County, West Virginia.

The Senate Committee on Human Resources, in introducing the Senate Bill to amend and extend the 1973 Rehabilitation Act, stated:

- In recognition of the recreational and social needs of handicapped individuals, the committee bill amends section 304 to authorize the secretary to make grants to states and public non-profit agencies and organizations for the purpose of initiating recreational programs for handicapped individuals.

- Recreation programs for handicapped individuals are greatly needed in order to assist them in developing their capacity for mobility and socialization. Unfortunately, existing programming for this purpose is limited; therefore, it is the committee's intent that this authority stimulate the development of and utilization of more community-based recreation programs.

- It is the committee's intent that handicapped individuals participate in existing regularly scheduled recreation programs to the maximum extent feasible; the committee realizes, however, that the specialized needs of handicapped individuals may necessitate adaptive equipment and programming and specially trained personnel. The committee therefore expects that such adaptive equipment and programming as well as specialized personnel attuned to the needs of handicapped persons will be an integral part of any recreation program initiated under this authority. It is further expected that such recreation programs should be coordinated with other recreational activities offered in the community. (Senate Report, 1978)

From a legislative funding perspective, recreation services to special populations have fared quite well. As a result of the amendments to the Rehabilitation Act of 1978 (PL 95–602), with reference to Sections 311 and 316, approximately $9 million have been allocated through the two sections to various agencies to make recreation facilities and programs accessible to disabled individuals.

Section 311 provides grants to public or nonprofit agencies and organizations to pay part or all of the costs of special projects and demonstrations for . . . operating programs and, where appropriate, renovating and constructing facilities to demonstrate methods of making *recreational* activities fully accessible to handicapped individuals.

Any project or demonstration assisted by a grant under this section that provides services to indivduals with spinal cord injuries shall . . . (4) demonstrate and evaluate methods of community outreach for individuals with spinal cord injuries and community education in connection with the problems of such individuals in areas such as housing, transportation, *recreation*, employment, and community activities.

Section 316 provides grants to State and public nonprofit agencies and organizations for paying part or all of the cost of initiation of *recreation* programs to provide handicapped individuals with *recreational* activities to aid in the mobility and socialization of such individuals. The activities authorized to be assisted under this section may include, but are not limited to, scouting and camping, 4–H activities, sports, music, dancing, handicrafts, art, and homemaking.

Two million dollars were allocated in 1984 through Section 316. In 1985, the National Recreation and Park Association (NRPA) urged the House subcommittee on Labor, Health and Human Services, and Education to support supplemental appropriations for Section 316. Over $2 million have been appropriated for Section 316 for fiscal year 1986. This type of legislative support, along with support from the Special Education Program (Office of Special Education and Rehabilitation Services) in personnel preparation and research will continue to contribute to the growth and development of the profession (Reynolds & O'Morrow, 1985).

Finally, a major new section added to the 1978 act expanded the number of persons with disabilities eligible to receive services and "recreational and leisure time activities." Title VII, entitled Comprehensive Services for Independent Living, made funds available for the development of comprehensive services to persons with disabilities.

EDUCATION LEGISLATION

Education for Handicapped Children Act of 1967, PL 90–170

Legislation having great influence on recreation services for children with disabilities has been the Education for Handicapped Children Act of 1967, PL 90–170, amended by PL 93–380 and by PL 94–142. PL 90–170 provided a considerable amount of federal funds for the professional preparation of recreation personnel working with children with disabilities. In 1967, Senator Edward Kennedy (D-Mass.) introduced an amendment that created specific authorization for funds in the areas of physical education and recreation. More specifically, Title V, Section 501(a) stated:

> It is authorized to make grants to public and other non-profit institutions of higher learning to assist them in providing professional or advanced training for personnel engaged or preparing to engage in

employment as physical educators or recreation personnel for mentally retarded and other handicapped children . . . or engaged or preparing to engage in research or teaching in fields relative to the physical education or recreation of such children.

Over the past 15 years, this legislation enabled many colleges and universities to educate hundreds of students to work with children with disabling conditions in a variety of recreational settings.

Education for All Handicapped Children Act of 1975, PL 94–142

The Education for Handicapped Children Act was amended by PL 94–142 (1975). The amended act was titled the "Education for All Handicapped Children Act." It read, in part:

> It is the purpose of this act to assure that all handicapped children have available to them, within the time periods specified in Section 612 (2) (B), a *free appropriate public education* (FAPE) which emphasizes special education and related services designed to meet their unique needs, to assure that the rights of handicapped children and their parents or guardians are protected, to assist states and localities to provide for the education of all handicapped children, and to assess and assure the effectiveness of efforts to educate handicapped children.
>
> The term "related services" means transportation, and such development, corrective and other supportive services (including . . . *recreation* . . .) as may be required to assist a handicapped child to benefit from special education. . . .

The regulations governing implementation of the law define recreation as including:

1. Assessment of leisure functioning
2. Therapeutic Recreation
3. Recreation in Schools and Communities
4. Leisure Education

The inclusion of recreation as a related service provided a rationale for the inclusion of recreation as part of the individualized education plan (IEP) and suggested a framework for the delivery of recreation services. This particular point is highlighted in a hearing in Massachusetts involving a female student, Sandra T. In this court hearing, provisions on access to, and equal opportunity to participate in, extracurricular activities in after-school hours that were offered to students without disabilities was a major issue. Dispute between the parties centered on whether Sandra's special needs indicated that an after-school therapeutic recreation/leisure education component should be included in her Individual Education Plan (IEP). In short, a decision (BSEA # 3231)* ordered Old Rochester Regional School District to provide an after-school program of related services for Sandra T, incorporating socialization, recreation, physical development, and leisure education objectives for a minimum of six hours per week. Additionally, it was stated: "an aide shall be designated to carry out the program and a therapeutic recreation specialist shall provide a consulting and in-service program to interested teachers, etc., as well as provide direct service to Sandra individually or in a small group for a minimum of one hour per week."

OTHER LEGISLATION

This section contains four other pieces of legislation that have impacted community recreation services for special populations.

Developmental Disabilities and Facilities Construction Act of 1970, PL 91–517

This act provided services to children and adults with developmental disabilities attributable to mental retardation, cerebral palsy, epilepsy, or other neurological conditions. This law was amended by PL 94–103, entitled "The Developmentally Disabled Assistance Bill of Rights Act of 1975," which added autism to the list of disabilities.

The developmental disabilities program does not provide direct services to individuals; rather, it is oriented toward the provision of grant funds to a grantee who, in turn, provides the direct service to a population as a result of the acquired funds. Monies are awarded according to priorities established in the annual state plan.

These grants are for planning, administration, services, and construction of facilities and are awarded through Titles I and II of The Developmental Disabilities (DD) Act. Title I provides funding under a Formula Grant, which is money allocated to the states on a formula basis to be distributed by state agencies. "Recreation" as a fundable activity is mentioned in the law as one of the specific supportive services under the formula grants. Recreation services are aimed at providing opportunities for recreation, physical education, and open space acquisition and development.

---

*This decision was issued pursuant to the requirements of M.G.L. C. 15, 31A, C. 718, The Education of All Handicapped Children Act (20 V.S.C. 1401–1461), The Rehabilitation Act of 1973, Section 502 (20 V.S.C. 794), . . . 1980.

Title II of the law is allocated for "interdisciplinary training programs in institutions of higher learning and for University Affiliated Facilities to house these programs." These facilities offer out-patient and in-patient services, provide training for service personnel, and improve the move toward integration and appropriate community services to developmentally disabled individuals.

In 1978, the DD Act was amended through passage of The Rehabilitation Comprehensive Services and Developmental Disabilities Amendments. This had an impact on the expansion of services for individuals with disabilities. It affected the Rehabilitation Act of 1973, the Developmental Disabilities Services and Facilities Construction Act, and The Developmentally-Disabled Bill of Rights Act of 1975.

The overall purposes of the act were:

1. To assist in the provision of comprehensive services to persons with developmental disabilities, with priority to those persons whose needs cannot be covered or otherwise met under the Education for All Handicapped Children Act, the Rehabilitation Act of 1973, or other health, education, or welfare programs;
2. To assist states in appropriate planning activities;
3. To make grants to states and public and private nonprofit agencies to establish model programs, to demonstrate innovative habilitation techniques, and to train professional and paraprofessional personnel with respect to providing services to persons with developmental disabilities;
4. To make grants to university-affiliated facilities to assist them in administering and operating demonstration facilities for the provision of services to persons with developmental disabilities, and interdisciplinary training programs for personnel needed to provide specialized services for these persons; and
5. To make grants to support a system in each state to protect the legal and human rights of all persons with developmental disabilities.

The implications of these amendments to the recreation field are numerous. They allow recreation professionals opportunities to develop and implement special services, training, and research projects in the area of developmental disabilities. Some of the possibilities include: (1) services necessary for community adjustment, such as counseling and educating the individual regarding leisure habits and resources for involvement in the community; (2) public awareness and educational programs to assist in the integration of handicapped individuals into the mainstream of society; (3) coordination of all available community resources; (4) training of specialized personnel needed to service delivery or for research related to developmental disabilities; (5)

development of demonstration techniques and/or projects to serve as a pilot for the expansion and continuation of innovative and successful programs; and (6) gathering and dissemination of information related to developmental disabilities.

The qualified recreation professional can actively involve himself or herself in the provision of quality services following acquisition of federal monies through grant writing. This law addresses the areas of facilities, research and training, demonstration projects, and special recreation programs.

Nationwide Outdoor Recreation Plan, 1963, PL 88–29

Public Law 88–29 was passed in 1963 and authorized the establishment of the Bureau of Outdoor Recreation (BOR), later to be referred to as the Heritage, Conservation and Recreation Service (HCRS) (terminated in 1981). One section of the Nationwide Outdoor Recreation Plan focused on the needs of handicapped individuals with particular attention to architectural barriers. In 1978 HCRS appointed a task force to update the recreation needs of the handicapped individuals. A report entitled "Recreation Needs of the Handicapped" identified nine important issues concerning recreation for handicapped persons. The issues identified included the following:

1. Accessibility of Facilities
2. Accessibility of Programs
3. Compliance
4. Consumer Involvement
5. Training
6. Technical Assistance
7. Research
8. Employment
9. Transportation

Park (1980) notes that "a synopsis of the issues addressed in the 1978 revised plan has been published in *The Third Nationwide Outdoor Recreation Plan*, December, 1979," (p. 13).

Comprehensive Employment and Training Act (CETA) of 1978, PL 95–524

CETA was signed into effect in 1973. Its purpose was to initiate new forms of manpower training and to increase employment. CETA was amended in 1977 (PL 95–44) and again in 1978 (PL 95–524). Section 306 of Title III of PL 95–524 called for special provisions for the establishment of programs to train people to provide the special supportive services and removal of architectural barriers. With respect to training personnel to work with and assist disabled individuals, the National Therapeutic Recreation Society, through its 750-hour training program, approved CETA-sponsored programs, namely, in the Commonwealth of Pennsylvania. CETA provided funds to support trainees in recreation programs for persons who were ill and disabled. Thus, this act had a substantial impact during the 1970s in terms of training paraprofessionals and in the development of community-based recreation programs and clinical programs. As a result of cutbacks, however, only a handful of training programs existed in the early 1980s.

Illinois Special Recreation Associations

In 1967, professionals in northern Illinois were aware that the leisure and recreational needs of special populations were not being met. As a result of two years of study and demonstration programs, members of the Illinois Senate and House pledged support of permissive legislation that allowed park districts and/or municipal recreation departments to join together to operate recreation programs for citizens with mental and physical disabilities. The legal base for all special recreation cooperatives is the result of Senate Bill 745 of the 1969 Illinois General Assembly. This bill made it possible for two or more park districts and/or municipal recreation departments to join together to provide recreation for the disabled members of their communities. Funding for these special recreation cooperatives was made possible through legislation passed in 1972, which allowed park districts and municipalities to levy up to $.02 of $100 assessed valuation for recreation services for individuals with disabilities. Later, in 1975, Senate Bills 220 and 221 were passed; these allow park districts or municipal recreation departments, which are members of a cooperative of two or more such agencies, by the use of a referendum-by-petition, to tax their local citizens up to but not to exceed $.02 per $100 of assessed valuation.

The first cooperative was the Northern Suburban Special Recreation Association (NSSRA), formed in 1970, and included eight local park districts in the northern Chicago metropolitan area. By 1973, there were a total of ten member agencies of NSSRA serving portions of a two-county area (Keay, 1976).

———————————— **SUMMARY** ————————————

This chapter presents and discusses legislative acts aimed at equal rights for special populations. Both federal and state legislation dealing with accessibility have made the public more aware of architectural barriers. Legislation has also made new and remodeled federal and state buildings more accessible to and usable by persons who are physically disabled, as well as elderly individuals with mobility problems. Specifications for making buildings and facilities accessible to and usable by persons with physical disabilities are part of the legislative acts and are becoming common knowledge among professionals in a variety of fields. The Rehabilitation Acts have provided monies and opportunities to hundreds of recreation students to become professionally prepared to work with persons who are disabled in a variety of leisure settings. In addition, the Education for Handicapped Children Act of 1967, PL 90–170, has provided a considerable amount of federal funding for the professional preparation of recreation personnel working with children with disabilities. The Developmental Disabilities Act (PL 91–517) has provided grants to recreation agencies so leisure services can be provided in community-based programs. The training and employment of recreators, particularly of paraprofessionals, was seen in the 1970s via CETA monies. The State of Illinois has passed legislation to allow park districts and municipal recreation departments to join together to operate recreation programs for individuals who are disabled.

All in all, legislation has had a profound impact on the delivery of recreational services to disabled children and adults. Acts have made buildings and other facilities accessible to and usable by people with disabilities. Appropriated monies have helped prepare professionals and paraprofessionals and have made direct services available via demonstration programs and construction projects.

Suggested Learning Activities

1. Discuss the implications of the various Rehabilitation Acts and Amendments on the field of recreation.

2. Go to the library or other source and outline all of the aspects pertaining to the Architectural Barriers Act in your state. Bring the information to class for discussion.

3. Review public law 94–142 and indicate the possible implications to community-based recreation programs for school-aged children who are disabled.

References

American National Standards Institute. *American National Standard Specifications for Making Buildings and Facilities Accessible to and Usable by Physically Disabled People.* New York: American National Standards Institute, Inc., 1980.

Keay, S. *Community Operated and Funded Recreation Programs for the Handicapped.* Report prepared on federally sponsored project under the direction of the Department of HEW. Highland Park, IL, 1976.

Park, D. C. *Legislation Affecting Park Services and Recreation for Handicapped Individuals.* Published and distributed in part by the U.S. Department of Education, Office of Special Education, Washington, D.C., and Hawkins and Associates, Washington, D.C., 1980, 28 pages.

Reynolds, R. P. and G. S. O'Morrow. *Problems, Issues and Concepts in Therapeutic Recreation.* Englewood Cliffs, NJ: Prentice-Hall, Inc., 1985.

Sessoms, H. D. "The Impact of the RSA Recreation Trainee Program, 1963–1968," *Therapeutic Recreation Journal* 14(1), 23–29, 1970.

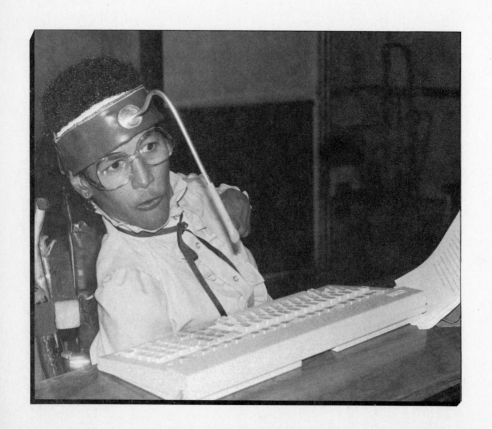

13

Trends in Special Recreation Services

In this chapter we will attempt to peer into the future to gain a glimpse of what may unfold in special recreation services. Knowing today's trends points the way to the world of tomorrow and provides us with visions of future realities.

We are living in a rapidly changing world of high technology. Computers, satellites, robots, space shuttles, rapid communication systems, and other signs of high technology are already a part of our culture. Naisbitt (1982) in his best seller, *Megatrends*, reflects on the rapid changes in our society when he stated: "Change is occurring so rapidly that there is no time to react; instead we must anticipate the future" (p. 18).

The world is rapidly changing. As Toffler (1970) discussed in *Future Shock*, some of the facts in almost all books are obsolete before publication. Because of the speed of change, it is difficult to forecast in any area, including community recreation for special populations. But as Toffler has aptly stated:

> In dealing with the future . . . it is more important to be imaginative and insightful than to be one hundred percent "right." Theories do not have to be "right" to be enormously useful. Even error has its uses. The maps of the world drawn by medieval cartographers were so hopelessly inaccurate, so filled with factual error, that they elicit condescending smiles today when almost the entire surface of the earth has been charted. Yet the great explorers could never have discovered

the new world without them. Nor could the better, more accurate maps of today been drawn until men, working with the limited evidence available to them, set down on paper their bold conceptions of the worlds they had never seen. (p. 6)

With this in mind, we reviewed the literature and questioned experts* for their thoughts regarding trends in special recreation programs. The resulting compilation of trends is presented with the admission that, as a wag has said, those who live by the crystal ball must learn to eat ground glass. We shall probably digest our share.

PROGRAM TRENDS

Outdoor Recreation Programs

Few activities cannot be entered into by persons with disabilities. Therefore, programs for special populations are likely to follow societal trends. The rising interest in outdoor recreation pursuits among persons with disabilities is evidence of a societal trend reflected in special recreation programs. Various terms, such as "outdoor adventure," "high risk," and "stress challenge," are used to describe programs that offer participants new and challenging experiences in the outdoors. Caving, rapelling, traversing rope courses, and backpacking are examples of adventure activities enjoyed by many persons. Cold climate pursuits such as ice skating and winter camping are gaining popularity, as is snow skiing. Many persons with visual and physical disabilities are discovering snow skiing as a recreation pursuit. In Canada, sledge hockey and ice picking, a form of speed skating, are developing (Sledge Hockey and Ice Picking, 1981). In Scotland, curling is a popular sport for persons with disabilities, including wheelchair users. Other outdoor recreation activities gaining participation include sailing, fishing, gardening, archery, riding, and nature study.

Indiana University's Bradford Woods (5040 State Road 67 North, Martinsville, IN 46151) is a trend setter in the provision of programming and training opportunities utilizing outdoor recreation experiences with persons who have disabilities. Among its programs, Bradford

---

*Experts included Barbara "Sam" Browne, Cincinnati Recreation Commission, Cincinnati, Ohio; Mary Crooks and Dorthy Lougee, Park and Recreation Department, Lincoln, Nebraska; John McGovern, West Suburban Special Recreation Association, Elmwood Park, Illinois; Lawrence Reiner, Northeast DuPage Special Recreation Association, Elmhurst, Illinois; Lynn Rourke, Courage Center, Golden Valley, Minnesota; Byron Welker, Central State Hospital, Indianapolis, Indiana.

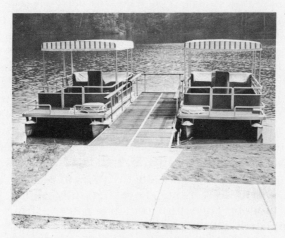

Figure 13–1. Boat dock at Bradford Woods.

Woods offers extensive camping and outdoor adventure activities for persons with disabilities. In addition, a number of training opportunities are provided through Bradford Woods. These include a variety of internships and an annual institute on innovations in outdoor recreation programming for persons with disabilities. In addition, within Bradford Woods is located the national headquarters of the American Camping Association (ACA). Both Bradford Woods and the ACA offer many resources that support the trend toward greater participation in outdoor recreation pursuits by individuals with disabilities.

Sport and Fitness

Competitive athletics continue to thrive under the auspices of traditional organizations such as the National Wheelchair Basketball Association, American Blind Bowlers Association, and Special Olympics. Recently, however, there has been an expansion in the types of sports associations. For example, the National Association of Sports for Cerebral Palsy (NASCP) was created in 1978 to sponsor events in everything from bowling to track and field. Additional organizations have been formed for wheelchair road racers, wheelchair marathoners, wheelchair softball and tennis players, and disabled skiers, among others.

While many of the athletic programs initially instituted were competitive sports for children and young adults, noncompetitive opportunities are beginning to develop for both children and adults. Many persons do not want competition but seek health and fitness through sport. Aerobic dance, karate, yoga, and weight lifting are some activities demanded by those in special recreation programs. Still others desire to learn lifetime sports through adult leisure education classes. For example, in Indianapolis bowling instruction is being provided to adults with disabilities under a program modeled after the President's Council on Physical Fitness and Sport.

A particularly unique sports and fitness program, which serves persons with disabilities, has been developed at the Vinland National Center (3675 Ihduhapi Road, Loretto, MN 55357). The Vinland program has been patterned after the Beiostølen Health Sports Center in Norway. Vinland emphasizes the concepts of high-level wellness and holistic health through sport and fitness activity. Examples of Vinland programs include swimming, riding, kayaking, snow skiing, ice sledding, and various outdoor adventure activities ranging from cooperative games and initiative tasks to high adventure experiences.

The Vinland National Center also presents a wide variety of training experiences for persons with disabilities, professionals, and students wishing to learn about Vinland's "healthsports." These training opportunities take the form of short courses, workshops, and student internships.

Goals of the Vinland Center are to:

- Assist individuals with categorical physical handicaps or other disabilities to achieve an optimal level of health and to assume increased responsibility for their own health.
- Provide training in healthsports and recreation as one component in a program designed to improve fitness and build confidence.
- Conduct health programs to effect positive changes in lifestyle.
- Provide social and psychological counseling for participants and their families.
- Implement outreach programs to reinforce participants upon return to employment and the community. (*Vinland National Center*, n.d.)

It is obvious that the Vinland National Center has established itself as a leader in the trend toward sports and fitness for persons with disabilities. It is likely that sports and fitness programming, such as those promoted by Vinland, will continue to grow in the future.

Travel Programs

Communities are developing a variety of travel programs for persons with disabilities. These are developing under a number of auspices. In some communities a single agency, or several cooperating agencies, may sponsor opportunities for travel. For example, the Association for Retarded Citizens in Lincoln, Nebraska, has sponsored sightseeing trips to Colorado, and camping trips to the Ozarks.

Also, the number of commercial travel agencies for persons with disabilities is on the upswing in the United States. In 1974, Galbreaith listed five such agencies from Hollendale and Delray Beach, Florida, on the east coast, to Indianapolis, Indiana, and Owatonna, Minnesota, in the midwest to Lynwood, Washington, on the west coast. In 1983, Weiss listed 14 travel agencies that specifically served clients with disabilities.

Galbreaith (1974) has extolled the virtues of travel arranged by commercial agencies for individuals who have disabilities. In her words:

> If you can pack a bag, put on a hat, and leave familiar surroundings, you can find yourself flying the skies or sailing the oceans, and sleeping in a different country every night if you choose.
>
> You ask, "How can this be?" First of all, much research and planning has been done and arrangements made so that all major facilities can be used by all travelers. You know beforehand that the restaurant in Paris is completely accessible, the hotel in Japan will pose no problems for you, and help is available to enable you [to] enjoy sightseeing. All the work is done for you—all you have to do is sit back and enjoy it. (p.136)

Opportunities for air travel should expand in the future. The first American barrier-free airplane, United Airline's Boeing 767, has initiated the "Age of Air Travel" for the 35 million Americans who have disabilities, according to Galbreaith (1983). She goes on to elaborate on the features of the 767.

> The 767's accessible features include an on-board wheelchair (aisle-chair); four aisle seats with movable arm rests for easy wheelchair-to-seat transfers; and a wheelchair accessible lavatory with manageable handles, grab bars with faucets, special lighting and signage for deaf passengers and an adjacent 10 square-foot privacy area.

Another indication of the concern for American travelers with disabilities was the publication, in 1984, of *The United States Welcomes Handicapped Visitors*. It contains basic travel and tourism information for travelers who have visual impairments, hearing impairments, physical disabilities, or developmental disabilities. This 48-page handbook was published by the Society for the Advancement of Travel for the Handicapped, in cooperation with Greyhound Lines.

It is obvious that there is a trend toward greater travel opportunities for persons with disabilities. It is likely that a large portion of this travel will be organized by leisure service delivery systems, as well as through commercial travel agencies.

Leisure Education and Leisure Counseling

A developing trend is toward leisure education to help build leisure skills and attitudes. For example, the Northeast DuPage Special Recreation Association near Chicago has designed curricula to help teachers provide leisure education to children with disabilities. These curriculum materials have been eagerly accepted and widely used by teachers of special education students. As special recreation programs grow, greater numbers of individuals and families will require leisure counseling. Professionals competently prepared with counseling skills and a knowledge of leisure will advance the field of leisure counseling far beyond the relatively simple level of today's leisure counseling programs. Leisure services agencies offering leisure counseling services for special populations will be at the forefront of this effort. Advances will include higher levels of counseling skills and innovations in the use of computers in leisure counseling programs. A computerized resource center is currently being used by the Northeast DuPage Special Recreation Association to match client interests with available community leisure resources. The computer will play a larger and larger role in both leisure counseling and leisure education as computer programs are developed to teach people about leisure opportunities, to assess interests, and to catalog leisure resources.

Programs for Individuals in Group Homes

There is a continuing trend to provide community living situations for individuals who have been hospitalized or institutionalized, or who need an alternative to living at home with their parents. Group homes have been established by both private firms and public agencies for persons who need supervised community living situations. Group homes offer supervised community living in houses located in residential neighborhoods in towns and cities.

Because of the advances of physical medicine, there is a growing population of persons with spinal cord injuries, head injuries, and developmental disabilities who require the community living opportunities offered by group homes. Some group homes are for individuals with physical disabilities who will reside in the homes on a temporary basis while building their independent living skills. Other homes provide more long-term living arrangements for adults who, while mentally retarded or otherwise disabled, can function relatively independently but who need some amount of assistance.

Some individuals residing in group homes need motor skill development. More common is the need to develop competencies related to social and leisure skills. Special recreation programs have been created to help those living in group homes to develop motor skills and to have positive social and leisure experiences. Often these programs take place in the evening since participants normally have employment in the community or in a sheltered workshop, or work in the group home. Some programs are conducted in the group homes, while others are offered in community recreation centers or human service agencies.

APPROACHES TO PROGRAMS AND SERVICES

Integration

The integration of persons with disabilities into regular, ongoing community recreation programs is a trend certainly worthy of development. Nevertheless, it can be difficult to get regular staff to accept their responsibility to integrate persons with disabilities into ongoing programs. Personnel may dismiss their responsibility because of the existence of special recreation program specialists. Or they may feel unprepared to deal with those integrated into programs. Therefore, regular staff, as well as the community as a whole, need to be educated on the necessity for integration. The keys to successful integration appear to be providing in-service training for regular staff, preparing participants and/or their parents for the integration process, and evaluating existing programs before making referrals to them. Where these elements have been considered, integration has proceeded in a smooth fashion. Certainly, integration is a trend that is here to stay.

Levels of Programming

There exists a definite trend to establish several levels of programs within community services for special populations. For example, the Cincinnati Recreation Commission has a four-level system encompassing teaching sensory-motor and self-help skills (Level I), instructing basic activity and socialization skills (Level II), developing advanced recreation and socialization skills (Level III), and providing relatively independent participation where staff act as facilitators, trainers, consultants, liaison persons, and advocates (Level IV). Following these levels of programming, participants may become integrated into ongoing programs of the department. Another illustration is a model proposed by Hunter (1981). This model has five levels: (1) institutional and home-bound one-to-one visitations, (2) developmental skill programming focusing on the acquisition of skills transferable to community recreation participation, (3) special interest groups where segregation is by choice for a particular activity such as wheelchair basketball, (4) integration with support (e.g., transportation, emotional support) to promote community involvement, and (5) direct independent participation in community leisure experiences. Throughout the five levels leisure counseling and leisure education services may be provided to facilitate the participants' involvement. As programs grow in sophistication, more and more communities will adopt multiple levels of programming.

Therapeutic Programs

Closely related to the trend to offer various levels of programs is a trend toward the provision of therapeutically orientated programs. Community-based therapeutic recreation specialists are offering purposeful interventions for clients needing goal-directed programming. The therapeutic recreation process (assessment, planning, implementation, and evaluation) is being employed by skilled therapeutic recreation specialists to reach specified client outcomes. While the primary thrust of community-based special recreation programs will remain recreation participation, more therapeutically orientated programs will develop as therapeutic recreation specialists are employed by community leisure service agencies.

Campus Recreation Programs

A growing area of programming is found on college and university campuses throughout the United States. Students who have disabilities have made their needs for special recreation services known to campus administrators, who have begun to respond with a variety of leisure services. These services have included wheelchair user and nonwheelchair user sports, outdoor recreation offerings, lectures, special events, and leisure counseling. Leisure services for students are sometimes administered by an office for handicapped student services but, more and more, are found in traditional campus recreational service systems, such as departments of recreational sports. The authors of this textbook project this trend will continue and that there will be increased campus/community cooperation between campus recreation providers and community park and recreation departments as the recreational needs of young adults, who are disabled, become more widely recognized.

High Technology

As previously discussed, computers will be used extensively in leisure education and leisure counseling programs. Beyond this, however, computers offer many possibilities to enhance services to special populations. A software explosion is now upon us. Computer programs for scheduling, participant registration, inventories, and so on are fast becoming available in parks and recreation. These will be applied to community special recreation services. Computer games will also find their way into special recreation programming. These games are no longer just for children. Innovations provide interactive computer games that are stimulating for adults and may be played by participants with even severe physical disabilities. For example, flight simulator games allow players to land (or crash!) at dozens of airports across the United States.

With expanding capabilities, television also offers a media to be tapped by leisure service agencies to reach those who have not traditionally been served. Videotapes will be produced on wheelchair sports and other activities for persons with disabilities. These will be made available through leisure service agencies.

Naisbitt (1982) has introduced the thought that as high technology becomes more a part of our lives, we will seek increased opportunities to be around other people in our leisure time. Naisbitt has termed this need for human contact as *high touch*, a reaction to *high tech*. Even though people will have access to computers and television in their homes, they will desire to socialize with others. Special recreation programs will meet this need by providing activities not only in traditional facilities, such as recreation centers, but in shopping malls and other areas where people congregate.

In the years ahead, technicians will also create new vistas for persons with disabilities through the production of innovative assistive devices. Already a number of devices have become available that enable persons with severe disabilities to grow toward independence. For example, a great deal of progress has been made in developing communication aids for nonverbal severely physically disabled individuals. Several of these devices are described in an extensive catalog of assistance equipment published by the Wisconsin Vocational Studies Center (Gugerty et al., 1981). One, the Autocom, has a portable board that is built into a wheelchair lap tray. A handpiece or headstick is used to point to vocabulary items on the board's surface, with a message appearing on an LED display or printed onto a paper roll. In England, Possum sells the Communicator, a device much the same as the Autocom. A father and mother whose 12-year-old son used a communication board reported to one of the authors that it had "opened new worlds" for the boy who, for the first time, was able to readily communicate with others.

Other devices send typed messages via telephone for profoundly deaf individuals. Computer terminals print in braille and speak in full-word synthetic speech. Electronic control systems allow severely disabled persons the use of the telephone and control of the television, radio, lights, and other appliances by means of a puff on a tube. Wheelchair control systems are directed by means of the chin, joystick, or puff-sip device (Gugerty et al., 1981). In addition, the availability of computerized banking and shopping from the home in some areas of the country is expanding independent living opportunities to persons with severe mobility impairments.

Today's assistive devices, and others in the planning stage, hold great potential to enhance the lives of persons with severe disabilities. We are, however, a long way from such aids being within the financial means of most persons. Nevertheless, recreation professionals need to begin contemplating the possible effects of assistive devices, computers, television, and other types of new technology on programs and services. They are a certain part of the future.

Changing Views Toward Sexuality

Traditionally, disabled and aging individuals have not been perceived by human service professionals to have sexual feelings or sexual activity. The traditional view has been that disabled and aging persons are basically asexual. In recent years, however, professionals have been undergoing substantial change in their views toward the *sexuality* of both groups. Perhaps the "sexual revolution" has inspired a healthier view. Or it may be that a number of special population groups are beginning to be seen as persons with feelings and desires similar to others. Whatever the reason, it seems there is a definite trend toward perceiving both persons with disabilities and individuals who are aging as sexual beings who have needs to express their sexuality.

A handbook on sexuality and disabled persons, edited by Cornelius and others (1982), states: " . . . sexuality can be defined as an integration of physical, emotional, intellectual, and social aspects of an individual's personality which expresses maleness or femaleness" (p. 1). Cornelius and his colleagues go on to state:

> People do not express their maleness or femaleness only in the
> bedroom. Sexuality is a part of all the activities in which a person
> engages: work, socialization, decoration of one's home, telephone
> conversations, political discussions, expressions of affection, arguments,

eating a meal, child rearing, walking down the street, watching a movie, etc. Sexuality, then, is an expression of one's personality and is evident in everyday interactions. (p. 1)

Recreation professionals are recognizing that persons with disabilities and individuals who are aging should be free to express their sexuality, just like anyone else. For example, progressive recreation professionals do not treat mentally retarded adults like children who are to be protected from their sexuality. Instead, these adults are offered opportunities for learning and practicing social skills necessary to deal with their sexuality in appropriate ways. These professionals also realize that the mere presence or absence of a disability does not influence the ability to enter into sexual relationships. A disabled person and nondisabled person may share much in common. On the other hand, two disabled people may have very little in common other than being disabled (Cornelius et al., 1982). Progressive professionals, therefore, offer opportunities for single adults and teenagers who are physically disabled to mix with others in typical recreation activities such as dances, parties, and co-recreational sports. Through such healthy recreation, disabled and nondisabled participants can express their sexuality. Similarly, progressive professionals provide older persons recreational opportunities through which they may express their sexuality in social interactions with others with whom they share common interests.

In sum, there exists a trend for human service professionals, including recreation professionals, to accept the sexuality of persons who are old or disabled. These professionals believe that individuals who are aging and those with disabilities deserve the same sexual rights as others enjoy and provide opportunities within their programs for the normal expression of sexuality.

Outreach Workers

Outreach workers are being used by at least one agency* to identify those who are homebound or for some other reason have not had the opportunity to become aware of programs and services for special populations. Outreach workers also develop referral systems with local hospitals and nursing homes that are returning clients to the community. Finally, these staff help refer those who contact the agency to appropriate programs and services. In short, it is the responsibility of the outreach worker to reach out to newly disabled persons and those

---

*The Northeast Dupage Special Recreation Association in Elmhurst, Illinois, employs outreach workers.

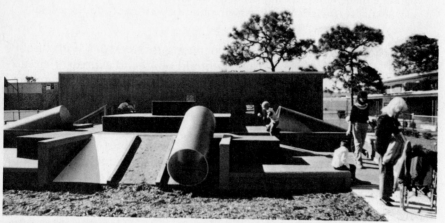

Figure 13–2. Modern playground in Tampa, Florida, designed to meet the needs of children with disabilities. Design by Dr. Lou Bowers.

not traditionally served so that they may have the benefit of special recreation programs and services. This may involve not only contacting and referring participants but also assisting clients to initially take part in existing programs. Outreach workers will become more widely utilized as agencies learn of their value.

Playgrounds

Traditionally, playgrounds have not been constructed to accommodate the needs of all children. Often barriers have excluded children with disabilities from playgrounds, creating feelings of social isolation. Today there is, however, a trend toward building and programming playgrounds to meet the needs of all children, including those with disabilities. Advancements in playground design are discussed in detail in Chapter 5. Far more will occur in playground design during the next decade as current knowledge becomes more widely disseminated and playground apparatus manufacturers include design features for children with disabilities.

TRENDS IN COMMUNITY RELATIONS

Community–Hospital Linkages

Community leisure service departments are building linkages between themselves and hospitals, institutions, and mental health centers. In doing so, networks are being developed to enhance the programs of all agencies involved. For example, the Cincinnati Recreation Commission has worked with state institutions to facilitate the return of clients to the community. The arrangement allows Recreation Commission staff to meet individuals before they are released from the institution. The need for a close working relationship between institutions and community programs will likely grow as institutions place more clients into alternative community living situations.

Another example of a community–hospital linkage is that of a community-based special recreation program and a private psychiatric hospital that have joined together, in west suburban Chicago, for the mutual benefit of their clients. The community program is the West Suburban Special Recreation Association (WSSRA), established as a cooperative venture by the Berwyn, Oak Park, and River Forest park districts. The psychiatric hospital is Riveredge Hospital located in River Forest. Since 1980, Riveredge adolescent patients have served as volunteers in WSSRA programs serving youth who are mentally retarded. The adolescents have assisted with swimming, bowling, track and field, day camps, and dance programs. Staff both at WSSRA and at Riveredge have been enthusiastic in their expression of support for the program (Schwartzel, 1983).

Volunteer Programs

Volunteers are extremely important to the success of special recreation programs. For this reason, the Cincinnati Recreation Commission has developed an awards program to formally recognize volunteers. Volunteers who give 50 hours of service are awarded an "I'm a TRiffic Volunteer" T-shirt. Other appropriate awards are given for all levels of service. Another trend is using special recreation programs participants as volunteers. In so doing, participants not only help the program but gain a sense of giving as well as receiving. Finally, strong advisory councils and parent's groups have become essential to establishing and maintaining high quality special recreation programs. The involvement of citizens is particularly necessary to securing appropriate community support and funding. It is likely that the trend toward expanded use of volunteers in many roles will continue and enlarge.

Cooperative Arrangements Among Leisure Service Agencies

The recent trend toward two or more leisure service agencies cooperating to meet the leisure needs of their special populations grew out of the frustrations of several progressive park districts and municipalities in Illinois during the late 1960s. Although efforts to serve persons with disabilities had been made in the form of summer camps and special events, the park districts and municipal recreation departments realized the limited nature of their programs and that they served only a small fraction of members of special population groups residing within their jurisdictions. While park and recreation personnel desired to enlarge their services for persons with disabilities, their efforts were hampered by financial restrictions, low incidences of some special populations in given districts, and a lack of trained professionals to design programs. Out of this situation arose the concept of pooling resources to establish special recreation cooperatives, each to be supported by several park districts and municipal recreation departments (Robb, 1976).

In March of 1970, the Northern Suburban Special Recreation Association (NSSRA) was formed by eight local park districts and community recreation departments in Cook and Lake counties. From the beginning it was clear that NSSRA was setting a trend for Illinois and the nation. Within the history section of the *Policy Manual of the Northern Suburban Special Recreation Association* (1977) it is stated:

> Since this was to be the first such organization in the country, N.S.S.R.A. realized that it must succeed not only for the population whom it was designed to serve in its own area, but also for special populations throughout the State of Illinois and the nation who would see it as a model for other similar agencies.

The special recreation cooperatives in the Chicago area are a vital part of each of their member districts and municipalities. This sentiment is expressed in the NSSRA *Policy Manual*, which states: "Rather than a separate program, the N.S.S.R.A. is an extension of its member agencies whose specific responsibility is to provide for the special population a program of recreation comparable to that which is offered the general public." Thus the cooperative associations are not "add on" programs, but are a means for each park district and community to provide a comprehensive recreation program for its entire population.

The Northern Suburban Special Recreation Association began the trend toward cooperative ventures by park and recreation jurisdictions to establish special recreation services. From these pioneering efforts of NSSRA has come a concept and model for cooperation that will continue to be applied throughout the nation.

FINANCIAL TRENDS

Fees and Charges

There exists a general trend within leisure service agencies to levy fees and charges. This trend is being followed within special recreation programs. Generally, fees charged for special recreation programs are comparable to those charged the general public. It is the feeling of administrators of special recreation programs that they should not place an unfair burden on their participants by charging them disproportionately higher fees than other citizens, even though special recreation programming is often more expensive to conduct. It is anticipated this trend will persist as long as leisure service agencies continue to depend on the collection of fees and charges.

Fund Raising

Fund-raising efforts have become widespread among special recreation programs. Approaches to fund raising are varied. Illustrative of fund-raising projects are those of the Cincinnati Recreation Commission, which has developed a gift catalog, sponsored various 10K runs, and raffled tickets for a hot air balloon ride with a local celebrity. The Northeast DuPage Special Recreation Association has established the Cabin Foundation to help support the Cabin Nature Program Center, which offers integrated nature programs.

The forementioned fund-raising projects are all positive efforts. Questionable fund-raising practices, such as promoting feelings of pity for children with disabilities, are on the decline. Positive, innovative means to fund raising will be important for some time to come as a means to supplement tax funds.

PROFESSIONAL TRENDS

Continuing Education

Continuing education is an area that is growing today and that will become larger in the future. General recreation staff will need to receive information on special recreation services. Among topics covered will be attitudes toward serving persons with disabilities and issues surrounding the integration of persons with disabilities into ongoing programs. Some staff will "retool" in order to conduct special recreation programs for specific types of participants. Programs on employee burnout will be provided for staff who need to develop new ways of coping with the demands of working intensively in special recreation programs.

Those concerned with continuing education will develop many alternatives to traditional staff workshops and state and national conferences. New types of training approaches, including computer programs, will replace conventional means to continuing education. Further, universities and private consulting firms will make available an abundance of training packages on special recreation programming to local leisure service agencies.

Field-Based Research and Evaluation

Local leisure service agencies are beginning to enter into joint efforts with universities in order to answer applied research questions and to systematically evaluate programs. Both faculty and graduate students with research and evaluation skills are being called upon by agencies to conduct studies that are important to the agencies. For example, a graduate student in therapeutic recreation has conducted a study of a pilot program of the West Suburban Special Recreation Association near Chicago. As special recreation programs multiply and grow in sophistication, it will become established practice to conduct cooperative agency-university research and evaluation studies.

Further Definition of Special Recreators and Therapeutic Recreation Specialists

There is an emerging trend toward an identified area of specialization in *special recreation*. Special recreators will become recognized for their expertise in providing programs directed toward leisure experiences for members of special population groups. Therapeutic recreation specialists will function in leisure service agencies only to conduct programs where therapeutic intervention is called for, and to assess participants referred to them. Both special recreators and therapeutic recreation specialists will continue to work with general recreators to integrate persons with disabilities into ongoing agency programs. Ramifications of this trend will be the establishment of at least one professional organization devoted to the concerns of special recreators and to the development of university professional preparation opportunities specifically designed for students desiring careers as special recreators.

Methods and Materials to Interpret Programs to Community Officials

Means to interpret community special recreation programs will be developed for utilization with elected and appointed officials and board members. Handouts, films, videotapes, and, perhaps, computer programs will become available to make officials sensitive to the leisure needs of persons with disabilities and knowledgeable of concerns in serving special populations. Since public officials continually change, and community special recreation services will remain a relatively novel concept, it will be necessary for agencies to have professionally prepared educational materials available for somewhile, interpreting special recreation services to policy makers.

National Park Service

During the early 1980s, the National Park Service (NPS) initiated a concerted effort to improve accessibility to its facilities and programs for visitors with disabilities. A Special Programs and Populations Branch was established, under the direction of David Park, to facilitate NPS accessibility efforts. This division was given the responsibility of working closely with all units of the Park Service to identify and eliminate barriers to accessibility.

As a result of the efforts of the Special Programs and Populations Branch, in 1983, a special directive addressing policies on accessibility was issued by the (then) Director of the National Park Service, Russell Dickenson. This communication made explicit policies guiding NPS efforts on accessibility to personnel in all of our national parks, with the instruction that policies were to become effective immediately upon receipt of the directive.

While the NPS has only begun to correct accessibility problems, actions within the park system are clear signs of a trend toward making all of our national parks accessible to visitors who are disabled. It is the opinion of the authors of this textbook that the positive stance taken by the National Park Service will serve as a model to enhance accessibility efforts at state and local levels as well. NPS policies will positively effect accessibility in parks throughout America.

Greater Acceptance of Special Recreation Programs by Local Leisure Service Agencies

Members of special population groups remain underserved by leisure service agencies. Yet there has been a constant growth in special recreation programs during the past decade. McGovern (1983) reported that the American Park and Recreation Society/National Therapeutic Recreation Society Committee on Special Populations has observed a positive growth trend in community leisure service programs for special populations. From just over 40 programs in the mid-1970s, the number of programs in 1983 had grown to approximately 300. There will be continued growth in the numbers of special recreation programs. It is difficult, however, to anticipate the extent of this growth trend. The trend does reflect greater acceptance of community special recreation services on the part of local policy makers.

─────────────────── **SUMMARY** ───────────────────

It is evident that the authors of this textbook strongly endorse the trend toward the provision of special recreation services for those with disabilities. Persons with disabilities have the right to the same recreation and leisure activities that are available to the rest of the community. Some would even make a stronger claim for the rights of persons who are disabled. The authors of *The Source Book for the Disabled* (Hale, 1979) have stated:

> There is actually a strong case of claiming that handicapped (disabled) people have more than an equal right. Participation in recreational activities may well be the easiest or even the only way for a person with disabilities to become part of the community, to make new friends, to break out of an institutionalized setting or an overprotected home environment, to give expression to energies and inclinations for which the able-bodied usually have a greater diversity of outlets. (p. 317)

While the *Source Book* is directed toward individuals with physical disabilities, the message of its authors applies to all special populations. All members of special population groups have the same right as others for meaningful leisure, and perhaps a greater need.

The Delivery of Leisure Services Today. The present period promises to be an exciting one in the history of community leisure service delivery systems in the United States and Canada. Progressive systems have already gone beyond the philosophical question of "Should we provide services for persons with disabilities?" to the question, "How can we best serve the needs of persons who are disabled?" Novel departures in programming have begun to evolve. New organizational models are being tested.

Yet change has not occurred as quickly as might be anticipated. Many communities have been slow to respond to the rights of persons with disabilities for leisure services. It is clear that special recreation services are needed and that progressive leisure service delivery systems have responded to the challenge of developing these services. Others must follow to ensure proper recreation and leisure services for all members of our communities.

Suggested Learning Activities

1. Within a small group, discuss the statement that: "Few activities cannot be entered into by persons with disabilities. Therefore, programs for special populations are likely to follow societal

trends." Agree or disagree with the statement. List reasons for your position. Then discuss these with the entire class.

2. Pick one type of activity listed in the chapter in which you have not previously taken part. Arrange to participate in this activity with persons who are disabled. Write a one- to two-page paper on this experience or give a report in class.

3. Survey several community park and recreation departments, or park districts, to determine the type and extent of leisure education and leisure counseling program serving persons with disabilities. These may be integrated or separate programs. Prepare a report on your findings.

4. Interview several persons with disabilities as to trends they see in programming. Then interview program directors or other recreation administrators from the same community. Compare the responses of the consumers and professionals. Report your findings in class.

5. Invite a therapeutic recreation specialist from a state institution into class to discuss the institution's community linkages. Question the specialist as to what would be ideal in terms of community linkages with leisure service delivery systems.

6. Debate the question in class as to whether participants in special recreation programs should pay fees equal to other citizens, even though special population programming is often more expensive to conduct.

7. Invite a therapeutic recreation specialist and a special recreator to class to discuss their roles and what they see as future directions for the therapeutic recreation profession.

8. Survey a region, or state, to determine the extent of programming for special populations by leisure service agencies. With the instructor's assistance, prepare an article on your findings for submission to your state park and recreation journal.

References

Cornelius, D. A., S. Chipouras, E. Makas, and S. Daniels. *Who Cares? A Handbook on Sex Education and Counseling Services for Disabled People,* 2nd ed. Baltimore: University Park Press, 1982.

Galbreaith, P. New airliner shows progress won by handicapped persons. In *Yes You Can. The Indianapolis Star.* Page 45. August 26, 1983.

Galbreaith, P. *What You Can Do For Yourself: Hints for the Handicapped.* New York: Drake Publishing, Inc., 1974.

Gugerty, J., A. F. Roshal, M. D. J. Tradewell, and L. K. Anthony. *Tools, Equipment and Machinery Adapted for the Vocational Education and Employment of Handicapped People.* Madison, WI: Wisconsin Vocational Studies Center, University of Wisconsin, 1981.

Hale, G., ed. *The Source Book for the Disabled.* New York: Bantam Books, Inc., 1979.

Hunter, J. C. Leisure education: Its role in the recreation integration process. *Recreation Canada*, Special Issue, 76–81, 1981.

McGovern, J. Personal communication. June 10, 1983.

Naisbitt, J. *Megatrends: Ten New Directions Transforming Our Lives.* New York: Warner Books, Inc., 1982.

Policy Manual of the Northern Suburban Special Recreation Association. Highland Park, Illinois, 1977.

Robb, G. M., ed. *Guidelines for the Formation and Development of Special Recreation Cooperatives in the State of Illinois.* University of Illinois at Urbana-Champaign: Office of Recreation and Park Resources, Department of Leisure Studies and the Cooperative Extension Service. 1976.

Schwartzel, M. *West Suburban Special Recreation Association/Riveredge Hospital Cooperative Volunteer Program Questionnaire Results.* Unpublished Report. May, 1983.

Sledge hockey and ice picking. *Recreation Canada*, Special Issue, 102, 1981.

The United States Welcomes Handicapped Visitors. Washington, D.C.: Society for the Advancement of Travel for the Handicapped, 1984.

Vinland National Center. 3675 Ihduhapi Road, Loretto, MN, n.d.

Weiss, L. *Access to the World.* New York: Facts on File, Inc., 1983.

A

Guidelines for Community-based Recreation Programs for Special Populations*

HUMAN RESOURCES
Population Over 1 Million

A. Employees responsible for implementation of the special populations program should have the title of director of special populations and be accountable for an administrative division.
   1. Person holding this position should have the following education and experience:
      a. Master's degree in recreation, with emphasis in TR, and 3 years of experience in community and/or clinical settings, preferably certification with NCTRC (see Appendix D), *or*
      b. Bachelor's degree in recreation, with emphasis in TR, and 5 years of experience in community and/or clinical settings, preferably certification with NCTRC (see Appendix D).

B. Area supervisor (program supervisor) should have a bachelor's degree in recreation and 2 years of experience, and be eligible for certification with NCTRC (see Appendix D).

C. Program personnel working with special populations should have the following qualifications:

---

*From: Vaughan, J.L. & Winslow, R. (eds.) *Guidelines for Community-Based Recreation Programs for Special Populations.* Arlington, VA: National Therapeutic Recreation Society, 1979.

1. Full-time employees should hold a bachelor's degree in recreation and have previously worked with special populations.
2. Part-time employees should have experience and/or in-service training in working with special populations.

D. Volunteers working with special populations should be provided ongoing in-service training the comprehensiveness of such training being dependent on the extent to which they are involved in the program, and the functional level of the handicapped persons with whom they are working.

E. An advisory board of parents, consumers, and professionals should be formed to assist the director of programs for special populations.

F. Job descriptions should include the following responsibilities and tasks:

1. *Director of special populations*
   a. Should correspond in position, title, and responsibilities to other program directors within the department
   b. Should serve as department liaison with other special populations agencies and associations within the community
   c. Should work closely with the special populations advisory committee in the coordination and implementation of the special populations program
   d. Should explore all available governmental and nongovernmental supplemental funding sources for the special populations program, for the alleviation of architectural barriers, and for the provision of transportation
   e. Should coordinate and provide in-service training in the area of special populations for all existing departmental personnel and volunteers

2. *Area supervisors* (program supervisor)
   a. Should correspond in position, title, and responsibilities to other program area supervisors within the department
   b. Should serve as a special populations liaison with other program area supervisors and personnel in the implementation of the special populations transitional and regular programs
   c. Should coordinate all special populations programs within the geographical area
   d. Should develop a close working relationship with other special populations agencies within the geographical area

      e. Should coordinate transportation services of the special populations program within the geographical area

      f. Should supervise all special populations programs within the geographical area

   3. *Program personnel*

      a. Should correspond in responsibilities to other program personnel within the department

      b. Should be directly responsible for the program leadership and implementation of the special populations program segregated classes, and should work closely with other program personnel in the implementation of the special populations program

      c. Should assist in the coordination and implementation of transportation services for the special populations program

   4. *Volunteers*

      a. Should correspond in program personnel responsibilities to other volunteer personnel within the department

      b. Should be provided with an ongoing in-service training program in the area of special populations

      c. Should be utilized for assistance in program leadership and transportation services

   5. *Advisory board/committee*

      a. Should work closely with and assist the special populations program director in the development, implementation, and evaluation of the special populations program

      b. Should provide assistance to the special populations program in the identification of handicapped consumers in the community, public relations for the special populations program, sources for program funding, and transportation services for the special populations program

Population 500,000 to 1 Million

A. Employee responsible for implementation of the special populations program should have the title of director of special populations and be accountable for an administrative division.

   1. Person holding this position should have the following education and experience:

      a. Master's degree in recreation, with emphasis in TR, and 3 years of experience in community and/or clinical settings, preferably NCTRC certification *or*

      b. Bachelor's degree in recreation, with emphasis in TR, and 5 years of experience in community and/or clinical settings, preferably NCTRC certification

B. Area supervisor (program supervisor) should have a bachelor's degree in recreation and 2 years of experience, and be eligible for NCTRC certification.

C. Program personnel working with special populations should have the following qualifications:

1. Full-time employees should hold a bachelor's degree in recreation and have previously worked with special populations.
2. Part-time employees should have experience and/or in-service training in working with special populations.

D. Volunteers working with special populations should be provided ongoing in-service training, the comprehensiveness of such training being dependent on the extent to which they are involved in the program, and the functional level of the handicapped persons with whom they are working.

E. An advisory board of parents, consumers, and professionals should be formed to assist the director of programs for special populations.

F. Job descriptions should include the following responsibilities and tasks:

1. *Director of special populations*
   a. Should correspond in position, title, and responsibilities to other program directors within the department
   b. Should serve as department liaison with other special population agencies and associations within the community
   c. Should work closely with the special populations advisory committee in the coordination and implementation of the special populations program
   d. Should explore all available governmental and nongovernmental supplemental funding sources for the special populations program, for the alleviation of architectural barriers, and for the provisions of transportation
   e. Should coordinate and provide in-service training in the area of special populations for all existing departmental personnel and volunteers.

2. *Area supervisors* (program supervisor)
   a. Should correspond in position, title, and responsibilities to other program area supervisors within the department
   b. Should serve as a special populations liaison with other program area supervisors and personnel in the implementation of the special populations special skills and mainstreaming programs
   c. Should coordinate all special populations programs within the geographical area

       d. Should develop a close working relationship with other special populations agencies within the geographical area

       e. Should coordinate transportation services of the special populations program within the geographical area

       f. Should supervise all special populations programs within the geographical area

   3. *Program personnel*

       a. Should correspond in responsibilities to other program personnel within the department

       b. Should be directly responsible for the program leadership and implementation of the special populations program segregated classes, and should work closely with other program personnel in the implementation of the special populations program

       c. Should assist in the coordination and implementation of transportation services for the special populations program

   4. *Volunteers*

       a. Should correspond in program personnel responsibilities to other volunteer personnel within the department

       b. Shoud be provided with an ongoing in-service training program in the area of special populations

       c. Should be utilized for assistance in program implementation and transportation services

   5. *Advisory board/committee*

       a. Should work closely with and assist the special populations programs director in the development, implementation, and evaluation of the special populations program

       b. Should provide assistance to the special populations program in the identification of handicapped consumers in the community, public relations for the special populations program, sources for program funding, and transportation services for the special populations program

Population 250,000 to 499,999

A. Employee responsible for developing and supervising special populations programs should have the title of supervisor and have the following qualifications:

   1. Master's degree in recreation, 3 years of experience, and eligibility for NCTRC certification, *or*

   2. Bachelor's degree in recreation, 5 years of experience, and eligibility for NCTRC certification

B. Supervisor should be assigned to the recreation division of the department.

C. Program personnel working with special populations should have the following qualifications:

1. Full-time employees should hold a bachelor's degree in recreation and should have previously worked with special populations.
2. Part-time employees should have experience and/or in-service training in working with the handicapped.

D. Volunteers working with special populations should be provided ongoing in-service training, the comprehensiveness of such training being dependent on the extent to which they are involved in the program, and the functional level of the handicapped persons with whom they are working.

E. An advisory board of parents, consumers, and professionals should be formed to assist the supervisor of programs for special populations.

F. Job descriptions should include the following responsibilities and tasks:

1. *Supervisor*
   a. Should correspond in position, title, and responsibilities to other program area supervisors within the department
   b. Should serve as a special populations liaison with other program area supervisors and personnel in the implementation of the special populations special skills and mainstreaming programs
   c. Should coordinate all special populations programs within the geographical area
   d. Should develop a close working relationship with other special populations agencies within the geographical area
   e. Should coordinate transportation services of the special populations program within the department's jurisdiction

2. *Program personnel*
   a. Should correspond in responsibilities to other program personnel within the department
   b. Should be directly responsible for the program leadership and implementation of the special populations program segregated classes and should work closely with other program personnel in the implementation of the special populations program
   c. Should assist in the coordination and implementation of transportation services for the special populations program

3. *Volunteers*
   a. Should correspond in program personnel responsibilities to other volunteer personnel within the department
   b. Should be provided with an ongoing in-service training program in the area of special populations

    c. Should be utilized for assistance in program implementation and transportation services

  4. *Advisory board/committee*

    a. Should work closely with and assist the special populations program supervisor in the development, implementation, and evaluation of the special populations program

    b. Should provide assistance to the special populations program in the identification of handicapped consumers in the community, public relations for the special populations program, sources for program funding, and transportation services for the special populations program.

Population 100,000 to 249,999

A. Employee responsibile for developing and supervising special populations program should have a title of supervisor and have the following qualifications:

  1. Master's degree in recreation, 3 years of experience, and eligibility for NCTRC certification, *or*

  2. Bachelor's degree in recreation, 5 years of experience, and ligibility for NCTRC certification

B. Supervisor should be assigned to the recreation division of the department.

C. Program personnel working with special populations should have the following qualifications:

  1. Full-time employees should hold a bachelor's degree in recreation and should have previously worked with special populations.

  2. Part-time employees should have experience and/or in-service training in working with the handicapped.

D. Volunteers working with special populations should be provided ongoing in-service training, the comprehensiveness of such training being dependent on the extent to which they are involved in the program, and the functional level of the handicapped persons with whom they are working.

E. An advisory board of parents, consumers, and professionals should be formed to assist the supervisor of programs for special populations.

F. Job descriptions should include the following responsibilities and tasks:

  1. *Supervisor*

    a. Should correspond in position, title, and responsibilities to other program area supervisors within the department

    b. Should serve as a special populations liaison with other program area supervisors and personnel in the implementation of the special populations special skills and mainstreaming program

c. Should coordinate all special populations programs within the geographical area

d. Should develop a close working relationship with other special populations agencies within the geographical area

e. Should coordinate transportation services of the special populations program within the department's jurisdiction

2. *Program personnel*

a. Should correspond in responsibilities to other program personnel within the department

b. Should be directly responsible for the program leadership and implementation of the special populations program segregated classes and should work closely with other program personnel in the implementation of the special populations program

c. Should assist in the coordination and implementation of transportation services for the special populations program

3. *Volunteers*

a. Should correspond in program personnel responsibilities to other volunteer personnel within the department

b. Should be provided with an ongoing in-service training program in the area of special populations

c. Should be utilized for assistance in program implementation and transportation services

4. *Advisory board/committee*

a. Should work closely with and assist the special populations program supervisor in the development, implementation, and evaluation of the special populations program

b. Should provide assistance to the special populations program in the identification of handicapped consumers in the community, public relations for the special populations program, sources for program funding, and transportation services for the special populations program.

Population 50,000 to 99,999

A. Employee responsible for developing and supervising special populations programs should have the title of supervisor and have the following qualifications:

1. Master's degree in recreation, 3 years of experience, and eligibility for NCTRC certification, *or*

2. Bachelor's degree in recreation, 5 years of experience, and eligibility for NCTRC certification

B. Supervisor should be assigned to the recreation division of the department.

C. Program personnel working with special populations should
have the following qualifications:
   1. Full-time employees should hold a bachelor's degree in
      recreation and should have previously worked with special
      populations.
   2. Part-time employees should have experience and/or in-service
      training in working with the handicapped.
D. Volunteers working with special populations should be provided
   ongoing in-service training, the comprehensiveness of such
   training being dependent on the extent to which they are
   involved in the program and the functional level of the
   handicapped persons with whom they are working.
E. An advisory board of parents, consumers, and professionals
   should be formed to assist the supervisor of programs for special
   populations.
F. Job descriptions should include the following responsibilities and
   tasks:
   1. *Supervisor*
      a. Should correspond in position, title, and responsibilities to
         other program area supervisors within the department
      b. Should serve as a special populations liaison with other
         program area supervisors and personnel in the
         implementation of the special populations special skills and
         mainstreaming programs
      c. Should coordinate all special populations programs within
         the geographical area
      d. Should develop a close working relationship with other
         special populations agencies within the geographical area
      e. Should coordinate transportation services of the special
         populations program within the department's jurisdiction
      f. Should write grant and foundation proposals.
   2. *Program personnel*
      a. Should correspond in responsibilities to other program
         personnel within the department
      b. Should be directly responsible for the program leadership
         and implementation of the special populations program
         segregated classes and should work closely with other
         program personnel in the implementation of the special
         populations program
      c. Should assist in the coordination and implementation of
         transportation services for the special populations program
   3. *Volunteers*
      a. Should correspond in program personnel responsibilities
         with other volunteer personnel within the department

    b. Should be provided with an ongoing in-service training program in the area of special populations

    c. Should be utilized for assistance in program implementation and transportation services

4. *Advisory board/committee*

    a. Should work closely with and assist the special populations program supervisor in the development, implementation, and evaluation of the special populations program.

    b. Should provide assistance to the special populations program in the identification of handicapped consumers in the community, public relations for the special populations program, sources for program funding, and transportation services for the special populations program.

Population 25,000 to 49,999

A. A full-time employee should be assigned to be responsible for developing programs for special populations.

    1. This person should have education and experience in TR and should devote 50% of his or her time to the development of special populations programs, *or*

    2. The person lacking such background should utilize the services of a TR consultant to devleop and implement special populations programs.

B. An advisory board of parents, consumers, and professionals should be formed to assist the full-time employee responsible for special populations.

C. Other volunteers working with special populations should be provided ongoing in-service training by either the full-time employee or the TR consultant, the comprehensiveness of such training being dependent on the extent to which they are involved in the program and the functional level of the handicapped persons with whom they are working.

D. Job descriptions should include the following responsibilities and tasks:

    1. *Full-time recreation employee*

    Same as program personnel for 1 million or over

    2. *Advisory board*

        a. Should act as the liaison for the department with all agencies serving the needs of the handicapped in the community

        b. Should work closely with and assist the special populations supervisor in the development, implementation, and evaluation of the special populations program

        c. Should provide assistance to the special populations

program in the identification of handicapped consumers in the community, public relations for the special populations program, sources for program funding, and transportation services for the special populations program

3. *Other volunteers*
   Same as listed under 1 million and over for this group of persons

Population Under 25,000

The same as 25,000 to 49,999, except TR consultant is optional

We feel that program guidelines are essentially the same for all communities, but we do realize there will be some variations with smaller size.

Program

A. The philosophy of the department should consist of making available all existing department programs (activities) and facilities to the entire handicapped population in the community.
B. Programs should be developed to meet the needs of those special populations that cannot be immediately integrated into existing programs.
C. All departmental personnel should participate in awareness sessions focusing on the leisure capabilities of special populations.
D. An advisory committee for the special populations program should be formed, composed of parents, handicapped consumers, interested citizens, and professionals. This committee would be responsible for assistance to the department in the identification of handicapped consumers in the community, public relations for the special populations program, sources for program funding, and advisement on program content.
E. The initial steps necessary to implement the department's special populations program should be as follows:
   1. Survey the existing department facilities to identify architectural barriers and accessibility limitations that would prevent the handicapped from participating in the recreation program.
   2. Identify existing schools within the community that serve special populations, and establish a positive working relationship with the administration of the identified schools.
   3. Identify agencies and associations within the community that advocate, serve, and/or represent special populations, make them aware of the department's desire to provide recreation services to special populations, establish a working relationship with these agencies, and enlist their support in identifying other community resources.

4. Form an advisory committee for the special populations program, which should be composed of parents, handicapped consumers, interested citizens, and professionals.
5. Utilize the identified schools, agencies, and associations for the location of special population citizens in the community to develop an accurate mailing list.
6. The special populations program director, the special populations program personnel, the advisory committee, and the existing departmental personnel should work together in the development of a special populations program.
7. Disseminate special populations program information via the developed mailing list, to identified schools, agencies, and associations, the advisory committee, and the local media.
8. Register the special population participants into existing recreation programs. For those special population participants who cannot participate in regular programs, develop and initiate transitional classes and register participants as in regular classes.

F. At the conclusion of each season or quarter, conduct a survey of program participants that can determine the effectiveness of the special populations program activities and can give direction for future programming.

G. The advisory committee and all schools, agencies, and associations with which a working relationship has been established should provide continuous feedback on the community's reaction to the department's special populations program.

H. The special populations program should consist of three types of classes: regular, transitional, and segregated.
   1. Regular classes are those that incorporate the disabled with the nondisabled participants.
      a. Nonspecial populations program personnel should teach these classes.
      b. The special populations program director or personnel should be available for program consultation, if necessary.
      c. Program goals for the disabled participants should be the same as for nondisabled participants.
   2. Transitional classes are those that provide the participant with skill development capabilities that will be necessary for participation in regular activities.
      a. Both the nonspecial populations program personnel and the special populations program personnel should teach these classes.

   b. The special populations program director or personnel
      should be available for consultation and in-service training,
      if necessary.
   c. Program goals for these classes are sensory, motor, and
      cognitive skill development, leisure education, socialization,
      improvement of self-image, and development of
      independence.
   d. Special activities and/or clinics can also serve the purpose of
      reaching the above objectives.
3. Segregated classes are those that provide, through adaptation,
   the more severely handicapped individual with leisure-
   oriented experiences.
   a. The special populations program personnel should teach
      these classes.
   b. Interagency cooperation and assistance can be utilized to
      implement and conduct these classes.
   c. Program goals for these classes are sensory, motor, and
      cognitive skill development, social skills development,
      improving self-image, developing independence,
      community awareness, and education.
   d. Participants in these activities may or may not acquire
      sufficient skills to be placed into the upper two levels of
      programming.

FINANCES/FUNDING
Population Over 500,000

A. Budgeting for the special populations program should be an
   integral part of the total park and recreation budget.
B. Fees and charges should be applied to all special populations
   programs when
   1. Participants in regular programs pay an established activity fee
   2. Participants in transitional programs are charged a fee
      comparable to fees paid for similar types of programs in the
      department
   3. Participants in segregated classes are charged a fee to cover the
      cost of materials or a portion of staff time (operating costs)
C. To supplement the operating cost of segregated classes and
   transitional classes, the recreation and park department should
   work closely with the special populations advisory committee to
   investigate and identify potential cooperative agreements with
   other agencies serving the handicapped in the community.
D. The special populations director should contact and explore the
   types of cooperative agreements that could be enacted with other

agencies serving handicapped individuals, that is, funding, facilities, staff, materials.

E. To develop the special populations program further, the recreation and park department and the director of special populations should explore all available governmental (federal, state, county) and nongovernmental (private foundations) supplemental funding sources.

F. The recreation and park department and the director of special populations should work closely with the city's research and development office (grant writers) in writing grant and foundation proposals.

G. The special populations advisory committee should investigate and establish avenues for financial support for special populations programs from individuals, service clubs, and other voluntary organizations within the community. Since the basic responsibility for funding the special populations program rests with the recreation and park department, other funding support should supplement, not maintain the program.

Population 100,000 to 499,999

The guidelines are the same as for over 500,000, except substitute "supervisor" for "director of special populations."

Population 50,000 to 99,999

The guidelines are the same as for 100,000 to 499,999, except that letter F should read: "The supervisor should write grant and foundation proposals."

Population 25,000 to 49,999

The guidelines are the same as for over 500,000, except substitute "responsible full-time employee" for "director of special populations." Also, letter F should read: "Recreation and park department should identify and apply for grants in support of the special populations program."

Population Under 25,000

Follow the guidelines for over 500,000 except for the following changes:

B. Fees and charges should be applied to all special populations programs when
   1. Participants in regular programs pay an established activity fee
   2. Participants in segregated classes are charged a fee to cover the cost of materials or a portion of staff time (operating costs)

C. To supplement the operating cost of segregated classes, the recreation and part department should work closely with the special populations advisory committee to contact and explore potential cooperative agreements with other agencies serving the handicapped in the community.

D. Delete this guideline
E. To develop the special populations program further, the recreation and park department, the responsible full-time employee, and the advisory committee should explore all available governmental (federal, state, county) and nongovernmental (private foundations) supplemental funding sources.
F. Delete this guideline.

TRANSPORTATION
Population Over 1 Million

A. Although some handicapped individuals can utilize traditional forms of transportation, a significant number must utilize special modes of transportation because of physical and/or mental limitations.
B. The special populations director should explore and investigate all avenues for potential transportation support and pursue those sources that will provide transportation for special population participants to attend recreation and park programs (activities).
   1. Recreation and park department vehicles should be utilized, when at all possible, for transportation during the initial developmental stages of the special populations program.
   2. Parents, participants, and friends should be encouraged to provide their own transportation and, where possible, develop car pools.
   3. Identified community agencies with appropriate vehicles should be contacted for assistance in providing transportation for participants (schools, for example).
   4. Service clubs and private foundations should be educated to the need for barrier-free vehicles and encouraged to donate such vehicles for the special populations program.
   5. The special populations director should pursue with the recreation and park department provisions for accepting and utilizing donated vehicles such as gas and maintenance.
   6. Mass transportation agencies (governmental and private) should be contacted in regard to current transporting policies for special populations and future plans to make their services accessible to all citizens of the community.
   7. The special populations director should explore all available federal, state, or county grant funding sources available for underwriting transportation costs.
C. The special populations advisory committee should assist the director of special populations in identifying potential

transportation sources and act as an advocate with mass transportation agencies to provide barrier-free transportation to the handicapped within the community.

Population 100,000 to 1 Million

The guidelines are the same as for over 1 million, except substitute "supervisor" for "special populations director."

Population 50,000 to 99,999

Follow the guidelines for 100,000 to 1 million except for the following changes:

B. 4. Service clubs and private foundations should be educated to the need for barrier-free vehicles and encouraged to work together to donate such vehicles for the special populations program.

B. 6. Delete this guideline.

C. The special populations advisory committee should assist the supervisor in identifying potential transportation sources.

Population 25,000 to 49,999

Follow the guidelines for 100,000 to 1 million except for the following changes:

B. 1,4,5,6. Delete these guidelines.

C. The special populations advisory committee should assist the supervisor in identifying potential transportation sources.

Population Under 25,000

Follow the guidelines for 100,000 to 1 million except for the following changes:

B. 1,4,5,6. Delete these guidelines. Substitute "advisory committee" for "supervisor."

C. Delete this guideline.

Project INSPIRES's Competency Identification Survey Results*

The following professional competencies/skills have been identified as being important for an undergraduate student majoring in *community* recreation and seeking an entry-level position. The rating for each skill is the combined average of our survey participants—college recreation educators and professional recreators who work with special populations.

**Orientation to Recreation for Special Populations:
Philosophy, History, Concepts**   Average Rating

- Understand continuum of recreation service to special populations including therapeutic recreation service.   4.14
- Develop a personal/professional philosophy of recreation for special populations in community settings.   4.25
- State a rationale for the provision of community recreation for special populations.   4.24

---

*From: Austin, D. R., and L. G. Powell, Competencies needed by community recreators to serve special populations. In Austin, D. R. ed., *Directions in Health, Physical Education, and Recreation, Therapeutic Recreation Curriculum: Philosophy, Strategy, and Concepts.* Bloomington: Indiana University School of Health, Physical Education, and Recreation, 1980, pp. 44–47.

	Average Rating
▪ Know role of recreation services for special populations in the community recreation department.	4.48
▪ Understand ways in which recreation can help to serve developmental needs of special populations.	3.98
▪ Develop awareness, on the part of special populations, for use of meaningful leisure.	3.80

Characteristics of Special Populations

▪ Understand the implications of sexuality to disabled populations.	2.72
▪ Understand terminology used by practitioners in human service disciplines.	3.59
▪ Understand psycho-social implications of acquired versus congenital disabilities.	2.99
▪ Given that the student understands normal human growth and development, recognize the impact of disabilities on the growth and development of the handicapped.	3.79
▪ Identify the nature and etiology of the major disability groups, contrasting them with normally developed individuals.	3.42
▪ Recognize the potential psychological impact of disabilities on individual's recreation participation.	3.87
▪ Recognize the potential sociological impact of disabilities on individual's recreation participation.	3.91
▪ Recognize the potential physiological impact of disabilities on individual's recreation participation.	3.78

Attitudes

▪ Understand how positive attitudes toward the handicapped may be developed within recreational programs.	4.66
▪ Demonstrate awareness of personal attitudes toward ill, handicapped, and disabled individuals.	4.46
▪ Understand parents' attitudes toward the handicapped child (over-protection, etc).	4.21

	Average Rating
■ Understand various societal attitudes toward special populations.	4.31
■ Understand how the handicapped individual's attitudes about self influence recreational behavior.	4.15
■ Understand the handicapped individual's attitudes toward other handicapped persons within, and outside of, his/her disability group.	3.79

Mainstreaming

■ Understand concept of mainstreaming.	4.56
■ Understand concept of normalization.	4.38
■ Describe approaches to mainstreaming special populations in community recreation.	4.31
■ Describe the phenomenon of labeling.	3.57
■ Discuss your personal feelings concerning labeling.	3.18
■ Explain possible consequences or effects of labeling.	3.62

Leadership and Supervision

■ Know principles of instruction useful for executing recreation activities for special populations (e.g., blind, hearing impaired, mentally retarded).	4.31
■ Analyze activities for their functional elements to determine their appropriateness for various handicapping conditions.	3.80
■ Specify the principles relevant to activity adaptation.	3.85
■ Select activities to serve developmental needs of special populations.	3.69
■ Know how to facilitate integrated recreational groups (create an atmosphere conducive to mainstreaming).	4.24
■ Understand the impact you, as a leader, can have on a handicapped individual.	4.38
■ Recognize the importance of considering individual needs and interests during program leadership.	4.63
■ Know competencies required of community recreation personnel working with special	

populations at a leadership/supervisory level (i.e., entry-level).

	Average Rating
	4.23

- Identify activities that are appropriate to age and functioning level of the handicapped person. — 4.22
- Describe typical information that should be found in a program application form for a handicapped individual. — 3.52

Program Design

- Know current trends in recreation program design for special populations. — 4.01
- Evaluate various models for the delivery of community recreation service for special populations. — 3.26
- State general objectives for recreation programs for special populations. — 4.23
- Know guidelines for programming recreation for special populations. — 4.12
- Identify the social and behavioral factors common to handicapped individuals, which have the potential for influencing programming. — 3.45
- Describe the importance of consumer input in program development. — 4.18
- Understand the importance of developing departmental policies, procedures, and practices which incorporate the department's philosophy of community recreation for special populations. — 4.14
- Know organizational structures (models) which might be utilized in community recreation services for special populations. — 3.76
- Know steps in organization of community-based recreation for special populations. — 4.14

Facility Design and Accessibility

- Identify resources available on the design of barrier-free recreational environments. — 4.13
- Describe physical barriers to accessibility and how they can be eliminated. — 4.14
- Describe attitudinal barriers to accessibility. — 4.20
- Understand the frustrations experienced in an inaccessible environment. — 4.37
- Know the basic design features to facilitate recreation experiences of the handicapped. — 4.03

Equipment and Supplies	Average Rating
■ Illustrate equipment adaptations appropriate to recreation programs for the handicapped.	3.85
■ Identify and evaluate supplies and equipment for recreation programs for the handicapped.	3.43
■ Know principles involved in selecting regular, adaptive, or alternative equipment.	3.80

Aids, Appliances, Assistive Techniques

■ Demonstrate the use of basic mechanical devices (including use of wheelchairs, crutches).	3.61
■ Knows first aid and safety procedures and practices as these relate to special populations (transfers, epilepsy).	4.67
■ Demonstrate the use of a variety of adaptive aids, devices, and techniques that will make activities available to clients with specific disabilities (e.g., card holders).	3.51
■ Demonstrate proper assistive techniques in the ambulation of blind individuals.	3.76

Resources and Services

■ Be familiar with the various leisure-oriented organizations for special populations (e.g., National Wheelchair Athletic Association, U.S. Association for Blind Athletes).	3.52
■ State general functions of local, state, and national organizations related indirectly to recreation for special populations (BEH, NTRS, UCP, Easter Seals, Kennedy Foundation, etc.).	3.10
■ Determine when the services of a therapeutic recreation consultant are needed in the provision of community recreation services for special populations.	3.63
■ Know methods of cooperative planning of leisure services for special populations with other community agencies.	4.18
■ Know human service agencies found in the community, including those established to deliver health care.	3.70
■ Discuss the role of the public leisure services agency in coordinating services for special populations.	3.82

	Average Rating
■ Know potential community resources (human and physical) that may be utilized for recreation for special populations.	4.30

Leisure Education (Being a Resource)

■ Understand the role of the community recreator as a liaison between the community and the disabled individual and his family.	4.60
■ Be able to assist special populations in identifying approprate leisure services in the community.	4.27
■ Identify levels of leisure counseling.	3.22
■ Recognize resources such as inventories and other methods that may be employed in leisure counseling.	3.11

Advocacy and Legislation

■ Discuss advocacy as it relates to the recreational needs of the handicapped.	3.67
■ Discuss the implications of legal liability that must be considered in the planning and implementation of a recreation program for special populations.	3.53
■ Know legislation related to delivery of leisure services to special populations (PL94-142, 504).	4.06

Funding Sources

■ Know local, state, and federal funding agencies and the procedures used to procure these funds for the development of recreation services for special populations.	3.27
■ Identify non-governmental (e.g., foundations) funding sources for recreation services to special populations.	3.24

Professionalism

■ Recognize professional societies, associations, and organizations related to the therapeutic recreation field (e.g., NTRS).	3.90
■ Understand various roles performed by the therapeutic recreator.	3.94
■ Compare functions of the community and the therapeutic recreator.	3.61

Average Rating

- Identify journals and other sources that could be used to improve the quality of recreation service for special populations.   3.72

Training

- Outline *considerations* for in-service training sessions for staff working with special populations.   3.63
- Outline *considerations* for orientation and training sessions for volunteers working with special populations.   3.69
- Discuss volunteer recruitment and selection (e.g., sources, use of handicapped).   3.62
- Apply the knowledge, understanding, and skills in actual supervised work experiences in recreation programs serving special populations.   3.99

Trends and Issues

- Know current social issues and how they affect recreation services to special populations.   3.55
- Know current trends in human service delivery systems and their impact on community recreation services for special populations.   3.68
- Know current trends in program development for community recreation for special populations.   4.19
- Know the extent to which communities are providing recreation programs for special populations.   3.95
- Discuss financial aspects of special population programming in comparison to other community recreation programs.   3.82

C

Selected Organizations Concerning Persons with Disabilities

American Association of Mental Deficiency, 5201 Connecticut Avenue, N.W., Washington, DC 20015

American Association of Retired Persons, 1225 Connecticut Avenue, N.W., Washington, DC 20036

American Diabetes Association, 18 E. 48th Street, New York, NY 10017

American Foundation for the Blind, Inc., 15 W. 16th Street, New York, NY 10011

American Orthotic and Prosthetic Association, 1440 North Street, N.W., Washington, DC 20005

Arthritis Foundation, 1212 Avenue of the Americas, New York, NY 10036

Council for Exceptional Children, 1920 Association Drive, Reston, VA 22091

Disabled American Veterans, P.O. Box 1403, Cincinnati, OH 45214

Epilepsy Foundation of American, 4351 Garden Drive, Landover, MD 20785

Helen Keller National Center for Deaf/Blind Youths and Adults, 111 Middle Neck Road, Sands Point, NY 11050

Muscular Dystrophy Associations of America, Inc., 810 Seventh Avenue, New York, NY 10019

National Association of the Deaf, 814 Thayer Avenue, Silver Springs, MD 20910

National Association of the Physically Handicapped, 2810 Terrace Road, S.E., Washington, DC 20020

National Association for Retarded Citizens, 2709 Avenue E East, Arlington, TX 76011

National Easter Seal Society for Crippled Children and Adults, 2023 W. Ogden Avenue, Chicago, IL 60612

National Multiple Sclerosis Society, 205 E. 42nd Street, New York, NY 10017

United Cerebral Palsy Associations, Inc., 66 E. 34th Street, New York, NY 10016

D

Athletic and Recreational Organizations for Persons with Disabilities

American Athletic Association of the Deaf, 3916 Lantern Drive, Silver Spring, MD 20902

American Blind Bowlers Association, 150 N. Bellaire Avenue, Louisville, KY 40206

American Library Association, Library Services to the Blind and Physically Handicapped, 50 E. Huron Street, Chicago, IL 60611

American National Red Cross Program of Swimming for the Handicapped, 17th and D Streets, N.W., Washington, DC 20006

American Printing House for the Blind, 1839 Frankfort Avenue, Louisville, KY 40206

American Wheelchair Bowling Association, 2635 N.E. 19th Street, Pampano Beach, FL 33062

Amputee Sports Organization, 11705 Mercy Boulevard, Savannah, GA 31406

Association of Handicapped Artists, 1034 Rand Building, Buffalo, NY 14203

Blind Outdoor Leisure Development, 533 E. Main Street, Aspen, CO 81611

Disabled Sportsmen of America, Inc., P.O. Box 26, Vinton, VA 24179

International Committee of the Silent Sports, Gallandet College, Florida Avenue and Seventh Streets, N.E., Washington, DC 20002

International Wheelchair Road Racers Club, Physical Therapy Department, Jackson Memorial Hospital, 1611 N.W. 12th Avenue, Miami, FL 33136

National Amputee Skiing Association, 3738 Walnut Avenue, Carmichael, CA 95608

National Association of Sports for Cerebral Palsy, P.O. Box 2874, Amity Station, New Haven, CT 06525

National Committee, Arts with the Handicapped, 1825 Connecticut Avenue, N.W., Washington, D.C. 20009

National Foundation for Wheelchair Tennis, 3855 Birch Street, Newport Beach, CA 92660

National Theatre of the Deaf, 1860 Broadway, New York, NY 10023

National Track and Field Committee for the Visually Impaired, 4244 Heather Road, Long Beach, CA 90808

National Wheelchair Athletic Association, 3617 Betty Drive, Suites Colorado Springs, CO 80907

National Wheelchair Basketball Association, 110 Seaton Center, University of Kentucky, Lexington, KY 40506

National Wheelchair Bowling Association, 2635 N.E. 19th Street, Pompano Beach, FL 33062

National Wheelchair Softball Association, P.O. Box 737, Sioux Falls, SD 57101

North American Riding for the Handicapped Association, Inc., P.O. Box 100, Ashburn, VA 22011

Special Olympics, Joseph P. Kennedy, Jr., Foundation, 1701 K Street, N.W., Washington, DC 20006

United States Deaf Skiers Association, 2 Sunset Hill Road, Simsbury, CT 06070

Assistive Sports Resources*

ARCHERY

Shooting Release. Enables individuals with limited finger/hand functioning to draw bow string to anchor point. Total Shooting Systems, Inc., 419 Van Dyne Rd., North Fond Dulac, WI 54935.

Splints, Braces, Cuff. Applied Technology for Independent Living; 2008 Lowry Ave. N.E., Minneapolis, MN 55418.

BILLIARDS

Billiards Accessories. Flaghouse, Inc.
18 West 18th Street
New York, NY 10011

Rollers/Cuffs. Applied Technology for Independent Living
2008 Lowry Avenue N. E.
Minneapolis, MN 55418

---

*Adapted from a handout prepared by Lyn Rourke, Sports, Physical Education and Recreation Department, Courage Center, Golden Valley, Minnesota.

BOWLING AIDS

Bowling Ball Holder. For wheelchair bowlers. Safely holds ball while moving chair up to foul line. Nelson Medical Products, 5690 Sarah Ave., Sarasota, FL 33583.

Bowling Ball Pusher. A long-handled device for pushing and guiding bowling ball down alley. Use from wheelchair or standing position. Extension handle lengthens for use. Shortens for transportation. Maddak, Inc., Pequannock, NJ 07440.

Bowling Ball Ramp. Allows disabled person to participate in the regular game of bowling. The ramp guides the ball toward the pins with minimal skill and effort by player. Easily stored and quickly set up. J. A. Preston Corp., 71 Fifth Ave., New York, NY 10003.

Bowling Ramp. Ideal for persons with little or no use of their arms. The ramp is placed in front of the lane, and an assistant places the ball on the frame. Maddak, Inc., Pequannock, NJ 07440.

Bowling Stick. Aluminum construction with adjustable handle. Swivel floor guides remain level for smoother delivery of the ball. Swivel nylon pads form a vee that keeps the ball centered for greater accuracy. Nelson Medical Products, 5690 Sarah Ave., Sarasota, FL 33583.

Third Hand. For wheelchair bowlers. Safely holds ball while moving chair up to foul line. Has steel ring and heavy duty aluminum attachment. No nuts or bolts. Attaches to most chairs. Maddak, Inc., Pequannock, NJ 07440.

Handle Grip Bowling Ball. Unique handle permits bowler to grasp ball without the usual finger-hold grip. Simply grasp the handle, roll the ball, and the handle retracts when released. Maddak, Inc., Pequannock, NJ 07440.

Bowling Ramp. Robert E. Lee, Lee's Lanes, RFD #2, Mason City, IA 50401.

Bowling Equipment. Recreation Unlimited, 830 Woodend Rd., Stratford, CT 06497, (203) 348-0802.

Mahler's Standard Bowling Rail. Serves as a bannister guide for blind bowlers. Type four balls fit in formed metal bars. Comes in two parts. No attachments to alleys for return racks are necessary. Replacement parts available. American Foundation for the Blind, 20 W. 17th Street, New York, NY 10011.

Bowling Sticks. Phillip Faas, 3226 Bayou Placido Blvd. N. E., St. Petersburg, FL 33703.

Ball Holders. George Snyder, 5809 N. E. 21st Ave., Ft. Lauderdale, FL 33308.

Snap Handle Bowling Balls. Barker's Bowling, Inc., 2659 E. 75th St., Chicago, IL 60649.

Bowling Aids. North American Recreation, P. O. Box 430, Fairhaven Station, 315 Peck St., New Haven, CT 06513, (800) 527-7415.

Bowling Aids. Flaghouse, Inc., 18 W. 18th Street, New York, NY 10011.

FISHING

One-Hand Fishing. Lightweight harness acts as a second hand. Two adjustable straps. Works for either right or left hand. Aluminum. Fashion Able, Rocky Hill, NJ 08553.

Left Hand Reel. Sepcially produced with crank on left. Thumb only casting. Fashion Able, Rocky Hill, NJ 08553.

Computer Control Fishing Reel. Miya Epoch, 1635 Crenshaw Blvd., Torrance, CA 90501, (213) 320-1172.

Garcia Handi-Gear. A small, light aluminum harness designed to function as the fisherman's second hand. Vargas Fishing Aid Rod-holder Co., 5453 Norwalk Blvd., Whittier, CA 90601.

TABLE TENNIS

Cuffs. Applied Technology for Independent Living, 2008 Lowry Ave. N.E., Minneapolis, MN 55418.

Tables. Flaghouse, Inc., 18 West 18th Street, New York, NY 10011.

Tables. North American Recreation, P. O. Box 430, Fairhaven Station, 315 Peck Street, New Haven, CT 06513, (800) 527-7415.

TRICYCLES

Adult Tricycle. For handicapped adults and grown children. All standard full-sized bicycle components including ball-bearing wheels. Handlebar brakes and extra-large seat. Rear platform supports a large basket. J. A. Preston Corp., 71 Fifth Ave., New York, NY 10003.

Chain-Drive Tricycle. Similar to a regular tricycle with standard bicycle-type chain and chain guard. All wheels have safety rims. Handbrake mechanism on right handle bar. Available with or without body support and foot attachments. J. A. Preston Corp., 71 Fifth Avenue, New York, NY 10003.

Direct Drive Tricycle. Aids in strengthening and coordination exercises for the lower limbs. Adapted foot pedals and torso support available in a variety of sizes. Med, Inc., 1215 S. Harlem Ave., Forest Park, IL 60130.

Irish Mail. An appealing substitute for children who are unable to pedal a standard tricycle. The Irish Mail moves when the handle is pumped back and forth. Comfortable front bar for resting feet. Extra large vinyl seat with a body support to ensure correct posture. Available without body support. J. A. Preston Corp., 71 Fifth Ave., New York, NY 10003.

Irish Mail. In child and adult sizes. Rugged vehicle has padded, tractor-type seat. Offers development exercise involving arm, upper torso, and leg movements. Adjustable seat. Body torso support and special pedals available. Other models also. Beckley-Cardy, 114 Gaither Dr., Mt. Laurel, NJ 08054.

Lo-Boy Trike. Low center of gravity plus the ample use of pre-lubricated ball bearings requiring little effort in pedaling makes this an ideal tricycle for handicapped child. Adjustable seat, no spokes to bend or break. Constructive Playthings, P. O. Box 5445, 1040 E. 85th Street, Kansas City, MO 64131.

Maddacycle Hand Propelled Tricycle for Handicapped Children. Seat tricycle with chair drive and steering mechanism. Rear wheel is an independent swivel wheel. Motive power is transmitted from the hand cranks to the front wheels. Suitable for indoor use for children from two to seven years of age. Maddak, Inc., Pequannock, NJ 07440.

Rifton Tricycle. Valuable aid to the mobility of the handicapped child. Includes adjustable handlebar, seat, and padded backrest with belt, a pair of upright handles and a pair of sandals. Community Playthings, Rifton, NY 12471.

Torso Support Tricycle. Has motorcycle-style back support made of steel tubing. A curved foam backrest with a broad nylon belt gives adjustable support. Available with standard or upright handlebars. For children who require such support. G. E. Miller, Inc., 484 South Broadway, Yonkers, NY 10705.

Trainer Bicycle. Has adjustable wheels for various stages of balance ability. Equipped with adjustable spring saddle-seat, handlebars, coaster brake and puncture-proof tires. Available with or without body support and foot attachments. J. A. Preston Corp., 71 Fifth Avenue, New York, NY 10003.

Kids Pedals. Specially designed pedals to keep kids' feet on pedals. Abbey Rents, 2220 Lyndale Avenue South, Minneapolis, MN 55405, (612) 374-4680.

WATER SKIING

Sitz-Ski: Mission Bay Aquatic Center
1001 Santa Clara Point
San Diego, CA 92109
ATTN: Catherine Wilkinson

Ski-Seat: Water Sports Industries
10230 Freeman Avenue
Santa Fe Springs, CA 90670

WHEELING

Indoor Wheeling Machine. Liberation Concepts
2675 Cleveland Ave., Suite 7
Santa Rosa, CA 95401
(707) 576-7074

Wheelchair Rollers. State Aluminum
P. O. Box 987
Paramount, CA 90723
(213) 634-4083

Electric Fishing Rig. Roger Irving, 8115 E. Paradise Dr., Scottsdale, AZ.

Fishing Cuffs. Applied Technology for Independent Living, 2008 Lowry Ave. N. E., Minneapolis, MN 55418.

HAND-CYCLES

Unicycle. Orthopedic Systems, Inc.
RR 1—Box 136A
Nelsonville, OH 45764
(614) 753-4155

Janssen
2885 S. Santa Fe Drive
Englewood, CO
(303) 781-8589

New England Handcycles, Inc.
228 Winchester Street
Brookline, MA 02146
(614) 277-3035

The Palmer Handcycle,
Palmer Industries
P. O. Box 707
Endicott, NY 13760

Unicycle (1982), Inc.
C. P. 276, Station N
Montreal, Quebec H2X 3M4
(514) 845-6757

Debbie Bike Company, Inc.
529 N. W. 9th Street
Chisholm, MN 55719
(218) 254-2020

Para Bike
Doug Schwandt c/o Rerand
VA Medical Center
3801 Miranda Avenue
Palo Alto, CA 94304

SNOW SKIING

Forearm Crutch Outrigger. This accessory is for amputees interested in skiing. Designed to fit adult, junior, and child crutches. Precision Grinding and Mfg. Co., Inc., 8019 Flood Rd., Baltimore, MD 21222.

Wheel-Ski. Designed for the physically impaired athlete, this device provides the user with the comfort and security of using his own wheelchair as part of his skiing equipment. Includes stabilizing skis, rear braking and a steering shaft lock that locks the position of the steering ski while the user moves forward with ski poles. Controls are on steering wheel. Has regulation skimobile skis. Easily transported on standard auto. A.P.E., Inc., P. O. Box 47, Madison Heights, MI 48017.

Outriggers. P.S.I., 124 Columbia Court, Chaska, MN 55318, (612) 448-6987.

SWIMMING

Floatation Devices. DanMar Products, Inc., 2390 Winewood Avenue, Ann Arbor, Michigan 48103, (313) 761-1990.

Swimming Cuffs. Applied Technology for Independent Living, 2008 Lowry Ave., N. E., Minneapolis, MN 55418.

VISUAL IMPAIRMENTS

Basketball

Audible Basketball. Official size and weight basketball with bell inside. Sturdy and durable for all weather play. American Foundation for the Blind, 20 W, 17th Street, New York, NY 10011.

Goal Ball

Men's Goal Ball. Bell fixed inside ball. Also available as women's goal ball. American Foundation for the Blind, 20 W. 17th Street, New York, NY 10011.

Biking

Buddy Bar. Enables a blind person to ride a bike side by side with a sighted partner. The Funway Co., 15940 Warwick Rd., Detroit, MI 48223.

"Cricket". Battery powered mechanism that emits a series of sounds enabling a blind person to follow a sighted person. Western Electric Co., Hawthorne Works Medical Engineering Division, Cicero and Cermak Rd., Chicago, IL 60650.

Name Index

Subject Index